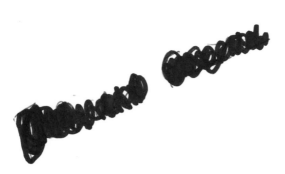

CULTURALLY COMPETENT PRACTICE WITH IMMIGRANT AND REFUGEE CHILDREN AND FAMILIES

Social Work Practice with Children and Families
Nancy Boyd Webb, Series Editor

Culturally Competent Practice with Immigrant and Refugee Children and Families

Edited by

ROWENA FONG

Series Editor's Note by
NANCY BOYD WEBB

THE GUILFORD PRESS
New York   London

© 2004 The Guilford Press
A Division of Guilford Publications, Inc.
72 Spring Street, New York, NY 10012
www.guilford.com

Printed in the United States of America

This book is printed on acid-free paper.

Last digit is print number: 9 8 7 6 5 4 3 2 1

Library of Congress Cataloging-in-Publication Data

Culturally competent practice with immigrant and refugee children
and families / edited by Rowena Fong.
     p.   cm. — (Social work practice with children and families)
Includes bibliographical references and index.
   ISBN 1-57230-931-8 (hardcover : alk. paper)
  1. Social work with children—United States. 2. Immigrant
children—Services for—United States. 3. Refugee children—Services
for—United States. 4. United States—Emigration and
immigration—Social aspects. I. Fong, Rowena. II. Series.
   HV741.C787 2004
   362.87′532′0830973—dc22

                                                    2003019178

To my parents, Owen and Wing Chung Fong;
to my husband, Lee;
and to my children, Naomi Siu-Mei and Daniel Mun-Wah

About the Editor

Rowena Fong, EdD, MSW, is a professor at The University of Texas at Austin. A graduate of Harvard University (EdD), the University of California at Berkeley (MSW), and Wellesley College (BA), she is the daughter of immigrant parents from Hong Kong and the People's Republic of China. She has also taught at the University of Hawaii at Manoa, Ohio State University, Bethel College, and Nankai University in Tianjin, China, where she did her dissertation research on China's One-Child Policy.

Dr. Fong is coeditor or coauthor of three books: *Culturally Competent Practice: Skills, Interventions, and Evaluations* (with Sharlene Furuto); *Children of Neglect: When No One Cares* (with Margaret Smith, in press); and *Multisystem Skills and Interventions in School Social Work Practice* (with Edith Freeman, Cynthia Franklin, Gary Shaffer, and Elizabeth Timberlake). She has two more books in progress: *Intersecting Child Welfare, Substance Abuse, and Family Violence* (with Ruth McRoy and Carmen Ortiz-Hendricks) and *Culturally Diverse Human Behaviors and Social Environments.*

Dr. Fong's teaching, writing, and research concentrate on children and families, specifically child welfare, immigrant children and families, and culturally competent practice. Widely published, she has done consultation and training in the People's Republic of China on foster care, adoptions, and social work curricula. Prior to her academic career, Dr. Fong was the founder and director of a Chinese bilingual, bicultural preschool in the San Francisco Bay area and has been actively involved in the Chinese immigrant communities in Boston, San Francisco, and Hawaii.

Contributors

Alfred S. Bednorz, MDiv, LMSW-AP, received his bachelor's degree in philosophy from Immaculate Conception College, Conception, Missouri, in 1973; his master of divinity degree from Oblate College of the Southwest, San Antonio, Texas, in 1976; and an associate degree in applied science–mid management, from Amarillo College, Amarillo, Texas, in 1986. Prior to becoming Executive Director of Catholic Family Services, Inc., Amarillo, Texas, in 1989, Mr. Bednorz worked primarily with refugee families as supervisor of that organization's refugee program from 1979 to 1989. He has worked as a consultant to the resettlement camps in Thailand and Bataan, the Philippines.

Kathy Caldwell, MSW, LSW, attended The University of Texas at Austin and graduated with her bachelor's degree in social work in 1980. Later, she returned to The University of Texas at Arlington and was awarded her master of science degree in social work in 1997. Ms. Caldwell has worked primarily with women and families and has been employed by Catholic Family Services, Inc., since September 1988. During her tenure with the agency, she supervised the Adoption and Foster Care division for 10 years, then the Refugee and Citizenship division. In 1998, Ms. Caldwell became Associate Director of Catholic Family Services.

Shalini Chaudhuri, MSW, received her master's degree (with specialization in family and child welfare) from Tata Institute of Social Work, Mumbai, India. She worked in the Department of Rural Development, Government of India, as a project officer evaluating and training community-based organizations in rural India to execute rural infrastructure development programs. Currently she is a full-time PhD student, with special focus on immigrants and refugees, at the School of Social Work, Howard University.

Edgar Colon, DSW, is a professor of social work at Southern Connecticut State University, New Haven. He teaches social policy, social welfare management, and clinical practice with vulnerable populations. Dr. Colon has published extensively on social welfare management, diversity, and substance abuse. He coauthored *Diversity, Oppression, and Social Functioning: Person-in-Environment Assessment and Intervention.*

Rowena Fong, EdD, MSW (see "About the Editor").

Sharlene B. C. L. Furuto, MSW, EdD, is a professor in the Social Work Department at Brigham Young University in Laie, Hawaii. She coedited *Social Work Practice with Asian Americans* and *Culturally Competent Practice: Skills, Interventions, and Evaluations*.

Melissa Goodman, MS, CSW, is Program Coordinator for the Sexual Assault and Violence Intervention Program (SAVI) at Mt. Sinai Hospital in Queens, New York. She received her master's degree in social work from the Shirley M. Ehrenkranz School of Social Work (New York University) and an MS in journalism (science communication) from Boston University.

Tamar Green, CSW, is Coordinator of the Mobile Crisis Unit, a component of the Comprehensive Psychiatric Emergency Program at Elmhurst Hospital Center in New York. She practices as a psychotherapist in Queens, New York, and has taught graduate-level courses at the Wurzweiler School of Social Work, Yeshiva University, New York, and at the University of Hawaii. She received her degree from New York University.

Altaf Husain, MSW, received his master's degree (with specialization in community organizations and nonprofit management) from Case Western Reserve University, Cleveland, Ohio. He worked as a project coordinator at Senior Outreach Services in Cleveland, Ohio, and as a counselor to Vietnamese refugees residing at the Sungei Besi Refugee Camp in Kuala Lumpur, Malaysia. He is currently a doctoral candidate at the Howard University School of Social Work in Washington, DC, specializing in Muslim immigrant and refugee family adaptation to the United States.

Gwat-Yong Lie, PhD, is an associate professor in the School of Social Welfare at the University of Wisconsin–Milwaukee. She teaches courses in social work methods and intimate partner violence, and has done research and published in the areas of intimate partner violence, multicultural social work practice, and women's issues, including those concerning Asian American women.

Flavio Francisco Marsiglia, PhD, is an associate professor at Arizona State University School of Social Work, where he serves as the lead instructor of the cultural diversity sequence and as the Principal Investigator of the Drug Resistance Strategies—AZ Project (DRS-AZ). DRS-AZ is an NIDA/NIH-funded prevention research grant involving more than 5,000 students and their teachers at 42 middle schools in Phoenix. The main purpose of the study is to identify and test culturally grounded prevention strategies. Dr. Marsiglia has authored many publications and has presented research papers at numerous professional meetings and seminars in the United States, Mexico, South America, and Europe.

Cecilia Menjívar, PhD, is a sociologist and an associate professor in the School of Justice Studies at Arizona State University. Her interests include immigrant families, social networks, gender relations, intergenerational dynamics, and religious institutions in immigrant communities. Recent publications include *Fragmented Ties: Salvadoran Immigrant Networks in America*.

Kalyani Rai, PhD, is an assistant professor at the Center for Urban Community Development, University of Wisconsin–Milwaukee Outreach. She has more than 10 years of experience working with Milwaukee's diverse communities, particularly southeast Asians, and has received a number of community-based research grants from state, federal, and private foundations.

Fariyal Ross-Sheriff, PhD, is a professor and Director of the PhD Program in Social Work at Howard University. She works with displaced populations, including refugees, immigrants, disaster victims, and the homeless. Among her publications are articles on adaptation of South Asians and Muslim women to U.S. society. She has served in several leadership positions, including the Chair of the Asian and Pacific Islander Caucus of the Council on Social Work Education, Secretary to the Steering Committee of the Group for the Advancement of Doctoral Education, and as a member of the International Commission on the Council on Social Work Education.

Gisela Sardinas, MSW, LCSW, is a senior clinical social worker within the Mid-State Behavioral Health System at the Milford Mental Health Center, Milford, Connecticut. Ms. Sardinas has extensive experience working with Latino children and families.

Sung Sil Lee Sohng, PhD, is an associate professor at the University of Washington School of Social Work, where she has taught participatory action research, cultural diversity, and social justice for over 10 years. Currently, she is the principal implementor for the Partnership for Integrated, Community-Based Learning Program, a major curriculum transformation at the University of Washington School of Social Work, focusing on community-based research and services. She serves as a co-director for the Institute of Intergroup Dialogue Research and Practice at the University of Washington, and is currently carrying out an international comparative study examining the partners in government not-for-profit health and social service organizations of Mie Prefecture, Japan, and Seattle, Washington.

Kui-Hee Song, PhD, an assistant professor at California State University, Chico, comes from the Department of Social Work at the University of Texas–Pan American. She received her doctorate in clinical social work at Loyola University Chicago, and has a BA in social work from Catholic University of Korea and an MA in social welfare from Seoul National University, Seoul, South Korea. Prior to applying for doctoral studies, she worked at the Family Therapy Institute of Korea as a professional clinical social worker and family therapist for over 7 years and taught social work courses at several universities in Seoul for 3 years. She has also done clinical work at the Family Service Center in Illinois. Her current research focuses on community needs assessments for immigrants and refugees in rural northern California.

Zoila Tazi, CSW, is a bilingual certified social worker with over 15 years' experience working with children and families. She has been a director of several children's programs, including private day care and a Head Start Child Development Center. Her clinical experience includes work with children as a primary therapist in a psychiatric setting and as a school social worker. She has worked the past 6 years servicing immigrant children and families, and is currently coordinator of a family literacy program, First Steps/Primeros Pasos, in her school district. Founder of Proyecto ALCANCE, an association of Spanish-speaking parents, Ms. Tazi has presented papers at several conferences on issues related to the Latino immigrant community. In 2002, Ms. Tazi received the Bilingual Support Person of the Year award from the New York State Association of Bilingual Education.

Carmina P. Tolentino, PhD, holds a bachelor's degree in social work from the University of the Philippines and a master's and doctorate in social work from the University of Illinois at Urbana–Champaign. Her professional experience includes serving as a social worker and supervisor in the Philippines and as a psychiatric social worker at the County of Santa Clara, California.

Pa Y. Vang, MS, is an Associate Outreach Specialist at the Center for Urban Community Development at the University of Wisconsin–Milwaukee. She is currently working on a project designed to develop and implement a culturally competent evaluation and assessment tool for the marketing of refugee programs. In addition to her work at the Center, she is the President of the Board of Directors, Wisconsin Coalition Against Domestic Violence, and a member of the Milwaukee Commission on Domestic Violence and Sexual Assault. In recognition of her work in welfare reform in the Hmong community, Ms. Pa is also a member of the W-2 Monitoring Task Force in Milwaukee.

Pahoua Yang, MSW, is the Coordinator and therapist at the Hmong Mental Health Institute, Children's Service Society, in Wasau, Wisconsin. She was actively involved in organizing a town hall meeting attended by juvenile court judges, law enforcement officers, and social service providers (including child welfare professionals) working with Hmong youth, in an attempt to elicit a coordinated, community-wide response to issues otherwise perceived as "Hmong problems."

Maria Zuniga, PhD, has been a professor of social work at San Diego State University for the past 16 years and has taught for 11 years at Sacramento State University. For 3 years she directed a gang prevention program in San Diego. She received a 3-year grant from NIMH to train bilingual/bicultural Spanish-speaking social work students to work with the Latino mentally ill population. As a Board of Directors member of the Council on Social Work Education, she cochaired the First Task Force on Cultural Competency held at the University of Michigan School of Social Work, and is coediting a text based on this conference. Dr. Zuniga has published numerous articles and chapters on how to intervene competently with Latino families and individuals, with a special focus on immigrant Latino populations.

Series Editor's Note

Tens of thousands of immigrants and refugees come to the United States each year seeking a better life for themselves and their families. Most are leaving their countries for economic or political reasons and hope to prosper in this new environment. Many are totally unprepared for the stresses and extreme hardships they will encounter in a new country, where opportunities for employment and success are limited because of language and cultural differences, in addition to discrimination and prejudice. The hoped-for better life may actually prove to be a life of back-breaking work and disappointment.

Culturally Competent Practice with Immigrant and Refugee Children and Families offers social workers a framework for assisting immigrants and refugees through the process of understanding and building on the clients' own cultural values. Using a strengths-based empowerment model as the basis for helping, the book offers diverse approaches to working with clients to find solutions that are culturally congruent and viable.

Rowena Fong has assembled an impressive group of authors who are experts on more than 14 different cultural groups. All contributors review the history of their immigrant group's migration to the United States, discuss the specific issues that apply to children and families, analyze the group's indigenous strategies for coping, and recommend strategies for assessing and intervening with families in a "culturally friendly" manner. Despite the great diversity among the different groups, common themes emerge regarding these people's efforts to adapt to the new environment. These challenges include dealing with poverty and discrimination, trying to function with a new language, and obtaining housing, employment, and schooling for the children. Many of the groups subscribe to values of interdependency and mutual help, leading them to depend on their families and communities rather than on outside sources when in need. Mental health services are distrusted and avoided, because the recognition and discussion of "problems" with an outsider creates fear of exposure and associated stigma.

Fong's introductory and concluding chapters present her theoretical and philosophical position on the importance of cultural competency for social workers. She appropriately expects practitioners to understand the impact of immigrants' histories of trauma and loss, in addition to their many other current stresses. Intergenerational conflicts and tensions in the new environment sometimes reflect the ongoing influence of these past unresolved traumas, together with the greater inclination of younger family members to disengage from their past experiences and to adapt in the present. Brief case vignettes poignantly describe both painful transitions and successful adaptations. The beauty of this book is that it provides practitioners with methods for joining with their prospective clients in a manner that respects the clients' beliefs and uses these to create a "bicultural blend." Doing this work competently requires a major shift in thinking and practice for the social worker who, in this model, encourages the client to be the teacher and the expert in conveying his or her culturally based beliefs. Using the client's values as the necessary context for practice, the social worker helps identify and implement interventions that will be effective in the new environment. The client and the social worker each learn and benefit during this creative helping experience.

NANCY BOYD WEBB, DSW

Preface

As the eldest daughter of Chinese immigrant parents, I grew up with many of the problems described in these chapters. Because my parents could not speak English and my three younger brothers were too young to help, I translated for my parents and cared for my brothers, while missing out on my own childhood. Brought up with Chinese values of receiving the best education possible and of filial obedience to my parents, I went to Ivy League schools but had difficulty transitioning from my home environment—ironing shirts in a laundry with my Chinese-speaking parents—to college with classmates whose parents were presidents of countries or executives of major corporations.

This book is the culmination of much thought about the experiences of immigrant children and families. I hope social work practitioners will listen with their hearts as the voices in these pages describe the difficulties immigrant families regularly face in a new culture—even members of the second generation, like myself. Despite the different backgrounds of people from Asia and the Pacific Islands, Central and South America, the Caribbean, Africa, and Europe, the perils and travails they experience are strikingly similar and merit a deeper level of understanding. This book acknowledges that each immigrant and refugee person's experience may vary from another's, since there are many differences within and between the various immigrant and refugee groups. While there are many ethnic groups, not all are covered here. The intent was not to slight or minimize importance, but to begin to maximize awareness.

This book was made possible in various ways by the assistance of many. Many thanks to the chapter authors for their steadfast work and their dedicated commitment to immigrants and refugee families. Support and words of encouragement from colleagues at the University of Hawaii at Manoa, Drs. Noreen Mokuau and Colette Browne, were greatly appreciated. In every enduring project, there are the vital individuals who help with the logistics of putting a book together. My warmest appreciation goes to Hisae Tachi and Herbert Lee at the University of Hawaii, who were endlessly patient with the details of typing and correcting the manuscript. I am grateful as well for the guidance, feedback, and support from Series Editor Nancy Boyd Webb and Senior Editor Jim Nageotte of The Guilford Press. Although all of these people played important parts in creating the book, the person critical in making it happen was the man who loved me, encouraged me, believed in me, and got me through to the end of the project. Thank you, Lee. Without you, it would not have been possible.

Contents

CHAPTER 1

Overview of Immigrant and Refugee Children and Families

ROWENA FONG

The fabric of American society is being embellished as recent immigrant and refugee families weave themselves into the social warp and woof of the nation. Potocky-Tripodi (2002) states, "In the United States, there are more than 28 million foreign-born persons in 2000. This represents approximately 10 percent of the U.S. population" (p. 20). However, the terrorist attacks of September 11, 2001, brought again to the fore the unease of many Americans with immigrants and refugees, prompting a national reassessment of attitudes and commitments to this population. Ensuing changes have added stressors for immigrants and refugees already in the United States and for those waiting to come. Legal immigrants join undocumented immigrants, refugees, and asylees who worry about their fate in seeking new opportunities and freedoms in America.

Bearing the stresses associated with the decision to emigrate, and then the journey itself, many immigrant and refugee children and families experience adjustment problems entering their new home environments (Ager, 1999; Berger, 2000; Canino, Earley, & Rogler, 1988; Chen, 1994; Foner, 2001; Gutierrez, 1996; Mupedziswa, 1997; Ong, Bonacich, & Cheng, 1994; Seller, 1981). Suarez-Orozco and Suarez-Orozco (2001) report the difficulties of remaking identities and the marginality of two cultures: "Immigrants are by definition in the margins of two cultures. Paradoxically, they can never truly belong either 'here' nor 'there' " (p. 92). Immigrant

1

children making attempts to adapt, according to Suarez-Orozco and Suarez-Orozco, link identity formation to contexts and social mirroring: "A new identity is forged, one that incorporates selected aspects of both culture of origin and mainstream American culture" (p. 103).

The process of moving from one context to another is described by Segal (2002) as a "push–pull" experience; she states that "immigration scholars have identified two phenomena that interact to provide the catalyst for migration: a 'push' from the country of origin and a 'pull' to the country of immigration" (p. 12). These push–pull experiences have other forms of interaction besides these two points of coming and going. Migration journeys for many refugees, asylees, and undocumented immigrants may be still more harrowing as a result of elements of force and exertion. Refugee families have experienced camps; adult asylees and families have languished in unfamiliar transit countries; and undocumented immigrants have endured sometimes desperately grim passages on boats. These transitional experiences can both directly and indirectly impact the identity formation of children and the coping adaptations of families.

Social workers addressing these transitional experiences need to first be aware of, and then be competent in assessing, the various contexts and social environments encountered in the emigration journey and understanding their influences on the adaptation behaviors of the clients. Kemp, Whittaker, and Tracy (2002) contend that there has been an "unrealized commitment" to the person-in-environment. They also maintain that "the ability to fully read the environment is an essential component of effective practice" (pp. 17–18). O'Melia and Miley (2002) emphasize the importance of contextual social work practice and of taking environments into account in empowering clients. Culturally competent social workers need to know more about the social environments and contexts of their clients' migration experiences.

This introductory chapter focuses on the influence of contexts and social environments, especially macro-level societal and cultural values, on the transition and adjustments of immigrants and refugees to their new places of residence. The social and political values of the home environments of recent immigrants and refugees are often so different that social workers neglect to "fully read the environments" and consider the magnitude of the changes their clients confront settling into America. Although contextual social work practice, specifically, person–environment practice (Kemp et al., 2002; O'Melia & Miley, 2002) is essential, the cultural competency component needs to be revised to incorporate cultural values and indigenous interventions.

In original home environments, immigrant and refugee children and families had quite functional cultural values and practices that operated as strengths and bound them to their countrymen. But in journeying to a new host country, many of these cultural values have been reevaluated, because the receiving country's culture either fails to understand them or disagrees with their priority. Fadiman (1997) describes such conflicts in the experiences of a Hmong family, the Lees, who already had 13 children by natural childbirth in Laos and Thailand. When their 14th child, Lia, was born in a community medical center in California, they clashed often with doctors and nurses, who neither understood nor valued indigenous Hmong practices. Their new host/home environment's different belief system compelled the Lees to reconsider some of those traditional cultural practices.

Not every conflict is resolved merely by a reevaluation, however, and social workers must not force immigrants and refugees to give up their cultural values, beliefs, and practices, except when they conflict with the law. Practitioners ought not only to acknowledge that cultural values of clients are strengths but also learn to use them in social work assessments to guide treatment planning and intervention implementation. This chapter champions the importance of the clients' cultural values, yet also aims to help social workers discern which macro-societal values from another country might collide with American values. For example, Muslim Asian Indians are unlikely to celebrate Christmas. The culturally competent social worker would need to be informed not only about Asian Indian culture but also Islam. So informed, a social worker could discern that the source of tension between the parents and children might be because of the tenets of the Muslim faith, and not Asian Indian culture.

Workers also need to be aware of the difficulty immigrant and refugee children and families have in sorting their cultural values from their native homes pertinent to their own ethnicity and religion, which may become compounded when they need to learn new values and practices in the new environment. A process of sorting and sifting which values play a more dominant or receding role in daily and long-term functioning of the immigrant and refugee families is necessary knowledge for culturally competent social workers. Consequently, this chapter also reviews that concept of the "intersectionality of cultural values," offering guidelines for culturally competent social work practice.

Although immigrant and refugee children and families, like the Hmong family, the Lees, mentioned earlier, had a problem-solving method of coping and using indigenous interventions in their countries of origin, social workers commonly prefer that clients adapt to and use Western interventions. Whereas their desire may be understandable and convenient, insisting on such an approach may be impossible with some cultures, or simply self-defeating. For example, mental health issues for many Serbs, Croats (as noted in Chapter 15), and Hmong (as explained in Chapter 7) either do not manifest themselves or are not treated the same in their home countries as in the United States. To expect or demand that immigrant and refugee clients be forthright in acknowledging and/or coping with posttraumatic stress disorders (PTSD) issues by attending support groups or participating in family therapy may be inappropriate and even detrimental to the client systems. Social workers need the tools that will equip them to better discern what did work in problem-solving approaches in clients' countries of origin and to supplement those with complementary interventions compatible with cultural values.

Social work literature does discuss preferred theoretical or treatment approaches for ethnic minorities, immigrants, and refugees (Bemak, Chung, & Pedersen, 2003; Ho, 1987; Jung, 1998; Lee, 1997). Some authors recommend a systems approach (Lee, 1997; Jung, 1998); others recommend specific theoretical orientations to family work (Falicov, 1998; Flores & Carey, 2000; Logan, Freeman, & McRoy, 1990). However, what remains is how to combine indigenous interventions with Western ones, choosing those compatible with the macro-level cultural values of the social and political environments of the clients' home and host countries. Kemp et al. (2002) promote "plac[ing] renewed emphasis on interventions that actively connect with and mobilize key factors in clients' environmental contexts" (p. 20). This chapter advocates the biculturalization of interventions (Fong, Boyd, & Browne, 1999), but for immigrants and refugees, both the societal macro-values of the home country and the personal cultural values of the client need to be taken into consideration. The assumption made is that, for some immigrants and refugees, the macro-level societal values may not be congruent with the personal cultural values, and value differentials may need to be acknowledged by practitioners. For example, for the Soviet Jew in the former Soviet Union, the macro-societal values are socialist, Russian, and Jewish. To assume that these Jews will be comfortable with interventions predicated on Jewish values may be an error; Green, in Chapter 16, reminds us that Russian culture often superceded Jewish culture. This introductory chapter concludes by highlighting differentials in values as a result of differing social environments and the impact on the social workers' assessment and intervention planning skills, which, according to Raheim (2002), is "adapting practice to the cultural context of the client" (p. 102).

CULTURAL COMPETENCE IN UNDERSTANDING CONTEXTS

Although immigrants have traversed the oceans to America since the 16th and 17th centuries (Daniels, 1990; Pedraza & Rumbaut, 1996), many waves of immigrants have come since then, and it is generally acknowledged that a "new immigrant" population has been coming to the United States since the Immigration and Nationality Act was amended in 1965. The amendments emphasized family reunification and "offered more visas and ... less stringent visa requirements" (Hing, 1993), enabling larger numbers of immigrants and refugees to enter.

Like their predecessors, these "new immigrants" have had to adjust to a new way of life, giving up aspects of the old life, whether good or bad, from their native countries. By immigrating, many who come surrender their professional status and their security in family ties and kinship communities. Others come without documents, and many, especially in the aftermath of events such as the bombing of the World Trade Center in New York City, must contend with the possibilities of mistaken identity and harassment. Immigrant and refugee populations face extraordinary adjustment challenges and warrant more understanding and support of their cultures and practices.

Despite this plea for understanding, the mixed attitudes of Americans toward the new immigrants is well described by Cafferty and McCready (1994)

> Central as immigration is to our national identity, we have always been ambivalent about the "new immigrants." These newcomers threaten us because they bring with them foreign languages, dress, customs, and religions. The new immigrants represent diversity, which make for the focal point of how much diversity is good for society. (p. 33)

How much diversity is good for society was central to the conversation about America even before Europeans bound for the New World had left the Old World. Several of England's New World colonies were, in fact, the result of quarrels over how much religious diversity was acceptable in English society. As a practical matter, those preparing for the trans-Atlantic voyages also debated how much diversity among social classes was desirable; too many soft-handed gentlemen or idle beggars, and too few sturdy farmers and craftsmen, meant starvation and ruin. Settlers grappled with racial and ethnic diversity when they met the colonies' indigenous inhabitants and, again, upon the arrival of slaves. And when tolerance for political diversity became unbearable during the American Revolution, thousands of loyalists departed for Canada. The conversation about diversity has yet to abate.

Typically, immigrants meet an uncertain welcome because they are different, create economic competition, and occasionally challenge government policies. In the seesaw between welcome and alarm, the 1996 Work Opportunity and Personal Responsibility Act cut off welfare benefits to naturalized citizens, including the elderly, then, after much political wrangling, benefits were restored. Whereas some legislation occasionally improves the position of immigrants, other legislation frequently negates those benefits and depends on the reception of the host country (the United States) (Segal, 2002). This legislative ambivalence toward immigrants and refugees reflects the problematic treatment of immigrants over the past half-century despite the improvements wrought in the Immigration Act's 1965 amendments.

However, it would be a mistake to suppose that all immigrant difficulties are merely the consequence of government policy. Immigrants and refugees have come to the United States in different cohorts and periods of time. Ambivalence about the most recent arrivals characterizes large immigrant communities themselves, where conflicts develop between newcomers and those who preceded them. Bevin (2001) notes such divisions among old and new Cuban immigrants, where "the most recent arrivals have proven difficult for Cuban Americans to accept or understand" (p. 187). Immigrants who have become well-established themselves may no longer be able to relate to the recent immigrants or refugees. Segal (2002) makes the point that newer immigrants may not be as welcome by either the government or immigrant communities when resources are scare in the host country, despite the best-intentioned policies.

For such reasons as these, contextual social work practice is important in the work with immigrants and refugees. Contextual social work practice considers immigrant backgrounds, the probability and degree of trauma, and the resources available to and among the clients. Lum (2003), for instance, speaks of the importance of social and environmental contexts. He maintains that social context "is an increasingly important theme in the worker–client relationship," concluding that "the life stories of the person are the basis for understanding contextual behavior" (p. 35).

Kemp, Whittaker, and Tracy (1997) write also of contexts advocating for person–environment practice. They contend that there are several environments to consider: physical, sociointeractional, institutional–organizational, cultural, and sociopolitical. Social workers need to be better informed and thus clearer in their understanding of the multiple social environments affecting immigrant and refugee families, and in their analysis of how their clients function in each social environment. A refugee family leaving a war-torn country has several environments to negotiate before it settles in the United States: the native country of origin, perhaps a series of refugee and transit camps, the journey to the United States, and often several temporary residences on arrival. Kemp et al. (1997) summarized: "We emphasize (1) the ideological and cultural messages and assumptions embedded and encoded in environmental experiences, including the ways in which spacial arrangements reflect and reinforce relations of social power; (2) the meaning, or symbolic significance, of the environment to individuals and groups, and (3) dialectical relationship between social space and physical space, including the ways in which the environment shapes and is shaped by human experience" (p. 22). All in all, more attention should be directed toward the contexts and social environments to enhance culturally competent practice.

CULTURAL COMPETENCE AND TERMINOLOGY

Cultural competence in the past has been defined as "the set of knowledge and skills that a social worker must develop in order to be effective with multicultural clients" (Lum, 1999, p. 3). However, part of the knowledge and skills that needs to be developed for working with immigrant and refugee clients is the understanding that many social environments and cultures intersect, and an effective social worker needs to know about all of them. An extension to Lum's definition is Fong's (2001) proposal for a conceptual shift toward multiculturalization. She argues that "to be culturally competent is to know the cultural values and indigenous interventions of the client system and use them in planning and implementing services" (p. 6). Cultural values are usually associated with beliefs related to race and ethnicity. Immigrant and refugee families in new environments may cling to their cultural values with a fresh intensity in reaction to the fear of losing the old culture in the new environment. Yet they necessarily go through a process of sifting which cultural values to emphasize and which to deemphasize. Thus, as immigrants and refugees move from their home environment to their host environment, some cultural values are retained and some are lost through the sieve. An extension of the cultural competence definition should include cultural values and beliefs, and the intersection of these values based on environmental contexts. The guiding principle that the cultural values of the home country may be retained or lost is based on the client's need to intersect the compatibility of old and new environments. This process of selecting, intersecting, and harmonizing values involves the intersectionality of value choice.

Intersectionality Framework for Cultural Values

The intersection of macro-level variables such as ethnicity and religion reflects cultural values. Many immigrants, for instance, are guided in their thinking and decision making by values based on religious beliefs, yet the literature has neglected religion as a major factor in shaping the social environment of immigrant and refugee children and families. Confucianism has often been cited as fundamental to traditional Chinese social values (Chung, 1992; Fong, 1992; Hsu, 1981; Sung, 1987), but little has been done to analyze the religious aspects of Confucianism and its influence on the social environment of the child and family. Conservative, Reform, and Hasidic Jews present markedly different faces of Jewish cultural identity. Asian Indian families may be Hindu, Muslim, Sikh, Jain, Parsi, or Christian, and whoever fails to grasp the differences among these faiths will not likely understand the profound differences within the Asian Indian immigrant population.

Ethnicity and religion are two intersecting factors affecting cultural values; another combination is ethnicity and the political systems under which the client has lived. Orleck (2001) describes the dilemma of Jewish children from the former Soviet Union, who grew up knowing more of mainstream Russian culture than Jewish culture. The public observance of Jewish religion and culture that was discouraged in the former Soviet Union was freely allowed in the United States. Thus, a child in the former Soviet countries may be Jewish by birth but not upbringing. Indeed, the ethnicity deriving from Judaism may be different not only as a result of being from the former Soviet Union or the United States, but also as a result of being an Orthodox, Conservative, Reformed, or even nonobservant Jew.

Culturally competent practice means that the social worker knows the many cultures the client brings (ethnicity, religion, political systems, etc.) and realizes how each has impacted the client's social functioning and behaviors. To operationalize this knowledge, the social worker must do multiple assessments focusing on the macro-level to get a context for the client's social environment. Although these various assessments are discussed further in Chapter 3, it would be good to start with a differentiation of terminology.

Terms and Definitions

The terms "immigrant" and "refugee" are often mistakenly used as synonyms. "Asylum seekers," "migrants," and "documented" and "undocumented" workers are also sometimes confusing terms but should become familiar to social workers. Fong and Mokuau (1994) noted in their literature review that differentiations between immigrants and refugees were absent, and that social workers who do not have information specific to the needs of either group may make inaccurate generalizations. Potocky-Tripodi (2002) has terms and definitions such as "alien," "asylee," "deportable alien," "immigrant," "legalized alien," "national," "nonimmigrant," "parolee," "principal alien," and "refugee." The many terms exemplify the complexity of the systems ascribing status and conditions of treatment. These statuses reflect the varieties of emigration experiences and affect the ways individuals adapt to the United States.

"Immigrant" usually refers to foreign-born persons who have left their nation of birth to dwell in another country. According to Suarez-Orozco and Suarez-Orozco (2001) 20% of all youth in the United States currently are from immigrant families. These scholars describe immigrant children as those who have migrated to the United States with parents or other adults and are not born in the United States. Children of immigrants, on the other hand, are "both foreign-born and American born" youth who have immigrant parents. The distinction between immigrant children and children of immigrant parents is worth making, as is the distinction between an immigrant and a refugee.

As defined by the United Nations in the 1951 Convention Relating to the Status of Refugees, a refugee is a person who,

> owing to a well-founded fear of being persecuted for reasons of race, religion, nationality, membership of a particular social group, or political opinion, is outside the country of his nationality, and is unable to or, owing to such fear, is unwilling to avail himself of the protection of that country. . . . (*http://www.unhcr.org/*)

Immigrants, refugees, asylum seekers, and migrants can be either documented or undocumented. Legal or documented immigrants have received the official papers that allow them to enter the country legally. Legal immigrants may work if employment can be found, though some categories of foreign-born residents—students, for instance—may be restricted in their freedom to accept employment. Refugees and asylum seekers may have temporary protective status (TPS) that allows them short-term legal entry and residence in the United States, while their petitions for permanent asylum are being considered. While those with TPS cannot be deported, Suarez-Orozco and Suarez-Orozco (2001) report that children whose parents are asylum seekers nevertheless experience uncertainty and tension.

The term "immigrant" has usually connoted legal immigrants, but there are also undocumented immigrants who have no legal status. Adult persons, children, and any other family member without legal documentation, have no legal status in the United States. Refugees may also be undocumented, and the lack of legal status has a definite impact on child and family functioning.

DEMOGRAPHICS AND DIVERSITY WITHIN ETHNIC GROUPS

Foreign-born people account for 1 out of 10 persons in the United States. The breakdown of the foreign-born population is as follows: Latin America, 51.0% (Central America, 34.5%; Caribbean, 9.9%; South America, 6.6%); Asia, 25.5%; Europe, 15.3%; and other, 8.1%. In the United States, half of the Latin American population and one-fourth of the Asian population are foreign-born.

The Latin American population is the largest ethnic minority group in America, yet half of these people were not born in the United States. Every fourth Asian person here has come from another country and faces the adjustments of immigration and adaptation to a new social environment. The many immigrant populations come from diverse social environments that produce unemployed, semiliterate tribal refugees, as well as high-tech entrepreneurs. Good social work practice would take into account such a range of functioning and examine the diverse social environments that have shaped these immigrant and refugee groups.

SOCIAL ENVIRONMENTS AND HUMAN BEHAVIORS

The human behavior and social environment (HBSE) literature is an expression of the belief that human behavior is affected by social environments (Ashford, Lecroy, & Lortie, 2001; Longres, 1995; Schriver, 2001; Zastrow & Kirst-Ashman, 2001). Immigrants' and refugees' behaviors have also been, and continue to be, affected by the social environments from which they came. A person-in environment ecological model looks at the impact of macro-level societal values and stressors on the individual's and family's functioning. For example, to understand refugees who seek political asylum in the United States, it is also necessary to understand their experiences with and attitudes toward government. Governments of socialist countries, such as the former Soviet Union, the People's Republic of China, and Vietnam, have controlled housing, jobs, medical care, and other commodities, allocating them to the population. Adults from these nations may arrive assuming that government here in the United States will exercise a similar paternalistic function, which presents another hurdle in their adjustment process. Green, in Chapter 16, speaks of the difficulties Soviet Jews from the former Soviet Union have had in adjusting to the American governmental welfare practices.

Schriver (2001) notes that the basis of understanding human function is understanding that the social environment affects human behavior. The ecological model of person-in-environment is appropriate; the challenge is to see the immigrant and refugee from the viewpoint of environment of origin and monitor their adaptation to the new environment. In that process, as we have seen, caution is necessary to avoid assuming that immigrants of the same ethnic group come from identical social environments. A Chinese immigrant speaking a Shanghai dialect may still feel quite alien in the Cantonese-speaking community of American-born and first-generation Chinese. The social environments in China and Chinatown are very different in political, religious, educational, and other arenas.

Working with immigrant and refugee populations requires some knowledge of their social and cultural environments, especially macro-level issues. They will look for elements of their social and cultural environments from their native lands in their new environments. Although they may think it is obvious that they will have to make adjustments, they will also want to replicate what is familiar. Thus, social workers need to be familiar with the native social environments, because in working with immigrants and refugees, the experiences of their migrations may need to be taken into account in social work practice.

MIGRATION EXPERIENCES AND ADAPTATIONS

In examining migration patterns, Sowell (1996) points out that immigrants usually migrate to a community of people who come from the same community back in the old country. He describes how, in New York City, specific tenements or streets would fill up with immigrants from the same village in Italy, in what he refers to as "chain" immigration. In such an immigration pattern, a few would emigrate, then others from the community would follow, so that immigrants from specific villages and districts of the old country would reestablish themselves as a particular community in specific places in the new country. This also has a bearing on the transition experience, because not much has been said about the fact that immigrants are not merely individuals directly confronted by "America," or even families directly confronting the host culture. Immigrants actually move into a community of countrymen, many of whom are relatives and familiar others from the old country. These old-timers are at least as powerful a part of the immigrant's social environment as anything in the host culture.

The journeys immigrants and refugees make to America are characterized by the same blend of patterns and differences as any of their other experiences. Traditionally, for a single family, immigration was not a one-time event but a succession of events. Family members arrived in three waves, according to their ability to survive independently. The first wave was the head of house or male relative, who immigrated and established himself, sending money back to support the family. The second phase characteristically included wives, couples, or intact families. The third phase brought older family members, children, or various combinations.

Before the 1965 Immigration Act, fathers, uncles, brothers, sons-in-law, nephews, and other male kin left for America to seek better employment, usually with the initial intention to return home. Separations may have been long and painful, but the decision to stay was a choice, not a forced imposition. The 1965 Immigration Act facilitated family reunification, and more skilled laborers were allowed into the United States. The situation for refugees seeking political asylum and for undocumented persons, however, was different. The possibility of being deported was a constant threat and stress. Although all left their homelands, some immigrants and refugees endured more trials and hostility than others. Immigrants and refugees left their countries at various times and for a variety of economic, political, social, and cultural reasons (Suarez-Orozco & Suarez-Orozco, 2001). Because immigrants left their native lands voluntarily, they had time to prepare and anticipate adjustments. Many refugees, on the other hand, left home countries disrupted by war and may have suffered separation, torture, rape, and trauma. Because their leaving was less voluntary, they tended to experience more fear and PTSD.

Adjustments and adaptations to the new environment are heavily influenced by the immigrants' experiences before and during migration, but little is written on the process of transitions after they have arrived in the United States. Life in the native country also receives scant attention, as if immigrants and refugees arrive in the new country a *tabula rasa*, having left all their knowledge and beliefs behind. What happens in the process of leaving the country and making adaptations? Documented and undocumented immigrants likewise have different transitional and adjustment experiences. How exactly does the migration experience affect adaptation? If an individual comes from a social environment of acceptance and security and transitions into another environment of rejection and insecurity, his or her resiliency may be tested or collapse altogether. McHubbin, Thompson, Thompson, and Fromer (1998) write of immigrant family resiliency:

> The immigrants and refugees migrated from native homelands important to them. To exclude their former home environments and to ignore their living conditions and family situations would be erroneous. They survived their home environment situations and the problems they encountered in adjusting to America. One needs to examine the strengths that allowed them to do it. The strengths come in the form of cultural values and indigenous interventions and coping strategies. To examine their strengths and means of coping, one needs to determine the problems they faced in coming to the United States.

It is important to distinguish between immigrants who left native lands voluntarily and looked forward to coming to the United States, and those whose decisions were forced and reluctant. The former class of immigrants experience adjustments, but stressors are more within their control than those for refugees and undocumented immigrants.

PROBLEMS ENCOUNTERED BY CHILDREN AND FAMILIES

Because immigrants and refugees come to the United States for different reasons, they have different problems. Some problems occurring at the macro-, meso-, and micro-levels are common to all immigrants and refugees, old and new. At the macro-level, poverty, discrimination, racism, language, immigration laws, and legal and illegal status characterize many of their experiences. At the meso-level, families often struggle with role reversal, husband–wife tensions, grandparent relations, and questions of abandonment and loyalty. At the micro-level, a father may encounter problems with his traditional role as the head of house and loss of authority, because he lacks command of the host-culture's language. At the micro-level, for the mother, accepting employment may introduce tension about her role as wife and mother. At the micro-level, for the child, tensions may be related to school and language deficiency. Children may also have conflicts due to illiteracy, the necessity to interpret for parents, and pressure to achieve and hurry through childhood.

Common assimilation problems for adults are finding employment/ work, retaining the native language, role reversal with children, voting, obtaining welfare benefits, lack of education/illiteracy, coping with immigration laws, and family separations. The problems for the immigrant children seem to be affected by variables such as the parents' status, the journey to the United States, and the age and gender of the child. Children who are undocumented may have problems with identity, play relationships, and age-appropriate social skills (Suarez-Orozco & Suarez-Orozco, 2001). They also frequently struggle with isolation and loneliness. When older, undocumented immigrant and refugee young adults sometimes attend college but cannot receive federal education aid. Their psychological problems may include PTSD, depression, and suicide. Social problems may include role confusion and social skills that are not age-appropriate. Emotional problems may include suppressed anger or anger manifested through gang involvement (Zhou & Bankston, 1998).

Although poverty is a common concern, immigrants and refugees regularly experience other economically related problems as well. Underemployment for immigrants from professional classes, or joblessness, is particularly worrisome for men. For women, the economic problems depend on their own employability, and children are affected if they have to sacrifice childhood and studies to add to the family income.

Immigrants leave a social network of family, friends, neighbors, and work associates for a social setting in which they are typically isolated by language barriers and perhaps not welcomed into the ethnic community with which they are most familiar. Men have problems when they are not welcomed into the community because of their status, or because they inherit the social problems of relatives who preceded them. Women experience problems when they are shunned or confronted by cliques. If they have been raped or physically abused, family members and relatives may distance themselves out of shame. Children can experience rejection from relatives and peers when they display poor language skills or inadequate acculturation processing.

Instances of culturally related problems for men may be the expectation to continue chauvinistic or patriarchal practices that are not well tolerated in the United States. Similar pressures to adhere to traditional roles that are not honored or accepted in the broader American culture complicate adjustments for women as well. Role reversal introduces culturally related problems for children, because those roles undermine the respect normally granted parents and elders.

Contending with the vagaries of immigration law, rulings, and enforcement adds another set of problems to the lives of immigrants and refugees. In the aftermath of the World Trade Center attacks in 2001, some feared deportation of all immigrants. Undocumented immigrants, naturally, have many more problems with the legal system than others. Documented or not, legal problems for men and women affect both their employability and their capacity to keep their families together.

Problems experienced by immigrants and refugees may be related to many variables, such as their gender, sibling order, political status, development, or ties to their native culture. These problems can also be explained by their different migration experiences. But at the core of their existence are the cultural values and indigenous strategies that are strengths, and that culturally competent social workers in the United States should heed in practice with this population.

CULTURAL VALUES AS STRENGTHS

Because cultural values are the expressions of important norms and attitudes in a society, they reflect the acceptable and expected behaviors of individuals and family members. Cultural values are supported by the community; thus, understanding cultural values is a way of understanding what holds that community together. Cultural values in their home environment allowed immigrants and refugees to survive. But some of the cultural values will have to change when they move to a new environment. How do social workers help clients transfer those values for survival in a new setting? Cultural translators are cultural values, attitudes, and norms that survive and are brought into a new host culture. When children acculturate faster than the parent, hierarchical authority is challenged. How does good social work help the parent and child survive? The family's strengths have contributed to how its members have adapted. How can culturally competent social workers continue to use their strengths to aid their adjustment?

Too often social workers assume that immigrant children and their families have experienced trauma by leaving lands with less economic opportunity and less political freedom than the United States. Whatever their difficulties in the old country, however, they had the strength to survive there for an extended part of their lives. These strengths should not be discounted as the immigrants move and transition to the United States. The literature does emphasize cultural values (Fong & Furuto, 2001; Lum, 1999, 2003; Mokuau, 1991; Webb, 2001) and the importance of respecting and promoting the transmission of these values. Yet culturally competent social workers need to take the values and incorporate them into assessments and interventions with immigrant children and families.

Some social workers assume that when people leave their native environments, they should also leave behind their cultural values, and that their primary need is to adopt Western values. Many immigrants and refugees cannot do this, and they ought not be forced to. Consequently, culturally competent assessments review the clients' norms and beliefs as expressed through cultural values, examine how the values have been incorporated in their indigenous strategies, and use appropriate indigenous strategies as empowerment tools.

INDIGENOUS STRATEGIES PROMOTING CULTURAL COMPETENCE

This book was written to help social workers become culturally competent in their understanding of cultural values and indigenous interventions. The goal is to prioritize and incorporate those values and interventions into Western assessments and interventions. It is assumed that the immigrants and refugees come from environments where their cultural values and indigenous interventions successfully helped them cope. In supporting their transition to the United States, it behooves the culturally competent social worker to adapt to the client's system of values and incorporate those values into their practice, instead of assuming that the client alone has to adapt to the American environment. In their research about practice experiences with immigrants and refugees, Russell and White (2001) found that "multiple connection pathways" were evident when

> social workers . . . rejected unidimensional definitions of culture and instead considered any one of numerous factors such as class, education, gender, language, country of birth, country of domicile, citizenship and religion when identifying similarities with clients. . . . While it is necessary for social workers to learn about different cultures, intellectual understanding alone may not be sufficient for productive interventions with such client population. Lived knowledge may be a prerequisite. (pp.79–80)

If a living experience is not possible, another way to achieve productive interventions is to choose interventions that are similar to or familiar with the norms and cultural values of the immigrant or refugee client. Fong et al. (1999) write of the biculturalization of interventions, which is based upon empowerment theory and strengths perspective. The purpose of biculturalization is to complement the ethnic group's indigenous interventions with compatible Western interventions, acknowledging the integrity of the group's cultural values. Social workers need to give more attention to what is normal and natural to the immigrant client or family, and use the strengths they already have, as manifested in their cultural values and indigenous interventions.

Because the immigrants or refugees come from different social environments, it is also vital to differentiate between the values of people within the same ethnic group and not assume all indigenous interventions would work for all persons within the ethnic group. For example, families arriving from the People's Republic of China, since the 1979 single-child policy went into effect, would be unlikely to subscribe to Chinese traditions valuing large extended families and lots of children. According to empowerment theory and strengths perspective, immigrant families have the traditional means to cope with the stressors in their lives. Because such families often resort to familiar cultural practices used in native homelands, these approaches should be recognized and utilized in culturally competent social work practice.

REFERENCES

Ager, A. (Ed.). (1999). *Refugees: Perspectives on the experience of forced migration.* New York: Pinter.

Ashford, J., Lecroy, C., & Lortie, K. (2001). *Human behavior in the social environment: A multidimensional perspective* (2nd ed.). Belmont, CA: Brooks/Cole.

Bemak, F., Chung, R., & Pedersen, P. (2003). *Counseling refugees: A psychosocial approach to innovative multicultural interventions.* Westport, CT: Greenwood Press.

Berger, R. (2000). When remarriage and immigration coincide: The experience of Russian immigrant stepfamilies. *Journal of Ethnic and Cultural Diversity in Social Work 8*(1/2), 75–96.

Bevin, T. (2001). Parenting in Cuban American families. In N. Webb (Ed.), *Culturally diverse parent–child and family relationships: A guide for social workers and other practitioners* (pp. 181–201). New York: Columbia University Press.

Cafferty, P., & McCready, W. (1994). *Hispanics in the United States: A new social agenda.* New Brunswick, NJ: Transaction.

Canino, I., Earley, B., & Rogler, L. (1988). *The Puerto Rican child in New York City: Stress and mental health.* New York: Fordham University, Hispanic Research Center.

Chen, S. (1994). *Hmong means free: Life in Laos and America.* Philadelphia: Temple University Press.

Chung, D. (1992). Asian cultural commonalities: A comparison with mainstream American cultures. In S. Furuto, R. Biswas, D. Chung, K. Murase, & F. Ross-Sheriff (Eds.), *Social work practice with Asian Americans* (pp. 27–44). Newbury Park, CA: Sage.

Daniels, R. (1990). *Coming to America: A history of immigration and ethnicity in American life.* New York: HarperCollins.

Fadiman, A. (1997). *The spirit catches us and you fall down*. New York: Farrar, Straus & Giroux.

Falicov, C. (1998). *Latino families in therapy: A guide to multicultural practice*. New York: Guilford Press.

Flores, M., & Carey, G. (2000). *Family therapy with Hispanics: Towards appreciating diversity*. Boston: Allyn & Bacon.

Foner, N. (2001). *New immigrants in New York*. New York: Columbia University Press.

Fong, R. (1992). History of Asian Americans. In S. Furuto, R. Biswas, D. Chung, K. Murase, & F. Ross-Sheriff (Eds.), *Social work practice with Asian Americans* (pp. 1–9). Newbury Park, CA: Sage.

Fong, R. (2001). Culturally competent practice: Past to present. In R. Fong & S. Furuto (Eds.), *Culturally competent practice: Skills, interventions, and evaluations*. Boston: Allyn & Bacon.

Fong, R., Boyd, C., & Browne, C. (1999). The Gandhi technique: A biculturalization approach for empowering Asian and Pacific Islander families. *Journal of Multicultural Social Work, 7*, 95–110.

Fong, R., & Furuto, S. (2001). *Culturally competent practice: Skills, interventions, and valuations*. Boston: Allyn & Bacon.

Fong, R., & Mokuau, N. (1994). Not simply Asian Americans: Periodical literature review on Asians and Pacific Islanders. *Social Work, 39* (3), 298–306.

Gutierrez, D. (Ed.). (1996). *Between two worlds: Mexican immigrants in the United States*. New York: Scholarly Resources.

Hing, B. (1993). *Making and remaking Asian America through immigration policy, 1850–1990*. Stanford, CA: Stanford University Press.

Ho, M. (1987). *Family therapy with ethnic minorities*. Newbury Park, CA: Sage.

Hsu, F. (1981). *American and Chinese: Passage to differences* (3rd ed.). Honolulu: University of Hawaii Press.

Jung, M. (1998). *Chinese American family therapy: A new model for clinicians*. San Francisco: Jossey-Bass.

Kemp, S., Whittaker, J., & Tracy, E. (1997). *Person–environment practice: The social ecology of interpersonal helping*. New York: Aldine de Gruyter.

Kemp, S., Whittaker, J., & Tracy, E. (2002). Contextual social work practice. In M. O'Melia & K. Miley (Eds.), *Pathways to power: Readings in contextual social work practice* (pp.. 15–34). Boston: Allyn & Bacon.

Lee, E. (1997). *Working with Asian Americans: A guide for clinicians*. New York: Guilford Press.

Logan, S., Freeman, E., & McRoy, R. (1990). *Social work practice with black families: A culturally specific perspective*. New York: Longman.

Longres, J. (1995). *Human behavior in the social environment* (2nd ed.). Itasca, IL: Peacock.

Lum, D. (1999). *Culturally competent practice: A framework for growth and action*. Pacific Grove, CA: Brooks/Cole.

Lum, D. (2003). *Culturally competent practice: A framework for understanding diverse groups and justice issues* (2nd ed.). Pacific Grove, CA: Brooks/Cole.

McHubbin, H., Thompson, E., Thompson, A., & Fromer, J. (Eds.). (1998). *Resiliency in Native American and immigrant families*. Thousand Oaks, CA: Sage.

Mokuau, N. (Ed.). (1991). *Handbook of social services for Asians and Pacific Islanders*. Westport, CT: Greenwood Press.

Mupedziswa, R. (1997). Social work with refugees. In M. Hokenstad & J. Midgley (Eds.), *Issues in international social work: Global challenges for a new century* (pp. 110–124). Washington, DC: National Association of Social Workers Press.

O'Melia, M., & Miley, K. (2002). *Pathways to power: Readings in contextual social work practice*. Boston: Allyn & Bacon.

Ong, P., Bonacich, E., & Cheng, L. (1994). *The new Asian immigration in Los Angeles and global restructuring*. Philadelphia: Temple University Press.

Orleck, A. (2001). Soviet Jews: The city's newest immigrants transform New York Jewish life. In N. Foner (Ed.), *New immigrants in New York* (pp. 111–140). New York: Columbia University Press.

Pedraza, S., & Rumbaut, R. (1996). *Origins and destinies: Immigration, race, and ethnicity in America*. Belmont, CA: Wadsworth.

Potocky-Tripodi, M. (2002). *Best social work practice with immigrants and refugees*. New York: Columbia University Press.

Raheim, S. (2002). Cultural competence: A requirement for empowerment practice. In M. O'Melia & K. Miley (Eds.), *Pathways to power: Readings in contextual social work practice* (pp. 95–107). Boston: Allyn & Bacon.

Russell, M., & White, B. (2001). Practice with immigrants and refugees: Social worker and client perspectives. *Journal of Ethnic and Cultural Diversity in Social Work, 8*, (1/2), 73–92.

Schriver, J. (2001). *Human behavior and the social environment: Shifting paradigms in essential knowledge for social work practice* (3rd ed.). Boston: Allyn & Bacon.

Segal, U. (2002). *A framework for immigration: Application to Asians in the United States*. New York: Columbia University Press.

Seller, M. (1981). *Immigrant women*. Philadelphia: Temple University Press.

Sowell, T. (1996). *Migrations and cultures: A worldview*. New York: Basic Books.

Suarez-Orozco, C., & Suarez-Orozco, M. (2001). *Children of immigration*. Cambridge, MA: Harvard University Press.

Sung, B. (1987). *The adjustment experience of Chinese immigrant children in New York City*. New York: Center for Migration Studies.

Webb, N. (Ed.). (2001). *Culturally diverse parent–child relationships*. New York: Columbia University Press.

Zastrow, C., & Kirst-Ashman, K. (2001). *Understanding human behavior and the social environment* (5th ed.). Belmont, CA: Brooks/Cole.

Zhou, M., & Bankston, C. (1998). *Growing up American: How Vietnamese children adapt to life in the United States*. New York: Russell Sage Foundation.

CHAPTER 2

Theoretical Perspectives for Culturally Competent Practice with Immigrant Children and Families

SHARLENE B. C. L. FURUTO

Immigrants have been coming to the United States for hundreds of years from all over the world. The first settlement of Filipino Americans in the Louisiana bayous was recorded in 1763 (Nimmagadda & Balgopal, 2000). Since then, Chinese, Asian Indians, Japanese, Europeans, Jews, and Africans have arrived. Some were taken as prisoners from their homelands whereas others willingly came "for a better life." Mexicans, Central and South Americans, Pacific Islanders, and others have also migrated to the United States.

When the 1965 immigration law abolished the national-origins quota system, a number of immigrants, particularly from the Asian countries, began entering the United States. Ten years later, when Vietnam, Cambodia, and Laos fell to Communism, thousands of Southeast Asian refugees fled and many resettled in the United States.

In the last 30 years, the number of immigrants has increased from 10 million in 1970 (5% of all Americans in the United States) to 28 million today (10% of the total U.S. population) (Camarota, 2000). Approximately 800,000 legal immigrants and several hundred thousand illegal immigrants enter the United States annually (Camarota, 2000). Immigrants have been coming primarily from Asia (37% of all immigrants) and Latin America (32%), followed by Europe (17%) (Hernandez & Isaacs, 1998).

Immigrants and refugees face a number of problems, such as poor health, language barriers, and poverty. Sixty-one percent of Hmong families, 42% of Cambodian families, and 32% of Laotian families are below the poverty level (Balgopal, 2000). In addition, difficulties affording food, crowded housing, and not having health insurance also continue to plague seriously children of immigrants compared to children of natives (Capps, 2001).

Social workers, at the forefront in helping immigrants and their families, should base their practice on a culturally competent theoretical background that includes the immigrant's "cultural values and norms, congruent with their natural help-seeking behaviors, and inclusive of existing indigenous solutions" (Fong & Furuto, 2001, p. 1).

This chapter reviews three theoretical approaches that are especially appropriate when practicing with immigrant children and families: ecological, strengths, and empowerment approaches. The breadth of the ecological approach fosters attention on influential immigrant and nonimmigrant groups in the immigrant's environment—family, peers, neighbors, and society—and factors such as a poor economy, high unemployment, high prejudice, high housing, and so on. At the same time, the strengths and empowerment approaches promote immigrants' and workers' personal knowledge, abilities, values, and beliefs as they collaboratively work towards mutually agreed-upon goals. The chapter ends with a discussion of stress factors particular to immigrant individuals and families, and culturally competent responses.

THEORIES AND APPROACHES USED IN SOCIAL WORK PRACTICE

Social work practice has been based on a number of theories and approaches, including psychosocial, problem-solving, task-centered, structural, and system methods. More recently, the process stage approach (Lum, 1999), ethnic-sensitive practice (Devore & Schlesinger, 1999), and social constructivism (Poulin, 2000) have been recognized, while the ecological, strengths, and empowerment approaches continue to receive attention. The strengths perspective and the empowerment approach, according to an analysis by Devore and Schlesinger (1999), are totally congruent with the ethnic reality. In addition, the ecological approach is considered by Devore and Schelesinger to pay major attention to ethnicity. Browne and Mills (2001), on the other hand, believe that "the conceptual framework provided by the ecological perspective, together with strategies and ideas from the strengths perspective and empowerment theory, has the potential to help social workers support the abilities and skills of individuals, families, groups, and communities to act on their own beliefs to improve their lives" (pp. 11–12).

THE ECOLOGICAL APPROACH

In 1970, Bartlett's reconceptualization of social work from the specialized practice terms "casework," "group work," and "community practice" to the generic term "social work practice" called for major changes in the social work profession. Social functioning interactions, in which individuals and their social environments meet, were identified as the central focus of the profession. The common domain included three essential concepts: people, interactions, and the environment, now known as the concept of person-in-environment. This reconceptualization of social work practice was the forerunner of several general social work practice conceptualizations during the 1970s and 1980s, including those of Middleman and Goldberg (1974), Pincus and Minahan (1973), and Germain and Gitterman (1980). Not long after the ecological or life model approach was developed by Germain (1979) and Germain and Gitterman (1980), social workers began accepting and using it to the point that it became the prevailing approach. Today, the ecological perspective has also been used in conjunction with other methods such as the solution-oriented model (Teall, 2000).

The ecological approach encourages the practitioner to consider the immigrant's current environment and life situation and also the environment and life situation prior to emigration when assessing and intervening. Social workers may need to review not only needs such as cultural values, intergenerational conflict, English-language limitations, ethnic misunderstanding, training for employment, health, traditional healing methods, and so on, but also perhaps the impact of immigrants' earlier experiences with war, fear of government, torture and physical suffering, starvation, loss of close family members, and so on, for a fuller understanding of the immigrants and best practice.

Concepts of the Ecological Approach

The ecological perspective had its beginnings in ecology, the science that studies the relations between organisms and their environments based on their relationships. Organisms need resources from their environment to survive, and they sometimes change their environment. The environment, on the other hand, can also impact the organism negatively or positively.

The ecological approach emphasizes understanding people and their environment, and the nature of their transactions. Important concepts of the ecological approach include transactions, good of fit between people and their environments, and adaptation. Transactions are continuous reciprocal exchanges that are integral to relationships in which people and environments influence, shape, and sometimes change each other. Exchanges that result in negative transactions are critical for social workers and consumers to understand and address, whereas exchanges that result in positive transactions normally do not require social work attention, because there is a good "fit." Human beings strive throughout life for the best person-in-environment "fit" between their needs, rights, capacities, and aspirations on the one hand, and the qualities of their environment on the other. If the fit is not good, then people may decide to change themselves or the environment, or both, and these changes are termed "adaptations." Adaptation is an active process of self-change or environmental change, or both.

Immigrant children and their families are best served by professionals who apply general knowledge about the immigrants' home country, traditions and values, family dynamics, and communication patterns, as well as the political, economic, and social circumstances, when working with them. For example, aware that mental health services are usually unavailable in much of the Philippines, and that Filipinos feel more comfortable in talking with medical doctors than with psychologists, the astute social worker would be more effective in referring the client to a medical doctor first rather than to a mental health worker for psychosomatic disorders.

Principles of the Ecological Approach

Some basic ideas of the ecological systems perspective follow (Germain, 1991; Hearn, 1979):

1. Social work practice is based on a dual focus, which includes the person and situation, and the system and its environment.
2. Social work practice occurs at the interface between the human system and its environment.
3. Transactions occur at the interface between the system and the environment.
4. In transactional relationships, both systems are influenced by change efforts.
5. Social work practice is best conducted when the transactions promote growth and development of the organism, while simultaneously being ameliorative to the environment, thus making it a better place for all systems that depend on it for sustenance.

It was Bronfenbrenner (1979) who adapted ecological systems theory from the physical sciences to human behavior. He discussed four different systems levels. The first one is the micro-system. The micro-system includes the roles and characteristics of a developing individual, such as gender, age, self-esteem, and so on. The second system, the meso-system, includes the settings with which the developing person interacts, such as the family, school, peers, church group, and so on. As children develop, they are influenced by the exo-system, or those settings with which the individual does not interact directly but that nonetheless have an effect on development, such as the neighborhood, friends of the family, the mass media, legal services, and so on. The final system, the macro-system, includes those cultural values and variables that exert an influence in terms of policies, resource distribution, values, and mores of the social environment (Corcoran, Franklin, & Bennett, 2000).

The ecological approach takes into account a holistic approach of the immigrant's status and transactions with other individuals and systems. When the consumer is the family, the practitioner needs to analyze the transactions between family members and other individuals, groups, organizations, and social institutions. Two assessment instruments that can be used with immigrant families are the eco-map and the genogram.

The eco-map is a major tool for studying the social context of families. The practitioner and consumer draw a map showing the major systems that are a part of the family's environment and the nature of the family's relationship with the various systems (Hartman & Laird, 1983; Sheafor, Horejsi, & Horejsi, 2000).

The genogram indicates the important emotional attachments of an individual or family and is an extension of the eco-map. The genogram provides a closer look at the family relationships and patterns for two or three generations and allows the examination of how these patterns affect members of the family (Congress, 1994; McGoldrick & Gerson, 1985; Sheafor et al., 2000).

Practitioners working with immigrant children and their families can use the eco-map and genogram to organize data, making for a more thorough assessment and effective treatment plan based on family members' transactions, goodness of fit, and adaptations in the home country and the United States. The culturagram, an assessment tool that focuses specifically on different aspects of culture, was developed to help practitioners better understand and empower culturally diverse families (Congress, 1994). Although generalizations about different ethnic groups have been helpful to family therapists in practice with culturally diverse clients (McGoldrick, Pearce, & Giordano, 1996), current practice with culturally diverse families has stressed the importance of individualizing families from different cultural backgrounds (Green, 1995).

The following is an example of how the ecological perspective can be used with Sophiap, a survivor of the Cambodian killing fields.

Case Vignette

Sophiap, 35, is a refugee woman from Cambodia. She suffers from severe somatic complaints in the form of intense physical pain throughout her body, extreme fatigue, and weight loss. These symptoms result in social suffering such as inability to work and low quality of life. Sophiap has been to a number of both Western medical doctors and Cambodian healers. Her current internist believes she should be able to work, and the Cambodian healers can't make the pain go away. Sophiap is constantly on painkillers. She doesn't understand why only she and not other survivors of the killing fields has such bad pain.

Sophiap has suffered cruel physical and mental punishment from the age of 9, when the Khmer Rouge forced her family to flee from their village. Since then, she has been beaten nearly to death several times, starved and dehydrated, and has witnessed family members dying violently, hidden between many dead corpses, and so on. The 6 years she spent in a Thai refugee camp were also difficult, and finally, in 1985, she arrived in the United States at 20 years of age. Since then, she has continued to have poor health, and no medical doctor, mental health professional, monk, or Cambodian traditional healer can offer her a plausible explanation. She thinks she may be sick due to "eating filthy things" rather than bad karma. Nevertheless, she can't understand why other survivors are now well and she is so tired and in such excruciating pain.

The social worker helping Sophiap needs to take a sound ecological approach by considering the client's environment in Cambodia and the impact on her then and now. For most of Sophiap's life, particularly since the Khmer Rouge took over Cambodia, there has not been a good fit between herself and her environment. Almost all of her exchanges with the Khmer Route resulted in unbearably negative transactions, and even today she does not have a good fit with her internist, monk, and traditional Cambodian healers. It has been very difficult for Sophiap to adapt well in her Cambodian, Thai, and U.S. environments. The social worker needs to focus on promoting Sophiap's growth and development by first addressing her physical needs. Perhaps the social worker and Sophiap will want to consider (1) a second internist's opinion or an "expert" opinion of someone familiar with her symptoms and culture; (2) psychotherapy, which may enable Sophiap to work through the intense pain and suffering she bore as a child and teenager without her family, school, village, religion, peers, culture, and so on; and (3) group sessions with others whose stories and issues may help Sophiap better understand herself and her personal health issues. By bringing together for Sophiap a holistic perspective, the social worker is better able to work with her in her reality.

THE STRENGTHS APPROACH

The social work profession made clear the importance of strengthening multilevel clients in the helping relationship when, in 1958, the Commission on Social Work Practice included as a main objective of the field to "seek out, identify, and strengthen the maximum potential in individuals, groups and communities" (Bartlett, 1958, p. 6). Today, the strengths approach guides practitioners in helping clients identify their competence, abilities, and strengths and then encouraging them to use these abilities, talents, potentials, and resources in the change process.

Leung, Cheung, and Stephenson (1994) indicate five components of the strengths approach: (1) developing positive attitudes toward clients, (2) focusing on family strengths rather than problems, (3) encouraging clients to engage in effective behaviors, (4) challenging clients to appreciate their own ethnic and cultural backgrounds, and (5) encouraging clients to locate their own resources.

Saleebey (1997) encourages the practitioner to "discover and embellish, explore and exploit clients' strengths and resources in the service of assisting them to achieve their goals . . . " (p. 3). The focus should be on mobilizing clients' strengths (talents, knowledge, capacities, abilities, skills, aspirations, and resources) rather than dwelling on problems, pathologies, weaknesses, diseases, and failures (Saleebey, 1997; Weick, Rapp, Sullivan, & Kisthardt, 1989).

Concepts of the Strengths Approach

The strengths perspective enhances concepts such as empowerment, membership, resilience, healing and wholeness, dialogue and collaboration, and suspension of disbelief. Empowerment indicates the intent and the processes of assisting multilevel clients to discover and expend the resources and tools within and around them. Practitioners need to create many opportunities for clients to have some control over their lives and make decisions that impact them.

Clients have membership in a community and need to be responsible and valued citizens. Even new members such as immigrants are entitled to the dignity, respect, and responsibility that comes with such membership. Resilience is also important in the strengths approach. People are resilient. Whatever the issue, people do go through the challenge and survive. Resilience is the continuing growth and articulation of capacities, knowledge, insight, and virtues that result from meeting the demands and challenges of one's life.

The strengths approach promotes healing and wholeness. Healing implies both wholeness and the inborn facility of the body and the mind to regenerate and resist when faced with disorder, disease, and disruption. Also important is dialog, the means by which we confirm to our clients their importance and value. As we dialog, we need to collaborate with our clients and become their agents or consultants in jointly developing resolutions. Practitioners need to collaborate and be open to negotiation and appreciate the input of their clients. Finally, we need to suspend feelings of disbelief, so as to promote client empowerment.

Principles of the Strengths Approach

The following are some principles that guide application of the strengths perspective, according to Saleebey (1997):

1. Every individual, group, family, and community has strengths. Even though it may sometimes be difficult to see strengths clearly, everyone has strengths from what they have have learned about themselves due to trauma, personal qualities and traits, what they know about the world around them, talents, cultural and personal stories and lore, and pride or "survivor's pride."
2. Trauma and abuse, illness, and struggle may be injurious, but they may also be sources of challenge and opportunity. When going through difficulties, clients do learn skills and acquire traits and capacities that preserve them and help them to face the future. Lessons can be learned from all crises and issues.
3. Assume that you do not know the upper limits of the capacity to grow, change, and take individual, group, and community aspirations seriously. Because we do not have sufficient knowledge to know clients' potential to grow and change, we should encourage them to do the best they can.
4. We best serve clients by collaborating with them. Our clients know themselves and their environment best. We can be most helpful by collaborating with them or serving as consultants.
5. Every environment is full of resources. There are individuals, associations, groups, and institutions that have something to give, something that others may need: knowledge, succor, an actual resource or talent, or simply time and place.

Traditional questions such as "What's wrong with this immigrant family?" and "Why is this ethnic immigrant mentally ill or delinquent or abusive?" should become "What are the strengths in this Hmong family that will help them grow and change?" and "What do the Cambodian immigrants need to develop into more creative and organized adults?" (Weick et al., 1989).

Other questions that help identify strengths in immigrants are as follows:

"What knowledge and skills help you as an immigrant 'make it' each day?"
"What kinds of things are important to immigrants?"

"When are immigrants happiest?"

"What kinds of things do you do to help other immigrant parents out?"

"Who are your heroes that are also immigrants?"

"If you awarded yourself a medal as an immigrant, what would it say?"

"What ethnic foods, ethnic exercises, and so on, do you use to stay healthy?"

In addition, there are also questions that promote the immigrant's involvement in the working relationship. Some questions that facilitate client involvement in the strengths approach are as follows:

"What do immigrant families from Laos do on a Sunday afternoon?"

"Where are the places you go in the Vietnamese community when you feel alone, nervous, or upset?"

"If you agree to work with me, what do I need to know about you as a Russian immigrant to be an effective helper?"

"What do Latino families like to do for fun?"

"When do you feel really good about yourself as a Filipino immigrant?"

"What was your favorite subject in school?"

"What do other immigrant teenagers do when they are bored?"

"What is your favorite ethnic food?"

"Who is your favorite author from back home?"

"What kinds of music from Nicaragua do you enjoy?"

"Who is your favorite Nicaraguan performer?"

(Kisthardt, 1997, p. 108)

The following is an example of how the strengths perspective can be used with Sergei, who was adopted by a couple who later divorced.

Case Vignette

A married couple with two biological children felt inspired and almost driven to adopt a child from Russia. During part of the 1990s, the Russians were allowing adoption of only children needing assistance that Russia could not offer. Sergei needed special education for undiagnosed learning difficulties, and mental health care for issues related to attachment and bonding, because he clung to his father and avoided his mother and two older siblings. Sergei also displayed restlessness, unpredictable behavioral outbursts, and inattention. Increasingly at odds with each other, the parents divorced, and the father gained custody of the Russian son.

The family used social work services in several ways: (1) The social studies for U.S. Immigration and Naturalization Services as well as U.S. and Russian adoption agencies required expert review by licensed authorities; (2) the family sought services for the adjustment of the adopted child, the siblings, the marriage, and the family unit; (3) when the marriage deteriorated, a new set of issues required intervention of the Family Court officers, several of whom were social workers; and (4) the developing child required assistance for education, mental health, and language development.

When working with Sergei and his family, various social workers displayed the following principles of the strengths approach: (1) identify individual and family strengths (workers identified an initially strong marriage, adequate finances, support of extended family and friends, ability to follow through on myriad details, and willingness to step into the unknown; (2) Using the difficulties of Sergei and his family members to teach them lessons and skills that now help them (struggles to get the adoption finalized, and, later, the divorce, which in hindsight actually strengthened each person and led to happiness); (3) encouraging family members to do the best they could (workers fostered this by displaying positive attitudes toward the family members, even while the parents were going through the divorce, and also focusing on family strengths rather than limitations); (4) collaborating with the husband and wife even while both were filing for a divorce; and (5) using resources in the environment (workers encouraged Sergei's parents to locate their own resources by first giving them some referrals to resources, then allowing them to locate others independently).

The strengths approach was used effectively with Sergei and his family to the point that, eventually, his adopted parents faced the reality of their unhappy marriage, divorced, and are now happier. Although most clients will not undergo the ultimate change of divorce, it nevertheless remains important that principles of the strengths approach be used when working with immigrants. Key questions that could help identify immigrant children and his/her family's strengths include the following: What are the strengths that will help him or her grow in this new country? What are his or her characteristics, talents, and abilities that are valued by the dominant society? What makes the parent or parents stand out as individuals or as a couple? How do siblings show their love for family members? What traumatic experiences did they go through prior to and upon arriving in the United States that have strengthened them? A third effective approach for work with immigrants is the empowerment perspective.

THE EMPOWERMENT APPROACH

Empowerment, a common term in social work education and practice, is sometimes used in conjunction with the concept of consciousness (Gutierrez, 1990; Lee, 1994) with powerless groups. Powerlessness, or the lack of empowerment of individuals, is based on indicators such as economic insecurity, absence of experience in the political realm, insufficient access to information, lack of training, physical and emotional stress, learned helplessness, and aspects of one's emotional or intellectual makeup. Oftentimes, those without power are part of the out- or stigmatized groups such as women; ethnic minorities; gays, lesbians, transgendered, and bisexual people; religious minorities; the aged; the poor, and so on. Beck (1983) believes that empowerment can be the keystone of social work.

Concepts of the Empowerment Approach

Empowerment has been defined by a number of authors. Browne (1995) believes that empowerment has been characterized in basically three ways: as an intervention and product, a skill, and a process. Gutierrez (1990) defines empowerment as a process from a political perspective: "Empowerment is a process of increasing personal, interpersonal, or political power so that individuals can take action to improve their life situations" (p. 149). Using the Gutierrez (1990) definition of empowerment, concepts such as consciousness and transformation are key to increasing power and moving toward social justice. Lee (1994) believes that practitioners need to help consumers be critically aware of their powerless status and raise the awareness or consciousness level of others. Gutierrez (1990) promotes developing group consciousness through fostering an awareness of how political structures affect individual and group experiences. Individuals are helped to see their powerlessness and focus their energies on the causes of their problems.

Principles of the Empowerment Approach

Some basic principles of the empowerment approach are as follows:

1. Power exists in various forms. Power can influence decision makers, buy goods and services, control a situation, enable people to make decisions, and enhance the circumstances for those with power.
2. Power is dynamic. Individuals, groups, and communities may gain or lose power. Those that have power are empowered, whereas others are powerless.
3. Powerless individuals, groups, and communities are sometimes stigmatized. Usually, consumers are powerless based on their ethnicity, gender, religious affiliation, sexual orientation, and/or physical and mental status.
4. Power can be gained through a variety of means: education, training, development of talents and resources, funding, political lobby-

ing, and so on. Those with power do not normally want to relinquish it.

5. Empowered individuals, groups, and communities have more control over their circumstances and are better able to solve their own problems.

The following is an example of how the empowerment perspective can be used with Tich Tien, a Vietnamese teenage male charged twice with auto theft.

Case Vignette

Tich Tien (who is also known as Tony by his peers), 17, is the son of Vietnamese refugees. He is not doing well in school, wants money to buy what others at school have, and is a gang member. Recently, he was caught twice with a stolen auto and is now on probation.

Tich Tien's parents suffered through the Vietnamese war, flight from Vietnam, refugee camp in Hong Kong, and resettlement in the United States. Currently, both parents are employed full- and part-time to support their family of five children and extended family members back home, leaving little time and energy for supervising and emotionally supporting their children.

Tich Tien is the oldest child, street smart, and one of the gang leaders. He wants name brand shoes and T-shirts, CDs, and electronic items such as a computer. At one time, he had a job at a fast-food vendor, but now he would rather steal to acquire status symbols. So far, Tich Tien has not been caught breaking probation rules, and he communicates regularly with his Probation Officer. Until middle school, Tich Tien did as well as could be expected in school and behaved appropriately.

Early on, the social worker needs to teach Tich Tien how to (1) maintain positive behaviors and take on additional appropriate behaviors in keeping the terms of his probation, being a model for his younger siblings, and refraining from gang activities; (2) prepare for part-time employment so that he can acquire the priority status items he values; (3) identify a balance and acceptance between being American by culture and Vietnamese by ethnicity; and (4) appreciate the predominance of Asians in the world and the richness of his Asian heritage. Tich Tien may also benefit from group sessions that redirect him toward appropriate goals such as high school graduation and employment, or a continuation of his education.

The social worker also needs to be involved in indirect practice by advocating and lobbying for social service programs that will help children of refugees such as Tich Tien. Ethnic minorities whose religious affiliation is unfamiliar with the general public are twice as powerless as members of the dominant society.

STRESS FACTORS PECULIAR TO IMMIGRANTS AND CULTURALLY COMPETENT RESPONSES

Immigrants are subject to several complex internal and external factors that may lead to stress and the need for social services: the cognitive, social, biological, psychological, spiritual, and cultural internal makeup of human behavior or the micro-system; the stage of the human life cycle of the client or the family life cycle, or the meso- and exo-systems; and the indirect external factors, or the macro-system.

On the micro-level, clients are at a cognitive, social, physical, spiritual, and cultural development or condition. Physical conditions such as ethnicity may in part lead to discrimination and oppress the immigrant searching for a job or low cost housing. Difficulties in securing a job that provides adequate income and obtaining affordable housing may cause financial problems, low self-esteem, and family disharmony, culminating in possible domestic violence and the need for social services.

In terms of cultural development, adherence to traditional cultural values and lifestyles without adequate adaptation to the host culture may result in a student being misdiagnosed "mildly retarded" or an employee being passed by for promotion because he or she "has no ideas" or "is a 'yes'man/woman." Immigrants continue to face these stressful situations.

Sometimes immigrant parents are not able to express themselves so that helping professionals understand them. School social workers must be diligent to know and understand fundamental values, lifestyles, and common behavioral patterns of immigrant and refugee students and their family members, so that ethnic students are diagnosed accurately; help immigrants identify their personal and cultural strengths, and encourage them to use these strengths while progressing toward empowerment; and encourage immigrants to adopt characteristics of the dominant society, such as assertiveness, to better "fit" in their new homeland.

The immigrant is always in a phase or transitioning into or out from a phase of the human life cycle. Ongoing developmental changes may also cause stress, and this discomfort could be compounded by the client's immigrant or refugee status or background. For example, a teenager whose parents fled Laos may be struggling in the adolescent stage with role identity. Difficult as this role confusion issue may be, it can be further exacerbated if the teenager is also struggling to be autonomous of traditional parents holding fast to their hierarchical parental position. Gang membership, drugs, and violence may be reasons for a parole officer to be involved with this refugee family. The parole officer may need to recognize the immigrant

family's strengths, such as respect for authority, religious ties, and preference for cooperation and nonconfrontation. A refugee family that holds
these values will work best with a parole officer that looks and sounds like
a professional helping person; includes the monk or priest in a supportive
role; and recognizes that tacit agreement does not necessarily indicate approval. The parole officer in this case may need to keep in mind the ultimate goal of helping this family become independent from social services
through attainment of education, resources, and opportunities, while seeking frequent feedback that silence is or is not an indication of approval.
Empowerment can only be achieved as the refugee family and social
worker both move forward collaboratively toward common goals that the
refugee family defines.

Macro-system external factors such as cultural values and variables
that influence policies, resource distribution, values, and mores of society
are also known to impact immigrants and refugees negatively. A failing
economy may mean that immigrants lose their menial jobs to poor whites;
the societal more to "marry your own kind" may keep the majority from
better understanding ethnic minorities and vice versa; and more education
dollars earmarked for upper-middle-class suburban schools, while neglect-
ing lower class, inner-city schools, may make it more difficult to prepare
immigrants and refugees living in inner cities for an adequate income and
lifestyle, let alone break through the glass ceiling. Social workers must help
immigrants and refugees learn English, pass citizenship or naturalization
tests, register to vote, meet candidates and become familiar with their positions, and vote as a block for candidates willing to fight for their needs.
Then, social workers may need to continue empowering immigrants and
refugees by teaching them to organize and lobby legislators for select bills
and amendments to help them gain equality and social justice. Political
power is a key macro means for broad changes that help ethnic groups empower and strengthen themselves.

Immigrants and refugees throughout much of their lives and in various settings face internal and external problems that keep them apart
from fair treatment, opportunities, and achievement. The total effect of
these challenges and issues oftentimes leadd to a cycle of despair, poverty,
and dependence on medical, mental health, and social services. More social workers must be better trained on many levels to address the social
and mental health issues of immigrant and refugee clients, based on social work knowledge, skills, values, and ethics in a culturally competent
context.

Hirayama and Cetingok's (1988) description of an empowerment
approach when working with Asian immigrants is still very relevant today. Goals such as bicultural attitude and behaviors, empowerment, and
increased coping and adaptational abilities of immigrants in families,

groups, and communities remain valid. Likewise, Asian values such as vertical relations, acceptance, interdependence, self-control, duty toward family and community, and obedience are still cherished by traditional Asians. Subsequent social worker tasks involve teaching the immigrant to learn new roles and characteristics, including when and how to use them while maintaining those qualities that are basic to functioning in more traditional settings.

The *Journal of Multicultural Social Work* devoted Volume 2, Number 1, in 1992 to a special issue, "Social Work with Immigrants and Refugees." Kelly (1992) describes the cultural appropriateness of systems practice with the Southeast Asian refugee population based in part on their emphasis on the family and community over the individual, and the less intrusive and more respectful nature of the approach complements the family's need for privacy relative to other issues that need not be discussed. Strategic therapy, the Milan systemic approach, genograms, and family maps are also considered to work well with the traditional Asian population.

Leung et al. (1994) proposes the following five components of a strengths approach when training ethnically sensitive child protective service workers: (1) developing positive attitudes toward clients, (2) focusing on family strengths and not problems, (3) encouraging clients to engage in effective behaviors, (4) challenging clients to appreciate their own ethnic and cultural backgrounds, and (5) encouraging clients to locate their own resources. They have also developed a lengthy list of questions regarding attitudes, knowledge, and skills to be asked throughout the problem-solving phases for a more culturally competent approach.

More recently, Fong and Furuto (2001) presented a comprehensive practice book that includes values and ethics, and micro-, meso-, and macro-assessments, interventions, and evaluations of Asians/Pacific Islanders, First Nations Peoples, Latinos, and descendants of African Americans—populations that include immigrants and refugees. The theoretical base of this book is the ecological, strengths, and empowerment approaches as applied to ethnic minority groups. All the practice chapters reflect use of these theoretical approaches when assessing, intervening, or evaluating micro-, meso-, and macro-ethnic populations.

Balgopal's book (2000) looks at micro-, meso-, and macro-levels of practice with immigrants and refugees. For example, Francis's (2000) description of Haitian men who traditionally believe that they "possess" their wives find it difficult to let them work in the United States. It is also stressful for parents when Haitian children behave more independently than they would back home. On the macro-level, Longres and Patterson (2000) promote the three macro-level social worker tasks to help ameliorate ethnic conflict and develop a unified multicultural society: (1) Change the circumstances that hinder the advancement of Latinos, (2) improve intergroup relations, and (3) reduce the physical and emotional stress associated with acculturation.

The following is an example of how the ecological, strengths, and empowerment perspectives can be used with José and his family as they adapt to the hardships of a life of poverty.

Case Vignette

José, 10 years of age, has recently moved to the United States from Mexico. He is having a difficult time adjusting to school and has been referred to the school social worker. He lives with his father, a seasonal crop worker, and his mother, who stays at home. Recently, his mom gave birth to her fourth child, and there were complications. His father is unable to pay the hospital bill for the Cesarean section, and other bills are mounting. His parents have been talking about just leaving all their troubles behind by moving on to another community.

The school social worker, in assessing José ecologically and holistically, considers his cognitive, social, biological, psychological, spiritual, and cultural makeup. She finds him to be fairly bright, reserved but somewhat friendly with other Mexican American children who speak Spanish, healthy, although his stature is smaller than most boys his age, of sound mind, religious-oriented, and traditional in his cultural outlook. He and his family are actively involved in a Mexican American farm community and Mexican American Catholic Church in Laredo, Texas.

By identifying the strengths of José and other Mexican American children, the school social worker is able to promote them in group sessions and in their Mexican sports and games activities. The intent is to make the immigrant children fit as well as possible in their new environment and have as many positive transactions as possible with their new friends and teachers.

The school social worker, who can perhaps best empower José by helping him make friends at school, learn the English language, and receive tutorial assistance, has designed a buddy program at school, whereby new students are paired up with similar peers or buddies who befriend them and help them adjust to the school system. José's buddy is Mario, and because both boys live in the same neighborhood, they are able to walk to and from school together. A major goal for José is that he do satisfactorily in school and graduate from high school. The afterschool tutorial program provides José with the opportunity for the one-to-one assistance he needs to learn the English language. Audiovisual and electronic learning technologies are also available.

The school social worker has just received some grant monies that will enable her to form a group for upper-elementary-level, Spanish-speaking boys new to school. The plan is that José participate. During some group sessions, the facilitator intends to invite model older students of Mexican American ethnicity to influence the group members positively, and during other sessions, the members will participate in activities that promote their Mexican heritage. At the end of the group sessions, the members will teach their classmates Mexican sports and games that bring the Mexican American and Anglo American children together.

CONCLUSIONS

This chapter has stressed the appropriateness of the ecological, strengths, and empowerment approaches when working with immigrants. The ecological approach takes a holistic perspective in assessment and intervention by focusing on transactions between the immigrant and his or her environment, including their goodness of fit and subsequent adaptations. The immigrant's past—a factor vital to understanding the goodness of fit in the present—is given attention in the ecological approach, as are eco-maps and genograms.

The strengths approach promotes the identification of strengths on many levels, the belief that trauma and difficulties can strengthen the immigrant; advises that we encourage our clients to attain their potential; recommends that practitioners collaborate with clients; and assures us that every environment has a number of resources. A number of questions that help identify strengths in immigrants and promote the immigrant's involvement in the helping process were cited.

The empowerment approach espouses that power exists in various forms and is dynamic. Powerless individuals, groups, and communities, such as immigrants, are sometimes stigmatized. These powerless groups can gain power by various means, and empowered immigrants have more control over their circumstances and can better solve their own problems. Case vignettes followed each of the three theoretical approaches, with descriptions of how social workers demonstrated each particular approach. The chapter proceeded with a discussion of multilevel internal and external stress factors particular to immigrants and culturally competent responses, then concluded with the case vignette of José with the school social worker using all three theoretical approaches.

When used together, all three theoretical approaches can be a powerful, holistic method for working with immigrants in their communities. The tritheoretical approach considers the transactions between the immigrant and the immigrant's unique environment, with a movement toward promoting those transactions that foster growth and development. Client strengths are identified and become fundamental for growth and development toward problem resolution in part by knowing how to locate and use community resources.

ACKNOWLEDGMENTS

I gratefully acknowledge Paula T. Tanemura Morelli and participants of the Cambodian American Health-Seeking and Social Networks Project and the National Research Center on Asian American Mental Health for use of the Sophiap case vignette; Ronaele Whittington for help with the Sergei case vignette; and the Kalihi–Palama Multi-Service Center for assistance with the Tich Tien case vignette.

REFERENCES

Balgopal, P. (Ed.). (2000). *Social work practice with immigrants and refugees.* New York: Columbia University Press.

Bartlett, H. M. (1958). Toward clarification and improvement of social work practice. *Social Work, 3,* 3–9.

Beck, B. (1983, February). *Empowerment: A future goal for social work.* Paper presented at the National Association of Social Work Conference, Boston.

Bronfenbrenner, U. (1979). *The ecology of human development.* Cambridge, MA: Harvard University Press.

Browne, C. (1995, May). Empowerment in social work practice with older women. *Social Work, 40*(3), 358–364.

Browne, C., & Mills, C. (2001). Theoretical frameworks: Ecological model, strengths perspective, and empowerment theory. In R. Fong & S. Furuto (Eds.), *Culturally competent practice: Skills, interventions, and evaluations* (pp. 10–32). Boston: Allyn & Bacon.

Camarota, S. (2000, December). Our new immigration predicament. *American Enterprise Institute for Public Policy Research, 11*(8), 26–29.

Capps, R. (2001, February). Hardship among children of immigrants: Findings from the 1999 National Survey of America's families. *New Federalism: National Survey of America's Families,* Series B, No. B-29. Washington, DC: The Urban Institute.

Congress, E. (1994). The use of culturagrams to assess and empower culturally diverse families. *Families in Society, 75,* 531–540.

Corcoran, J., Franklin, C., & Bennett, P. (2000). Ecological factors associated with adolescent pregnancy and parenting. *Social Work Research, 24*(1), 29–39.

Devore, W., & Schlesinger, E. (1999). *Ethnic-sensitive social work practice* (5th ed.). Boston: Allyn & Bacon.

Fong, R., & Furuto, S. (Eds.). (2001). *Culturally competent practice: Skills, interventions, and evaluations.* Boston: Allyn & Bacon.

Francis, E. A. (2000). Social work practice with African-descent immigrants In P. Balgopal (Ed.), *Social work practice with immigrants and refugees* (pp. 127–166). New York: Columbia University Press.

Germain, C. B. (Ed.). (1979). *Social work practice: People and environments, an eco-logical perspective*. New York: Columbia University Press.

Germain, C. B. (1991). *Human behavior in the social environment: An ecological view*. New York: Columbia University Press.

Germain, C. B., & Gitterman, A. (1980). *The life model of social work practice*. New York: Columbia University Press.

Green, J. (1995). *Cultural awareness in the human services*. Englewood Cliffs, NJ: Prentice-Hall.

Gutierrez, L. (1990). Working with women of color. *Social Work, 35*(2), 149–154.

Hartman, A., & Laird, J. (1983). *Family-centered social work practice*. New York: Free Press.

Hearn, G. (1979). General systems theory and social work. In F. J. Turner (Ed.), *Social work treatment: Interlocking theoretical approaches* (2nd ed., pp. 333–359). New York: Free Press.

Hernandez, M., & Isaacs, M. (1998) *Promoting cultural competence in children's mental health services*. Baltimore: Brooks/Cole.

Hirayama, H., & Cetingok, M. (1988). Empowerment: A social work approach for Asian immigrants. *Social Casework, 69*(1), 41–47.

Kelly, P. (1992). The application of family systems theory to mental health services for Southeast Asian refugees. *Journal of Multicultural Social Work, 2*(1), 1–13.

Kisthardt, W. (1997). The strengths model of case management: Principles and help-ing functions. In D. Saleebey (Ed.), *The strengths perspective in social work prac-tice* (pp. 97–113). New York: Longman.

Lee, J. (1994). *The empowerment approach to social work practice*. New York: Co-lumbia University Press.

Leung, P., Cheung, K. F. M., & Stevenson, K. (1994, November). A strengths ap-proach to ethnically sensitive practice for child protective service workers. *Child Welfare, 73*(6), 707–713.

Longres, J. F., & Patterson, D. G. (2000). Social work practice with Latino American immigrants. In P. Balgopal (Ed.), *Social work practice with immigrants and refu-gees* (pp. 65–126). New York: Columbia University Press.

Lum, D. (1999). *Culturally competent practice: A framework for growth and action*. Pacific Grove, CA: Brooks/Cole.

McGoldrick, M., & Gerson, R. (1985). *Genograms in family assessment*. New York: Norton.

McGoldrick, M., Pearce, J., & Giordano, J. (Eds.). (1996). *Ethnicity and family ther-apy* (2nd ed.). New York: Guilford Press.

Middleman, R., & Goldberg, G. (1974). *Social service delivery: A structural approach to social work practice*. New York: Columbia University Press.

Nimmagadda, J., & Balgopal, P. (2000). Social work practice with Asian immigrants. In P. Balgopal (Ed.), *Social work practice with immigrants and refugees* (pp. 1–29). New York: Columbia University Press.

Pincus, A., & Minahan, A. (1973). *Social work practice: Model and method*. Madi-son: University of Wisconsin Press.

Poulin, J. (2000). *Collaborative social work: Strengths-based generalist practice*. Itasca, IL: Peacock.

Saleebey, D. (Ed.). (1997). *The strengths perspective in social work practice* (2nd ed.). New York: Longman.

Sheafor, B., Horejsi, C., & Horejsi, G. (2000). *Techniques and guidelines for social work practice* (5th ed.). Boston: Allyn & Bacon.

Teall, B. (2000). Using solution-oriented interventions in an ecological frame: A case illustration. *Social Work in Education, 22*(1), 54–61.

Weick, A., Rapp, C., Sullivan, W., & Kisthardt, W. (1989). A strengths perspective for social work practice. *Social Work, 34*(4), 350–354.

CHAPTER 3

Contexts and Environments for Culturally Competent Practice

ROWENA FONG

The United States is becoming a place where people of diverse backgrounds are beginning to, and will continue to, dominate American society numerically and culturally, challenging social workers and other professionals to deliver more services and interventions that "start and get to where the client is." The social work profession has always strived to develop helping and meaningful relationships with clients, but with the immigrant and refugee population, we are still challenged to determine what is meaningful to them from their perspective. We seem to continue to label them as "strangers from distant shores" (Takaki, 1987), while not knowing exactly how to receive or service them. Since September 11, 2001, it is even more questionable whether they are welcome in the United States, or for those who live here, it is questionable whether they want to continue to live in an environment of mistrust and possible harassment.

The profession of social work through the Council on Social Work Education, 2002 Educational Policy and Accreditation Standards, mandates that social workers be prepared to address their clients' diversity and strengths, and offer services that are culturally relevant and effective for people from diverse backgrounds. Likewise, the National Association of Social Work, in 2001, passed Standards for Cultural Competence in Social Work Practice requiring practitioners to develop specialized and culturally competent knowledge, skills, and service deliveries. Although the mandates are necessary, there are still not enough theories, practice models, or interventions that adequately address the diversity among the five ethnic group-ings of Asians and Pacific Islanders, African Americans and Caribbeans, Euro-Americans, First Nations Peoples, and Latinos and Mexican Ameri-cans. Much expertise is offered in the awareness and knowledge-building stages of social work practice, but more information is necessary about how to provide services that are culturally effective to these populations. Too often, the approach is to service the immigrant and refugee population in the way it is always done in America, with some modification by having an interpreter involved in the process. This manner is becoming less effec-tive as immigrants and refugees require not merely the translation of words but, more importantly, the exchange of culturally different ideas and mean-ingful interventions.

As author Gwat-Yong Lie points out in Chapter 7, the traditional Hmong people do not have a concept that embraces mental illness. It is meaningless to talk about posttraumatic stress disorder (PTSD) to a first- or even second-generation Hmong person when it is only to the spiritual or the physical ailment that they can relate. If the shaman is the common heal-ing modality, then what will it take to have social work practitioners start with the shaman as the first treatment modality rather than the last resort?

The barriers to integrating indigenous practices need to be reexam-ined. If there is resistance to including them (shamans in the Hmong cul-ture, Buddhist priests in the Chinese, Japanese, or Korean cultures), then the minimally recommended treatment modality needs to be compatible with the values and practices of the ethnic culture. If Hmong people are worried about physical illness, then those symptoms cannot be dismissed and ignored. If depression is suspected in a Hmong family member who is not eating, treatment should initially focus on the hunger and how to in-crease the appetite. But the mental health assessments should not be ig-nored. Chinese social worker and psychotherapist, Marshall Jung, de-scribes in his book *Chinese American Family Therapy* (1998) his mother's somatization and his misunderstanding of it as hypochondria before fully realizing his error:

> Acceptance of psychosomatic medicine has been a part of the Chinese cul-ture. Traditionally, every organ has psychological meaning or symbolic functions. The heart is considered to be the seat of intellect; the lungs are the seat of righteousness; the gall bladder is symbolic of bravery; while kidneys produce ingenuity and power. Consequently, an exploration of somatic complaints needs to be a part of a family therapist's assessment of the prob-lems of his or her Chinese clients.
>
> As my mother grew older, she appeared to be plagued with an in-creasing number of physical ailments: headaches, back and stomach pains, and an inability to move various joints. One day, my brothers, Chester, Douglas, and I watched her coming out of the kitchen in the back of our grocery store. She was dragging one leg and had a right hand

on her forehead as she complained of having a severe headache. It looked so contrived it seemed comical, instead of eliciting feelings of empathy. We looked at each other, thinking that she was a hypochondriac. Later, I learned that to the Chinese somatization is a valid way of expressing inner conflicts and that physical, rather than psychological, complaints are an acceptable way to obtain attention. (pp. 46–47)

Physical complaints are an acceptable way to obtain attention from the Chinese son or daughter; physical complaints should also be an acceptable way for a non-Chinese practitioner to get information about the Chinese patient's psychological functioning. A parallel form of required symbolic interpretation is found in play therapy.

In play therapy there are many ways in which children's play is symbolic of their emotional or psychological state. Communication is difficult, for children do not know how to convey their emotions. Is it not possible in culturally competent, contextual social work practice that in some cultures in which expressions of mental health are cast in physical ailments, a language and framework of understanding and treating should be developed that reflect the client's indigenous culture? For children in play therapy, the color red is usually symbolic of anger; social workers need to know this work with children and interpret their play and artwork. In working with traditional Chinese immigrant families, the heart is symbolic of intellectual functioning; thus, social workers need to know how to interpret this symbolism of physical ailment in reference to cognitive and mental health functioning. This chapter focuses on frameworks, principles, and tools for culturally competent contextual social work assessments and interventions. It is based on the premise that strengths and solutions coming from the immigrant and refugee child and family clients have been underdeveloped. Strengths in their cultural values and solutions to problem solving using their indigenous interventions have been underutilized. This chapter presents a framework and practice principles for culturally competent contextual social work practice. It also addresses assessment practices that make distinctions in social environments and client statuses, and identify risk factors for immigrant and refugee children and families. It proposes use of cultural values as strengths and protective factors, with the conclusion that a solution-focused therapy framework needs to complement indigenous interventions.

CULTURALLY COMPETENT CONTEXTUAL PRACTICE

The knowledge and understanding of contexts make an enormous difference in how one approaches and offers social work treatment and services to immigrant and refugee children and families. Their myriad experiences are contextual, differing for individual children and family situations. O'Melia (2002) describes contextual social work practice as a means of empowerment, as evident in his chapter title "From Person to Context: The Evolution of an Empowering Practice." The goal of our work with immigrant and refugee children and families is to empower them, but it is better done when a conceptual framework focuses on contexts and an understanding of the cultural norm, values, and beliefs of their home countries is incorporated into social work practice. Thus, the components for culturally competent contextual social work practice are as follows (see also Table 3.1):

1. A theoretical framework of an ecological model of micro-, meso-, and macro-levels of person–environment practice.
2. A strengths-based orientation with macro-level societal and cultural values used in assessments and intervention planning.
3. The intersectionality of macro- and cultural values, and differential assessments.
4. An empowerment through a solution-focused therapy approach reflecting the biculturalization of interventions.

This book argues that the native social environment of the client plays a major role in the understanding of information collected during the assessment stage. In addition, intervention planning needs to include an approach that aims toward simulating a solution-focused attempt to refocus on the client's strengths and positive problem-solving experiences of how things were culturally handled before he or she came into contact with Western interventions. A simulation may not be totally possible, but at least the client will get the message that the social worker is interested in knowing what life was like when things were culturally comfortable for him or her.

As Balgopal (2000) challenges us, "Workers must be ethnically sensitive and skilled in helping these groups adapt to their new environments without losing their cultural heritage. The coping and adaptations of these 'new Americans' need to be seen as a dual process—learning new customs and lifestyles while retaining old traditions and values" (p. xi). The retention of values and traditions is critical and supports a strengths perspective.

Although the culturally competent social worker tries to help immigrants and refugees sustain old traditions and values, this is more easily done if the social worker's priority is to learn what the old traditions and values are and treat the cultural values as strengths. Each chapter in this book speaks to the values of the culture, and other works have also stressed their importance, arguing that cultural values are critical in understanding the multicultural client (Dhooper & Moore, 2001; Ho, 1987; Lum, 2003; Mokuau, 1991; Webb, 2001) and need to be better used in assessment

TABLE 3.1. A Framework for Culturally Competent Contextual Social Work Practice

Practice principles for assessment

1. Social workers need to have a knowledge of the context of macro-level environmental factors of the home country (macro-level societal value assessment).
2. Social workers need to know the cultural values and beliefs of the client in the home country (personal cultural value assessment).
3. Social workers need to determine and assess the impact of the intermediary environments (multienvironmental assessment).
4. Social workers need to discern when cultural values of home and host environment differ (differential cultural value assessment).

Practice principles for intervention planning and implementation

1. Social workers need to integrate the societal and cultural values of the client by utilizing the macro-level societal values assessments and the personal cultural value assessments in intervention planning and implementation.
2. Social workers need to use interventions based on clients' personal cultural values, and by using the differential values assessment, practitioners need to choose those treatments that do not clash with clients' cultural values.
3. Social work interventions need to reflect biculturalization of interventions, using cultural values as strengths.
4. Social workers need to take into account the different social environments and use the multienvironmental assessment in using a solution-focused approach to problem solving with the biculturalization of interventions.

planning and intervention treatment (Fong, Boyd, & Browne, 1999; Fong & Furuto, 2001; Fong, Sandau-Beckler & Haapala, 1994). Whereas there are universal cultural values such as love of family, respecting others, and so on, it is the challenge of the culturally competent social worker to understand the context of the value and operationalize it, so that it can actually be implemented as a tool or means to facilitate positive movement and activity in treatments and interventions.

Because ethnic groups vary markedly relative to one another and internal differences abound within single groupings, suggestions for assessments and interventions are proposed with the understanding that each immigrant and refugee family arrives with unique situations and experiences. Culturally competent practitioners must affirm that their clients' situations, though similar in some regards, are unique, and practice needs to be individualized to fit their circumstances. Although Latin Americans, Asians, and Caribbeans tend to currently dominate the census numbers, immigrant and refugee groups from other countries, such as the former Soviet Union, also need social services that reflect their unique circumstances of migration. Addressing current and future concerns and directions for culturally competent practice of contextual social work with recent immigrant and refugee families, four major areas come to mind in building a framework for assessments and interventions: (1) developing assessment practices that make distinctions in social environments and client statuses; (2) identifying and assessing risk factors for immigrant and refugee children and families; (3) utilizing cultural values as protective factors in indigenous strategies and interventions; and (4) ameliorating the impact of changing social environments through the use of culturally competent biculturalization of interventions.

MAKING DISTINCTIONS IN SOCIAL ENVIRONMENTS AND STATUSES

There are numerous terms affiliated with the immigrant and refugee population: legal permanent resident, migrant, asylee, undocumented alien, temporary protective status, trafficking victim, and so on. All of the terms imply a context and an affiliation with a social environment describing the conditions in which the immigrants or refugees left their home country and/ or entered or resided in the United States. Understanding these circumstances better is important for culturally competent contextual practitioners, because the diverse social environments of recent immigrants and refugees need to be factored into assessments and intervention planning. Culturally competent contextual social work practice assesses immigrants and refugees while emphasizing several factors:

- The assessment process begins at the macro-level, with societal and cultural values accounting for the differences in social environments and explaining difficulties in adaptation.
- The assessment process should take into account the different legal statuses, and political and economic circumstances of the social environments in the native countries that influence immigrants' and refugees' adaptations to the United States.
- The assessment process needs to reflect culturally competent contextual practice by the integration of differential legal statuses, transitioning in social environments, and adaptations in human behaviors.

Assessment and Treatment Planning with Macro-Level Societal and Cultural Values

Many recent immigrants and refugees left their native homes for better opportunities in the United States, whereas others were forced to flee for their physical safety and to avoid continued political persecution and economic duress. When assessing immigrants' and refugees' problems, the social worker needs to be aware that the time and reason for leaving the native county makes a difference in how they were and still are received in America, and how they adapt.

Recent immigrants and refugees are leaving their countries at a time when the United States is becoming skeptical of their presence. Since September 11, 2001, American white citizens, American-born people of color, and immigrants who came to the United States earlier are not always welcoming, and they may even be overtly resentful of these newcomers (Gold, 2000; McLemore, Romo, & Baker, 2001; Moore & Vigil, 2000; Waldinger, 2000). Although the 1965 Immigration Law allowed more immigrants to come to the United States and families to reunify, in addition to recent terrorist attacks, the tightening of monetary resources has contributed to skepticism at best and hostile discriminatory actions at worst toward immigrants and refugees. Segal (2002) warns that "in general, public immigration policy is closely bound to economic and national needs. Opportunities may be available to immigrants yet fraught with obstacles, mirroring the nation's ambivalence toward a particular immigrant group. The country's receptiveness is also reflected in the available programs for the immigrants. . . . The acceptance of a group is highly influenced by the country's openness to diversity and to ethnic specific variables" (p. 24).

These new immigrants may also be perceived are taking resources from older immigrants and sullying the good image the older immigrants have strived to create. In Chapter 11, Colon and Sardinas describes the *Marielitos* and *Balseros* as not receiving a warm welcome from earlier Cuban immigrants: "In the case of these Cuban immigrant groups, Cuban American leaders feared that their image and presence [the *Marielitos* and *Balseros*] would tarnish the Cuban American image as model individuals. " These newer immigrants also need federal assistance with language development, housing, and job training, but because of the lack of or minimal assistance available, the newcomers are resented by the older immigrants who may already have benefited from federal help (Erdmans, 2000; Fong, 2000; Trueba, Cheng, & Ima, 1993). Culturally competent contextual social work practice would include the understanding of the cohorts and time differences when immigrants arrive in the United States. The societal values and attitudes in the United States about immigrants' contribution to resource building through employment may change over time. The situation in 1965, when the law was passed allowing more skilled labor from foreign countries, is a far cry from the legalistic practices in 2003, when immigrant laborers, even skilled professionals, need be fearful of mistaken identities and endure mistrustful accountability procedures.

Another example of the importance of understanding in the assessment stage the differences in macro-values and their impact on adaptation is the situation of the Nicaraguans and Salvadorans. In Chapter 14, Marsiglia and Menjívar write about the understanding that Nicaraguans and Salvadorians had of promises for political asylum from the U.S. government. Awareness of this history hopefully ameliorates the blame imposed on these refugees, who may become asylees when living in the United

States. These refugees were promised support and have mixed expectations of governments (Harrold-Bond, 1999). They fled countries in which they experienced political persecution and entered the United States skeptical of government, because of the harsh practices they experienced in their home countries. It is not surprising that social work practice with these refugees should start by addressing their perceptions and experiences of the political systems of the two countries. They need to understand the macro-values of the United States and have them presented in a nonthreatening, educational manner, because too often, federal, state, and local rules and regulations are presented in a hostile, refugee-unfriendly manner rather than simply as a framework for solving problems.

In doing contextual practice, culturally competent social workers need to learn the macro-level values of the societies from which the immigrants come. For example, macro-level values surrounding politics, religion, and economics in the former Soviet Union, the Middle East, or Central America often differ greatly from those in the United States. Social workers assisting immigrants and refugees in transitioning from these social environments are better able to help when they know such differences exist. Fong (1997) wrote about assessment practice with immigrants from the People's Republic of China, advocating the necessity to understand and assess from the macro-level, then moving to the meso- and micro-levels. She maintains that worldviews and practices in a socialist, communistic country are very different, and clients from those countries need to be educated. Bemak and Chung (2002) write about the multilevel model (MLM) of counseling and psychotherapy with refugees, which has four levels. The therapist begins with Level I, in which the client is educated about mainstream mental health practices and interventions. Level II focuses on individual, family, and group, psychotherapy; Level III is aimed toward cultural empowerment; and Level IV focuses on indigenous healing, combining indigenous and Western interventions. In reviewing the MLM model, one would expect that its most effective use is to apply the levels simultaneously rather than sequentially. If it were sequential, cultural empowerment should be first not third. Part of the cultural empowerment would be to have the culturally competent social worker understand the macro level societal values of the home country of the immigrant or refugee client.

As to the meso- and micro-levels, whereas work with nonimmigrant clients usually starts at the individual microlevel, work with immigrants and refugees is usually best begun with an understanding of communities and families before undertaking work with individuals. Knowledge of the ethnic communities is crucial. Some communities of older immigrants need to be prepared to receive the new immigrants, and additional community resources may be needed to ease the burden if ethnic neighborhoods are already overcrowded and poor. An assessment approach that begins at the macro-level of understanding, then the family and community systems, and finally the individual system, is highly recommended for culturally competent contextual social work practice.

Legal Statuses Influencing Adaptation Behaviors

The 1965 Immigration law allowed many immigrants to seek employment and some to be reunified with their families. Many immigrants from south India (as stated in Chapter 9 by Ross-Sheriff and Husain) and other countries were able to come and establish themselves as professionals. Although many immigrants continue to come to America, however, there were and still are many immigrants who have illegal status because they lack documentation. These people come from many countries for a variety of reasons. Zuniga (Chapter 10) describes the undocumented migrant workers from Mexico, and Marsiglia and Menjívar (Chapter 14) mention the Nicaraguan refugees who come looking for temporary protective status but may not receive it, thus ending up as illegal immigrants. There are also foreign students whom when their educational visas expire, choose to remain in the United States as illegal residents. The lack of legality in their status, obviously, is a grave concern to many government officials and to many immigrant and refugee families who find themselves in that category. Their status affects health care, employment, and education for their children, and thus their adaptation to their resident environments. Many families may be separated because of a deported member. Even when reunification occurs, difficulties continue, because the uncertainty of deportation creates a pervasive tension in families and communities.

The status of undocumented immigrants has caused major problems for children and families. Undocumented families' fears of deportation and forced separation cause secrecy to occur. Unemployment is likely, as is the lack of health insurance. Children can attend elementary and secondary school, but as young adults, they are denied registration at college because of their status. Families who are reunified experience tensions over the unequal privileges of family members who are documented and those who are not. Undocumented immigrants cannot work legally in the United States and may also be resented by members of the immigrant community because of the scarcity of existing resources. Consequently, undocumented immigrants have a very difficult time transitioning to the United States, because there is really no permanent resolution in store for them. Their lack of a permanent residence may parallel that of children in multiple foster care placements—a lot of uncertain movement, with forced relationships in the guise of hopes for permanency.

The migration patterns of undocumented and refugee families are affected by the social environments they are leaving permanently or temporarily. The social environments in the refugees' countries of origin have usually included political strife, leading the refugees to find a new environment affording political freedoms and economic opportunities. These people seek asylum and may get legal permission to come to the United States and to receive temporary protective status. It is understood that they will not be returning to their native country. Children and families in these situations are susceptible to tension, trauma, uncertainty, grief and loss, possible violence and rape, and definitely PTSD issues (Ahern, Loughry, & Ager, 1999; Bemak, Chung, & Pedersen, 2003). Many refugees have spent extended time in camps and have had negative experiences with authority figures, experiences that still influence them in the United States and frequently prompt mistrust of persons in authority (Aptekar, 2003; Summerfield; 1999). Social workers need to accept that building trust will take a while.

Frequently, an additional barrier to effective treatment is the social worker's vague understanding of the different social environments that immigrant and refugee children and families are experiencing. When social workers only want to treat presenting problems and fail to do thorough assessments of each traumatic experience along the migration journey, interventions cannot get to the thorough healing that needs to take place. Lee (1997) proposes "Assessment Guidelines for Chinese American Immigrant and Refugee Families" and states that the following areas must be assessed: "ethnocultural heritage; family migration stress and relocation history; degree of loss and traumatic experience; postmigration experience and cultural shock; acculturation level of each family member; work and financial stresses; family place of residence and community support; family dynamics; family problems; family strengths; physical health and medication history; family's concept of presenting problem; help-seeking behavior, and treatment expectations" (p. 71). These categories are necessary, but there also must be others that reflect the experiences of undocumented immigrants and refugees. Segal (2002) speaks of the Asians who come to the United States as students and linger because of the prospects of better job opportunities. They come as students and are hired as full-time employees but may fail to formalize their documentation. Although there seems to be no mental or political persecution of this category of undocumented person, the fear and trauma of being separated from family members and sent away to another country, without any input at all, is just as great as for undocumented students as for migrants coming over the border from Mexico. Culturally competent contextual social work needs to factor into assessments the impact of the legal statuses upon the clients' adaptive or nonadaptive behaviors.

Culturally Competent Contextual Practice

While Census 2000 allows respondents to identify themselves by sixty-three different ethnic/racial categories, Hernandez and Charney (1998) reiterate the need to "distinguish . . . between [foreign-born] immigrant children [first-generation], U.S.-born children in immigrant families [second-generation], U.S.-born children in U.S.-born families" (p. 15). Racial and ethnic stratification need to be examined from an anthropological and psychological perspective as well as a sociological or political one. As noted in Chapter 1, one out of every 10 persons in the United States is foreign born. Among the foreign born, one-half are Latino and one-fourth are Asian. This poses many challenges. From a political and sociological perspective, policies and classifications of persons may overshadow the psychological and anthropological need to understand the immigrant or refugee situation.

Anthropologically, it is important to understand the culture and environment of immigrants' native lands. This may require more knowledge building of social workers in the geographic regions of countries. Northern and southern regions in the People's Republic of China have long emphasized their differences in cuisine, language, and customs; refugees from northern and southern China may reflect these differences. While taking care to avoid overgeneralizing, the social work literature needs be able to describe broad differences among ethnic immigrant and refugee groups. Similar attention needs to be given to the time period when clients arrived in the United States, and to the place and social environment from which they came.

To exercise cultural competence, social workers need to know the differences in the status and problems of immigrants and refugees, such as the simple but weighty matter of whether they are documented or undocumented. Old and new immigrants also face different adaptations and problems. An increasing number of refugees and migrants to the United States have problems that overlap those of immigrants. Social workers need to know the differences in legal status and in the ethnic groupings. In working with immigrants and refugees, culturally competent practice needs to be more contextualized. Lee (1997) states, "In discussing the family's postmigration experience, it is essential to assess the degree of cultural shock and its impact on the family. Many new Asian immigrants are placed in a strange and unpredictable environment. In addition to language barriers and homesickness, they have to adjust to physical changes, economic changes, cultural changes, political changes, and social relationship changes" (p. 18). These contexts, at least, need to factored in the following situations of most immigrants and refugees:

Context 1. The homeland situation
Context 2. The departure from the homeland
Context 3. The arrival experience in refugee camps or first site
Context 4. The initial landing in the United States
Context 5. The current home environment in the United States
Context 6. The continuous places lived in the United States for undocumented immigrants

Culturally competent contextual social work practice should include assessment questions that focus on each of the six different kinds of contexts and social environments that immigrants and refugees may experience in their migration journeys. These assessments should focus on the transitions between environments and determine whether additional stressors compound the existing ones. However, caution must be taken in seeking this information before a trusting relationship is established with the immigrant or refugee client. Practitioners warn that premature disclosure or pressure from the social worker may place the client at risk of further withdrawal and alienation, retreating into silences, or simply disappearing (Bevin, 2001; McAdoo, 2001; Shibusawa, 2001). Discernment of additional risk factors could help the social worker better plan for culturally appropriate treatments.

IDENTIFYING AND AMELIORATING RISK FACTORS

The Children's Defense Fund reported in 2000 that children and families are plagued with increases in child abuse and neglect, mothers in prison, homelessness, and children with absent parents (Children's Defense Fund, 2000). Many children from immigrant families have been separated from their parents for some period of time. Others have suffered from neglect. Suarez-Orozco and Suarez-Orozco (2001) report in their studies on immigrant children that some do well; others do not. Portes and Zhou (2000) report on the dilemmas faced by immigrants over whether to assimilate. Lynch and Hanson (1998) cite Guthrie (1975), who identifies five reasons for difficulties in understanding new cultures and making cultural transitions: "(1) Cultural understanding in one's first culture occurs early and is typically established by age 5; (2) children learn new cultural patterns more easily than adults; (3) values are determined by one's first culture and may have to be revised to be effective in another culture; (4) understanding one's first culture introduces errors in interpreting the second culture; and (5) long-standing behavior patterns are typically used to express one's deepest values" (pp. 24–27).

The risk factors for immigrant and refugee children and families are multifold, including the failure to rebuild support systems once in America, difficulties in gender-role reconstruction, and reluctance to share private family information with nonmembers. Health-related risks surface when a patient does not want to know an illness is terminal because of cultural beliefs or has no language to describe mental illnesses that manifest as spiritual or physical hurts. Intergenerational conflicts and underemployment also introduce additional risks.

Children are more at risk when they experience secondary trauma from their parents or are not allowed to socialize with American children,

American-born children, or children of their same ethnic background. Such is the case for some Muslim children growing up in America. They also bear the burden of conflicts with specific cultural values, such as when Hmong values regarding praise for children collide with American assumptions about self-esteem, or when traditional values about religion and ethnicity differ from those of the child's American peers. Reunification introduces its own array of risk factors, such as intergenerational conflicts, gender-role reconstruction, and role reversals of children that can result in hurriedness, overachievement, and underachievement, ultimately resulting in lost childhood.

Hurried Child Syndrome/Overachiever/Underachiever

Guthrie's (1975) cogent assessment of change endures despite a quarter-century of changes in immigrant and refugee groups. Problems for immigrant children and youth are manifold; many experience role reversal and "the hurried child syndrome," lapse into "overachiever" or "underachiever" categories, contend with being both undocumented and unentitled, or struggle to make sense of coming from multiple places and differing social environments. Because immigrant parents make sacrifices for their children's betterment, children are under pressure to excel. Many Asian Indian immigrants share an expectation that children will become highly educated professionals, creating stresses that rob some youth of their childhood. Immigrant children are sometimes forced to act as adult caregivers when parents are working and older children are caring for younger siblings. These children who bear adult responsibilities are rushed through childhood, and both they and the overachievers may experience what Elkind describes as the "hurried child syndrome" (2001). With their development unnaturally accelerated, these children become developmentally unbalanced. Yet immigrant children exposed to trauma may experience delays in developmental milestones. Some refugee children and most undocumented children have gone through traumatic experiences in emigrating. Being undocumented, these youth soon recognize that their futures are clouded by obstacles to future employment or education. Lack of documentation contributes to stressors not experienced by documented immigrants, such as the fear of constantly changing social environments to avoid deportation, which may resemble what children in the foster-care system experience in transitioning to multiple placements.

Changing Social Environments /Mirroring Multiple Placements

As in any other family system, stability and consistency are important to immigrant children and families. But many immigrant and refugee children and families have witnessed a multitude of changes in their social environments. This constant change might be analogous to what other children and families experience with the foster-care system and divorce. Both foster-care children, who endure multiple placements, and immigrant and refugee children have multiple environments called "homes." Immigrant children of undocumented parents are exposed to the vagaries of the legal system in a manner quite like foster-care children, whose parents no longer exercise parental rights. Some immigrant and refugee children who have been separated from parents also have attachment and reunification issues, and those whose parents have left them with relatives experience kinship care issues. Children who do not handle these transitions well are vulnerable to PTSD and additional risks in other areas of functioning.

Family Reunification / Mirroring Blended and Quasi-Divorced Families

Immigrant and refugee children and families grapple with myriad difficulties as they adapt to the United States. As noted earlier, major problems seem to surround the changes in parental status, gender roles, family reunification, and generational and multiple households sharing child-rearing responsibilities. Family reunification issues emerge when immigrant and refugee families, for whatever reason, choose to or have to break up the family. As families come together again, changes in roles, family structures, and expectations pose risks. These risks may revolve around unsuccessfully integrating two households into one and combining households that may have included, for instance, children raised in the native land by grandparents who employ different child-rearing practices than the parents. Reunification can then cause tensions to surface over both parents' and children's child-rearing expectations.

New immigrants who have left homeland environments in which they occupied a higher status than in the United States experience stressors of a different nature. Ross-Sheriff and Husain (Chapter 9) describe changes in status experienced over the course of three waves of Asian Indian immigration. The first and second waves comprised highly educated professionals, whereas the third tended to bring more shopkeepers and gas station operators. The abrupt tumble from respected, educated professional to non-English-speaking, unemployed or underemployed worker causes acute stress. Women may encounter comparably difficult adjustments in their changes in status, because some in their native lands were homemakers, subordinate to men, who were the primary breadwinners, yet have been forced by relocation to become the primary income earners themselves. As in divorced families, double-headed households require a close examination of roles and expectations for consistency to occur within the home environment.

To minimize the risk factors related to reunification or changes in multiple environments, it may help if social workers in the United States understand the problems of immigrants and refugees through the lenses of what happens to children of divorce with divided, blended, and reunification family issues with which to contend. The lens of the immigrant child going through multiple social environments is akin to the multiple placements of children in foster care where the goal is permanency and child well-being. Yet the risk factors are multifold, because each dynamic needs to be accounted for in culturally effective practices.

PROTECTIVE FACTORS OF CULTURAL VALUES AND INDIGENOUS INTERVENTIONS

In working with immigrants and refugees, some variables can serve as protective factors but are often neglected or not maximally used by social workers, including cultural values, religious beliefs, ethnic communities, immigrant networks, and cultural interactions. Protective factors can also be interventions—biculturalized interventions, culture-based family therapies, and solution-focused therapies. Cultural values of each ethnic grouping are strengths, but they are rarely maximized in assessment or treatment planning. Another underused empowering tool is the indigenous interventions, based on cultural values, used in native lands. In addition, an underdeveloped empowerment approach has been to use the framework and tenets of solution-focused therapy with immigrant and refugee families. Use of solution-focused interventions is a strengths-based approach that empowers the client to look at how situations were culturally solved prior to the problems identified in America. Immigrants and refugees can reveal what indigenous interventions were working for them, and the culturally competent social worker can then know what might be done to implement similarly congruent interventions based on cultural values.

Cultural Values as Protective Factors in Strengths Assessments

Researchers have discussed cultural values as strengths and indigenous strategies as primary interventions (Fong & Furuto, 2001; Mokuau, 1991, Webb, 2001). Immigrants and refugees have cultural values and beliefs that have allowed them to survive and thrive in home environments. Those values and beliefs have been protective factors, allowing the individuals to operate in familiar systems. Thus, it is important that culturally competent social services require the agency and staff to be aware and knowledgeable, and to continue their inductive learning about the values and needs of the different ethnic groups they serve.

Cultural values reflect philosophies and ways of living adopted by individuals, families, and societies. However, it has been noted that ethnic groups from other social environments may not have the same cultural beliefs as those within the same ethnic group. These differences may be due, for instance, to variations in political systems and structures. For immigrants and refugees from cultures in which religion has played a major role, as it has for some Muslims and Hindus, the values regarding religion need to be acknowledged. For example, the social worker with an Asian Indian Hindu client must be informed about Indian culture and Hinduism.

Other frameworks using cultural values as strengths are drawn from African American populations. McRoy (2003) notes that the terms "Africentricity"and "Afrocentricity" are used to describe "the cultural values of people of African American descent" (p. 234). Specific values are based on the "Nguzo Saba value system" and include unity, self-determination, collective work and responsibility, cooperative economics, purpose, creativity, and faith (p. 234). These values, especially the ones related to faith and cooperative economics, have been underused. For example, African American communities and churches should be a regular part of the social service delivery system. Harvey (2001) also draws attention to an Afrocentric approach to practice. Two principles he singles out are "to foster a sense of excellence, which consists of developing their creative genius; and to develop the uniqueness of the person in relationship to the development of their community" (pp. 234–235).

As one might expect, cultural values do not always transfer positively from one culture to another. Scheinfeld, Wallach, and Lagendorf (1997, p. 34) describe how values in both Cambodian and Vietnamese cultures clash with common Western values:

> Reluctance to praise one's children is rooted in the culture of the parents. Patriarchal values in Asian countries may have served a purpose for order and role definitions in native lands but may be restrictive in the United States where economics forces the immigrant woman to also seek employment. Praise and discipline measures need to be contextualized also.

To adopt a solution-focused approach with the goal of empowering clients and using their own solutions that are culturally familiar and positively received would help to contextualize practice and increase understanding of the strengths of cultural values and indigenous interventions.

Empowerment Interventions of Solution-Focused and Indigenous Approaches

Empowering our clients has been a priority in the social work profession. The goal advanced by this book is to empower clients and use treatments that are culturally appropriate, grounded in ethnic values, and indigenous-based. Although there is progress in acknowledging indigenous methods, the approach has usually been presented as an either–or choice. The paradigm shift espoused here is to operate in a multicultural dimension, with choices encompassing both Eastern and Western methods. The biculturalization of interventions forces us to integrate treatments and create empowerment interventions.

Biculturalization takes into account cultural values, or values compatible across cultures. In working with cultures that value oral traditions, several authors have recommended the combination with narrative therapies. Goodman, in Chapter 15, writes about the narrative therapies used with Balkan immigrants from the former Yugoslavian regions. Sohng and Song, in Chapter 5, describe the *haan* approach, which is verbally support of immigrants' retelling of the trauma, and unraveling the source and entanglement of dysfunctionalism in adapting to the United States.

Social service providers need to look for more indigenous interventions, but this cannot be an either–or situation. For example, even when using indigenous healers and shamans in the Vietnamese, Laotian, or Hmong cultures, there still needs to be a bridge, a biculturalization of interventions—a systematic and consistent approach to practice that looks for both indigenous and Western interventions. Bemak and Chung (2002) noted that "in 1992 the World Health Organization . . . described how the integration of indigenous healing practices with traditional Western healing practices can result in more effective therapeutic outcomes" (p. 225). For example, for family systems approaches in which family values of role and hierarchal structures are highly prioritized in many immigrant and refugee families, there needs to be more family group conferencing with structural family therapy. Doktor (1998) and Scheinfeld et al. (1997) discuss the use of art therapies in working with refugees and migrants. Immigrants often lack words that easily communicate their stories, but use of art to express trauma can be a bridge across languages. Colors and drawn figures of people can be translated in the understanding of stress and trauma.

Although Western interventions prevail in the United States, with the advocacy to add indigenous interventions in treatment, another approach to attaining knowledge of indigenous interventions is to use a solution-focused therapy framework. The philosophy of solution-focused therapy is to work with the individual's or family's strengths, resources, and competencies. An assumption of solution-focused therapy is

> that all people regardless of their functioning have strengths, resources, and competencies, although they many not be using them, may be underusing them, or may have forgotten they have them. Solution-focused therapy emphasizes the pragmatic utilization of client strengths, resources, and per-

sonal constructions to develop solutions and promote empowerment. . . . Solution-focused therapy is a specific type of conversation in which the clinicians "talk" with the client to develop new meaning and new realities through a dialogue of "solutions." . . . Solution-talk invites the clients to be the experts on their situations. Workers essentially consult with clients to discover strengths, competencies, and resources within clients and their cultures. (Greene & Lee, 2002, pp. 187–188)

Solution-focused therapy allows the social worker to help multicultural clients to find familiar and comfortable solutions, which for many immigrants and refugees may be found in their religions. But culturally competent social workers need also to understand the contexts of these religious strengths and their affiliated tensions. For example, tensions may exist between Muslims and Jews, Muslims and Christians, and Muslims and Hindus. Within the South Asian population, because people can be Hindus, Muslims, Buddhists, and Christians, clients from these different faiths have different worldviews and values; thus, it behooves the culturally competent social worker to know that religious belief of their Asian Indian client, and how it can be used as a strength.

The practice of social work will hopefully be able to utilize the strengths and the indigenous interventions that operated successfully for clients in their native environments. If practitioners view clients' indigenous interventions in the context of a solution-focused therapy approach, they might be better able to see the importance of blending Eastern and Western interventions, and using the solutions that were successful for clients in their native lands.

REFERENCES

Ahern, F., Loughry, M., & Ager, A. (1999). The experience of refugee children. In A. Ager (Ed.), *Refugees: Perspectives on the experience of forced migration* (pp. 215–236). New York: Pinter.

Aptekar, L. (2003). Cultural problems for western counselors working with Ethiopian refugees. In F. Bemak, R. Chung, & P. Pedersen (Eds.), *Counseling refugees: A psychosocial approach to innovative multicultural interventions* (pp. 208–224). Westport, CT: Greenwood Press.

Balgopal, B. (Ed.). (2000). *Social work practice with immigrants and refugees.* New York: Columbia University Press.

Bemak, F., & Chung, R. (2002). Counseling and psychotherapy with refugees. In P. Pedersen, J. Draguns, W. Lonner, & J. Trimble (Eds.), *Counseling across cultures* (5th ed., pp. 209–232). Thousand Oaks, CA: Sage.

Bemak, F., Chung, R., & Pedersen, P. (2003). *Counseling refugees: A psychosocial approach to innovative multicultural interventions.* Westport, CT: Greenwood Press.

Bevin, T. (2001). Parenting in Cuban Mexican families. In N. Webb (Ed.), *Culturally diverse parent–child and family relationships: A guide for social workers and other practitioners* (pp. 181–201). New York: Columbia University Press.

Children's Defense Fund. (2000). *Yearbook 2000: The state of America's children.* Washington, DC: Author.

Council on Social Work Education. (2002). *Educational policy and accreditation standards.* Alexandria, VA: Commission on Accreditation, Council on Social Work Education.

Dhooper, S., & Moore, S. (2001). *Social work practice with culturally diverse people.* Thousand Oaks, CA: Sage.

Dokter, D. (1998). *Arts therapists, refugees and migrants reaching across borders.* Philadelphia: Jessica Kingsley.

Elkind, D. (2001). *The hurried child* (3rd ed.). Cambridge, MA: Perseus.

Erdmans, M. (2000). Stanislaus can't polka: New Polish immigrants in established Polish American communities. In P. Kivisto & G. Rundblad (Eds.), *Multiculturalism in the United States: Current issues, contemporary voices* (pp. 395–408). Thousand Oaks: CA: Pine Forge Press.

Fong, R. (1997). Child welfare with Chinese families: Assessment for immigrants from the People's Republic of China. *Journal of Family Social Work, 2*(19), 33–48.

Fong, R., Boyd, C., & Browne, C. (1999). The Gandhi technique: A biculturalization approach for empowering Asian and Pacific Islander families. *Journal of Multicultural Social Work, 7,* 95–110.

Fong, R., & Furuto, S. (Eds.). (2001). *Culturally competent practice: Skills, interventions, and evaluations.* Boston: Allyn & Bacon.

Fong, R., Sandau-Beckler, P., & Haapala, D. (Eds.). (1994). *Empowering families: Papers from the Seventh Annual Conference on Family-Based Services.* Rapid City, IA: National Association of Family-Based Services.

Fong, T. (2000). The first suburban Chinatown: The remaking of Monterey Park, California. In P. Kivisto & G. Rundblad (Eds.), *Multiculturalism in the United States: Current issues, contemporary voices* (pp. 369–380). Thousand Oaks: CA: Pine Forge Press.

Gold, S. (2000). Israeli Americans. In P. Kivisto & G. Rundblad (Eds.), *Multiculturalism in the United States: Current issues, contemporary voices* (pp. 409–420). Thousand Oaks: CA: Pine Forge Press.

Greene, G., & Lee, M. (2002). The social construction of empowerment. In M. O'Melia & K. Miley (Eds.), *Pathways to power: Readings in contextual social work practice* (pp. 175–201). Boston: Allyn & Bacon.

Guthrie, G. (1975). A behavioral analysis of cultural learning. In R.W. Brislin & W.J. Lonner (Eds.), *Cross-cultural perspectives on learning* (pp. 95–115). New York: Wiley.

Harrold-Bond, B. (1999). The experience of refugees as recipients of aid. In A. Ager (Ed.), *Refugees: Perspectives on the experience of forced migration* (pp. 136–168). New York: Pinter.

Harvey, A. (2001). Individual and family intervention skills with African Americans: An Africentric approach. In R. Fong & S. Furuto (Eds.), *Culturally competent* practice: Skills, interventions, and evaluations (pp. 225–240). Boston: Allyn & Bacon.

Hernandez, D., & Charney, E. (Eds.). (1998). From generation to generation: The health and well-being of children in immigrant families. Washington, DC: National Academy Press.

Ho, M. K. (1987). Family therapy with ethnic minorities. Newbury Park, CA: Sage.

Jung, M. (1998). Chinese American family therapy: A new model for clinicians. San Francisco: Jossey-Bass.

Lee, E. (1997). Working with Asian Americans: A guide for clinicians. New York: Guilford Press.

Lum, D. (Ed.). (2003). Culturally competent practice: A framework for understanding diverse groups and social justice. Pacific Grove, CA: Brooks/Cole.

Lynch, E., & Hanson, M. (1998). Developing cross-cultural competence: A guide for working with children and their families (2nd ed.). Baltimore: Brookes.

McAdoo, H. (2001). Parent and child relationships in African American families. In N. Webb (Ed.), Culturally diverse parent–child and family relationships (pp. 89–106). New York: Columbia University Press.

McLemore, S., Romo, H., & Baker, S. (2001). Racial and ethnic relations in America. Boston: Allyn & Bacon.

McRoy, R. (2003). Cultural competence with African Americans. In D. Lum (Ed.), Culturally competent practice: A framework for understanding diverse groups and social justice (pp. 217–237). Pacific Grove, CA: Brooks/Cole.

Mokuau, N. (Ed.). (1991). Handbook of social services for Asians and Pacific Islanders. Westport, CT: Greenwood Press.

Moore, J., & Vigil, J. (2000). Barrios in transition. In P. Kivisto & G. Rundblad (Eds.), Multiculturalism in the United States: Current issues, contemporary voices (pp. 355–368). Thousand Oaks, CA: Pine Forge Press.

O'Melia, M. (2002). From person to context: The evolution of an empowering practice. In M. O'Melia & K. Miley (Eds.), Pathways to power: Readings in contextual social work practice (pp. 1–14). Boston: Allyn & Bacon.

Portes, A., & Zhou, M. (2000). Should immigrants assimilate? In P. Kivisto & G. Rundblad (Eds.), Multiculturalism in the United States: Current issues, contemporary voices (pp. 317–328). Thousand Oaks, CA: Pine Forge Press.

Scheinfeld, D., Wallach, L., & Langendorf, T. (1997). Strengthening refugee families. Chicago: Lyceum.

Segal, U. (2002). A framework for immigration: Asians in the United States. New York: Columbia University Press.

Shibusawa, T. (2001). Parenting in Japanese American families. In N. B.Webb (Ed.), Culturally diverse parent–child and family relationships (pp. 283–306). New York: Columbia University Press.

Suarez-Orozco, C., & Suarez-Orozco, M. (2001). Children of immigration. Cambridge, MA: Harvard University Press.

Summerfield, D. (1999). Sociocultural dimensions of war, conflict, and displacement. In A. Ager (Ed.), Refugees: Perspectives on the experience of forced migration (pp. 111–135). New York: Pinter.

Takaki, R. (Ed.). (1987). From different shores: Perspectives in race and ethnicity in America. New York: Oxford University Press.

Trueba, H., Cheng, L., & Ima, K. (1993). *Myth or reality: Adaptive strategies of Asian Americans in California*. Washington, DC: Falmer Press.

Waldinger, R. (2000). Who gets the "lousy" jobs? In P. Kivisto & G. Rundblad (Eds.), *Multiculturalism in the United States: Current issues, contemporary voices* (pp. 329–342). Thousand Oaks: CA: Pine Forge Press.

Webb, N. (Ed.). (2001). *Culturally diverse parent–child and family relationships*. New York: Columbia University Press.

CHAPTER 4

Filipino Children and Families

CARMINA P. TOLENTINO

The Philippines is an archipelago composed of 7,107 islands located in Southeast Asia. Filipinos first set foot in the United States during the 18th century through the Spanish galleon trade. Subsequent immigration, occurring in three distinct periods, has led to Filipinos becoming one of the most significant ethnic groups in this country.

In this chapter, I discuss the immigration history of Filipinos and their adaptation to the United States, examining the issues they face. The use of Filipino cultural values as strengths in assessment and intervention is examined. I analyze both indigenous and Western approaches to intervention, presenting culturally appropriate principles in the helping process. A case vignette is presented to exemplify cultural values as strengths and the use of culturally competent practices.

HISTORICAL BACKGROUND

The colonization of the Philippines by the Spaniards began in the 16th century and lasted for more than 300 years. Toward the end of the 19th century, the Spanish–American war was waged, resulting in the cession of the Philippines to the United States in 1892. In the period following the war, the United States needed cheap laborers for its agriculture. Oriental exclusion policies and the Immigration Act of 1924 had stopped the immigration of Chinese, Japanese, Korean, and Asian Indian nationals. Hence, from 1906 to 1934, about 120,000 young, single, Filipino males were recruited to work in Hawaiian sugar plantations, while 45,000 were employed on the West Coast for agricultural and manual services. Immigrants in this first wave were not allowed to become U.S. citizens or to bring in wives or family members. As their population in the United States increased, Filipinos suffered from racial discrimination and antimiscegenation laws. In 1934, the Tydings–McDuffie Act drastically limited the immigration of Filipinos.

The second wave of immigrants, between 1946 and 1964, comprised mainly Filipinos who served in the American armed forces or worked in defense factories during World War II, along with their families. From the early 1950s to early 1990s, Filipinos also came as recruits serving in the U.S. Navy.

With the passage of the Immigration Act of 1965, immigration of Filipinos to the United States again escalated. This third wave of immigrants comprised predominantly middle-class, college-educated, English-speaking professionals who integrated easily into U.S. society. They were allowed to become U.S. citizens and to petition family members in the Philippines.

According to the 1990 census, Filipino Americans had become the second largest Asian American group in the United States, next to the Chinese, and one of the fastest growing groups (U.S. Bureau of the Census, 1991). The 2000 census indicated that 1.9 million Filipinos were living in the United States, an increase of 24% over the 1.4 million in 1990. They are heavily concentrated in the West, with 50% in California. Of Filipino Americans, 1.46 million are foreign-born (U.S. Bureau of the Census, 2000).

Filipino Americans are presented as a "model minority" that is assimilated, acculturated, and economically upwardly mobile. They have relatively high educational attainment (Kao, 1995). There is a high level of labor force participation, particularly among women, and a large percentage of the population work as professionals (Cabezas, Shinagawa, & Kawaguchi, 1986). They have the lowest rate of poverty in the United States and California (Oliver, Grey, Stiles, & Brady, 1995; Rumbaut, 1995). Despite their significant number, the lack of research and knowledge about Filipino Americans affects service delivery and utilization.

ADAPTATION TO THE UNITED STATES

The ecological model views the immigration process as a reciprocal shaping of the individual and the environment. As Filipinos change to adapt to the American environment, the environment also changes as a result of the interaction of this group with the rest of American society.

Filipino immigrants go through major transitions. They leave behind employment, career, and social status in the Philippines. Obtaining employment commensurate with their education and experience in the Philippines is difficult (Okamura & Agbayani, 1991; Takaki, 1989). Language barriers decrease employability. Licensure exams or reenrollment in academic courses are a necessity for getting jobs in their field. Oftentimes, Filipinos have had to restart from the bottom professionally. A supervisor in the Philippines takes on an entry-level job in the United States. A successful doctor in the Philippines who is unable to pass the professional exams becomes a truck driver here. Occupation is very significant, because it is a key factor in determining one's placement in the Filipino social hierarchy. Loss of occupational status results in loss of self-esteem, disappointment, frustration, and even depression (Chan, 1998).

Filipino immigrants leave behind a tightly knit network of support (Tompar-Tiu & Sustento-Seneriches, 1995), including the nuclear family, extended kin, friends, household helpers, church members, godparents, and neighbors. In the process of immigration, it is common for the nuclear family to break up temporarily, such as when a parent pursues better opportunities abroad (Santos, 1983). In the home country, individuals are involved greatly in each other's lives and there is less possibility of isolation. Rebuilding or maintaining a support system becomes more challenging in the United States because of the demands of professions and parenting (Espiritu, 1994).

Economic pressures are another stressor. In the Philippines, Filipinos can rely on family members during times of financial need, but in the new environment, there is a push to become economically self-sufficient. Immigrants often feel obligated to send material help to family members in the home country (Chan, 1998). This is strengthened by a general belief in the Philippines that the United States is the land of milk and honey. Immigrants may also be lured into consumerist spending and incur many debts.

The ecological model posits that the individual attempts to achieve an adaptive balance of rights, needs, capacities, and goals within the environment to change oneself and the environment. The Filipino immigrant adjusts to the new culture in trying to achieve an adaptive fit with American society. This process can lead to difficulties, including a clash in value systems (e.g., submissiveness vs. assertiveness, restraint of feelings vs. open communication, interdependence vs. autonomy). Language barriers, including accent, difficulties with grammar and pronunciation, and idiosyncratic use of English, can create communication problems. Adapting to a new culture is especially hard for Filipinos with less exposure to Western orientation, such as those from rural areas and of lower educational attainment and socioeconomic class (Tompar-Tiu & Sustento-Seneriches, 1995). Coming from a largely homogeneous society, the immigrant becomes a racial minority in the new setting and might experience discrimination.

PROBLEMS FOR CHILDREN AND FAMILIES

Immigration is a stressful process. A relationship between acculturation and stress has been demostrated (Padilla, Wagatsuma, & Lindholm, 1985). Within the family, changes that take place both in the husband–wife and parent–child systems can create tension.

Traditionally, women have the main role in child rearing and home maintenance, whereas the husband focuses on the breadwinner role. Such is the case even when both spouses are working. In the Philippines, the task is made manageable with the aid of household helpers, extended kin, and even neighbors. In the United States, both members of most Filipino immigrant couples must work to survive economically. Gender-role restructuring becomes a necessity due to the lack of support with household tasks. There are Filipino husbands who are flexible and able to adapt, but others have greater difficulty. They may feel that their status as head of the family is diminished and therefore experience a sense of loss of power and authority. Others may resist change and maintain traditional roles, creating much pressure on the wife. The shifting of roles or resistance to change creates strain in the marriage.

Spouses may acculturate at varying levels and rates, which can lead to problems. They may disagree on the manner of raising their children. Pauline Agbayani-Siewert's (1988) survey of social service agencies serving Asian Americans in Los Angeles County identified changes in child-rearing practices and spousal sex-role expectations as a major source of marital role strain and domestic violence directed toward Filipino women.

In the Philippines, if the couple is not able to resolve conflict, partners may resort to the mediation of relatives or close friends. Oftentimes, this conflict resolution mechanism is not available in the United States, which can lead to breakdown in communication, escalation of conflict, and domestic violence. Divorce is not a socially acceptable option for the abused or unhappy spouse; this is taboo in the culture. Couples who do resort to divorce may experience shame and isolation.

In the intercultural marriage, cultural differences can become a source of conflict, such as differing views on the obligation to and role of the family of origin. In contrast to Americans, Filipinos' use of indirect communication of feelings through facial expression and subtle gesture can create communication problems. Language and cultural barriers may make it difficult for the Filipino spouse to integrate with the American spouse's social circle, leading to isolation or separation of social networks.

Likewise, the parent–child system goes through major changes that threaten its stability. Difficulties in raising children result from the absence of caretaking support. Because parents are often busy working, children may receive inadequate supervision, which can lead to behavioral problems. Heras and Revilla (1994) noted the rising incidence of high school dropouts (Azores, 1986–1987), university dropouts (Almirol, 1986), gang involvement (Domingo & Wong, 1990; Pulido, 1990), and teenage pregnancies (Aesquivel, 1990).

In the Philippines, physical forms of discipline are used. Because of child protective laws in this country, Filipino parents can no longer rely on the use or threat of physical discipline, and hence may feel a decreased sense of authority and control over their children. Lack of knowledge of alternative means of discipline can lead to absence of or minimal discipline. Some get involved with the child protective system because of their lack of awareness of laws in this country. Moreover, stress related to the immigration and acculturation process increases risk of child abuse and neglect.

Immigrant youth typically acculturate at a faster pace than their parents. Second-generation Filipinos are socialized into American culture. The result is an acculturation gap that becomes a source of conflict between parents and children. Because the children are more adapted to American culture, parents may experience a sense of loss of power and authority over their children. For example, a child might correct a parent's grammar or accent. This shames the parent, because in Filipino culture, parents are the authority, and children are not supposed to correct or challenge them.

Youth experience conflict between family expectations and those of peers and the wider society. Traditionally, the family is considered more important than the individual, whereas higher value is placed on individuality in American society. Filipino youth want more autonomy, like their American peers, whereas parents set many limits and expect them to be obedient and submissive. First-generation immigrants who want their children to hold on to traditional Filipino values are faced with resistance from their children. The lack of coherence in the youths' socialization process contributes to psychological maladjustment (Heras & Revilla, 1994).

Despite the relative success of Filipino American immigrants compared with other immigrant groups, research indicates that a significant proportion of the youth experience alienation, depression, poor self-image, and other problems. In Rumbaut's (1996) study among second-generation immigrant youth, a subsample of 818 Filipino students scored high relative to other ethnic groups in English and educational achievement but lower in self-esteem and higher in depression. A random survey of San Diego public high school students conducted in May 1993 under the auspices of the Federal Centers for Disease Control and Prevention showed that 45.6% of Filipino female students surveyed said they had seriously considered attempting suicide in the year preceding the survey. At least once in the preceding year, 23.3% actually attempted suicide. In Heras and Revilla's (1994) study, second-generation Filipino immigrants reported significantly lower self-esteem and poorer self-concept than the earlier generation of immigrants.

Whereas the family is a source of security and support for the immigrant youth, it can also be a source of stress. Diane L. Wolf's (1997) study among 22 Filipino second-generation students at the University of California at Davis identified some of the difficulties reported by these youth. Pressured by their parents to excel academically and to choose financially rewarding professions, they are expected to approach their parents for counsel and are discouraged from seeking help from outsiders—yet their parents lack sympathy and receptivity. Because they resisted going to counselors or friends for fear of gossip and shaming the family, the youth felt they had no one to turn to for help. This created intense feelings of loneliness, deep unhappiness, and, at times, despair.

Second-generation Filipino immigrants often have decreased familiarity with their country of origin, native language, and cultural heritage. This leads to a weakened ethnic identity and group identification, further contributing to their maladjustment (Heras & Revilla, 1994).

Female Filipino American youth appear to exhibit more signs of distress. In Rumbaut's (1996) study, Filipino female participants had consistently higher depression scores than their male counterparts. Wolf's (1997) interviews indicated that male and female children are treated differently, are given different messages about what it means to be Filipino, and react differently to their environment. Parental control over females' movements, body, and sexuality is greater. This differential treatment of children based on sex is related to the double standard in gender expectations in Philippine culture. For instance, men's extramarital affairs are tolerated, whereas women are expected to be self-sacrificial and stay loyal to their husbands. This inconsistency can breed resentment and rebelliousness in Filipino female youth, possibly contributing to the rise in teenage pregnancies.

Despite the problems faced by Filipino Americans, research suggests that they are underutilizing mental health services. In Los Angeles County, for example, Filipinos were estimated to comprise 26% of the Asian population in 1985. Only 19% of the Asians in the Los Angeles Public Mental Health System from 1983 to 1988, however, were Filipinos, indicating a considerable underrepresentation (Ying & Hu, 1994). This is supported by research that shows American-born Asian Americans have higher utilization rates and greater benefit from mental health services, whereas foreign-born Asian Americans are more likely to regard Western treatment methods as strange and are less likely to utilize and benefit from mental health services (Ying & Hu, 1994).

Stigma is attached to seeking treatment from a mental health center (Tompar-Tiu & Sustento-Seneriches, 1995). Filipinos are suspicious of counseling and prefer to get advice from relatives, religious people, or friends. They are hesitant to discuss emotions with health care workers (Baysa, Cabrera, Camilon, & Torres, 1980) and may avoid seeking help because they do not want to be a burden (McLaughlin & Braun, 1998). They tend to minimize the presentation of the problem or symptoms because of family loyalty and secrecy, and often seek help at an acute or chronic stage (Tompar-Tiu & Sustento-Seneriches, 1995).

CULTURAL VALUES AS STRENGTHS IN ASSESSMENT

The strengths perspective in social work practice assumes that all individuals have capabilities and strengths that may be marshaled to improve the quality of their lives and help them to survive difficult circumstances. Indigenous cultural values have helped Filipinos cope with stressors. Collectivism, support of family, spirituality, and resiliency have historically been key to their survival. These same values assist Filipinos in immigration and adaptation to their new environment.

Collectivistic Nature of Filipino Culture

Filipino culture is collectivistic in nature. The goals and well-being of the group are more important than those of the individual. The family, which is often defined as the extended kinship system, is the individual's group of identity. Enriquez (1993) identified *kapwa* as the core value of the Filipino personality, a shared awareness of identity with others that determines an individual's sense of self to the extent that "without *kapwa* one ceases to be a Filipino and human" (p. 162).

Harmony

Harmony and order are highly valued in Filipino culture. Maintaining peace and smooth interpersonal relationships (*pakikisama*) is of utmost importance. Submission and restraint of feelings are encouraged to maintain harmony. A child is taught sensitivity to the needs of others, agreeableness, recognition of subtle cues, and to cope with angry feelings without open expression (Carandang, 1979; Guthrie & Jacobs, 1966). Avoidance, withdrawal, or accommodation is used to handle conflictual feelings arising from the need to maintain smooth interpersonal relationships (Heras & Revilla, 1994). Conflict and confrontational methods, seen as improper, often are used only in anger. Indirect methods of communication are often utilized, such as euphemisms and subtle gestures (Roces & Roces, 1985).

Debt of Gratitude (Utang Na Loob)

Filipinos are taught to have a deep sense of indebtedness to someone who has bestowed kindness on them and are expected to repay the kindness when the opportunity arises. There is a Filipino saying, *Ang hindi tumingin sa kanyang pinanggalingan ay hindi makararating sa kanyang paroroonan.* ("He who does not look back at where he came from will not be able to reach where he is going.") Children are expected to provide long-term care to their parents as a reciprocal obligation for the care provided to them (Braun & Browne, 1998).

Self-Respect (amor propio)

Amor propio literally means self-love and is similar to the concept of self-respect or self-regard. This enjoins Filipinos to be sensitive to anything that threatens their self-respect or demeans their personal dignity (Jocano, 1997). Filipinos are very conscious of how they and their families are perceived by others and try to project a good image of themselves to outsiders. Problems are kept within the confines of the family to preserve the family's image. Social embarrassment, rejection, and loss of face (*hiya*) are avoided and serve as social sanctions. Shame is earned when the community's norms and standards are not followed. *Walang-hiya*, which literally means "no shame," is a big insult.

Respect for Authority

Respect for and submission to authority are sanctioned in Filipino culture. Authority is gained through age, placement among siblings, parenthood, occupational status, and socioeconomic standing. Words of respect are embedded in the language (e.g., *opo* and *oho* are polite versions of "yes"), and elders are addressed with respectful terms. At the same time, emphasis on duty, responsibility, and harmony prevents abuse of power and unfair use of authority (Ponce, 1980). Moreover, a family member can appeal to extended kin to intercede on his or her behalf.

Filipino collectivist values can be used as strengths in assessment. Emphasizing the benefits of the intervention on the family's well-being can potentially motivate members to participate. The value of maintaining harmony within the home and with the therapist might motivate the individual and family to cooperate in treatment, provide accurate information in assessment, and to be involved in treatment planning and implementation.

The value of reciprocity can become a tool for the helping professional. The sense of gratitude that family members have toward each other can be invoked to address problems. Feelings of reciprocity toward the professional for help extended can become an instrument in keeping the family involved in treatment.

Because of fear of social embarrassment, individuals and families might seek treatment to resolve the problem that can potentially cause shame. Talking about a "family secret" with an outsider might provide a safer, less threatening environment than discussing it with friends or extended kin who can spread the word. There are those who prefer non-Filipino therapists because of the fear of exposure to the community and loss of face. The professional can point out the repercussions of not pursuing treatment, especially in escalating the problem, to use the risk of social embarrassment as a motivating factor for the client to pursue help. Moreover, the principle of confidentiality needs to be emphasized to assuage fears.

Alignment with a person of authority in the family can be a positive factor in the intervention. This person can use his or her influence in getting the family to participate in assessment, treatment planning, and implementation. Such alignment must be done judiciously, however, to avoid antagonizing family members.

Central Role of the Family

The Filipino family is a bilateral extended kinship system (Ponce, 1980). Additionally, an intimate friend or person to whom one is indebted can be initiated into the family by serving as godparent in a child's baptism, confirmation, or wedding rites, thus becoming a *compadre* or *comadre* (literally, co-parent).

The family has a central role in the Filipino's life. The individual's identity is strongly linked with the family's identity. Members have a deep sense of loyalty and obligation to the family, and are expected to contribute to the family's goals and well-being. The success of the individual is viewed as the success of the family, and the failure and shame of the individual are regarded the family's own, too. Interdependence among members is encouraged, whereas individualism and independence are discouraged. Likewise, the family is the individual's primary source of nurturing and support, and is the first line of defense. The family cares for its ill, weak, or aged member.

The family serves to protect Filipino immigrants from the pains of acculturation. Heras and Revilla (1994) suggest that children who perceive their families as close and know that they can rely on them for support are more secure and have positive self-esteem.

Family orientation leads members to help each other and be a part of the treatment process. Perceived threats to the family equilibrium can mobilize the entire kinship system into action. When involved, extended kin can play an important role in providing information for assessment, participating in treatment planning, and facilitating the implementation. The helping professional can utilize the cultural expectation that the family system cares for its members in need.

Important Role of Spirituality

Filipinos are a spirituality-oriented people. They hold onto both religious and animistic beliefs. The Catholic religion has a significant influence in Filipino culture and tradition because Filipinos are predominantly Catholic.

Many believe in the existence and power of evil spirits and good spirits, and their constant interaction with the human world. Health problems and accidents are attributed to environmental factors, including punishment from God, curses, souls of the dead, or evil persons (Braun & Browne, 1998). There is a cultural belief that bad behavior leads to unfavorable outcomes and people get what they deserve (Baysa et al., 1980).

Filipinos' belief in the supremacy of a higher Being can lead them to view their situation as their destiny and, thus, to an attitude of resignation and complacency. This is embodied in the commonly used phrase, *bahala na*, derived from *Bathala na* which literally means "Let God." On the other hand, faith is a major source of hope and strength for Filipinos, which helps them in persevering and coping with difficulties.

Filipinos typically refer to their spiritual beliefs when talking about their problems with a helping professional. Their religious beliefs can be explored and potentially utilized to promote optimism and hope toward resolution of the problem. The fear of divine retribution can be a motivating factor in addressing dysfunctional behavior. Faith can encourage Filipinos to persevere in a bad situation and hold tightly to their families to avoid any breakdown in relationships. This persevering attitude can be used to focus the individual and family on what needs to be done to improve the situation.

The spiritual leader has an important role in Filipino culture. At the social level, a Philippine president often seeks advice from clergy in matters of state. The Church has played a major role in instituting changes in the sociopolitical situation in the country. For the family, the priest, pastor, or other spiritual leader or mentor is a source of advice and guidance in various situations. In assessment, this person can be an important source of information, with the client's consent. He or she can also complement the role of the therapist, such as reinforcing the therapist's input or performing family mediation when the therapist is unsuccessful. If the client or family is uncooperative, the spiritual adviser can intercede to encourage participation in treatment.

Traits of Resiliency

As a people, Filipinos have endured tremendous difficulties, including centuries of colonization, natural disasters, poverty, and underdevelopment. These have developed in them a high degree of tolerance and resiliency. They are creative in meeting needs and solving problems, and skillful in generating resources and finding a use for everything. Filipino Americans are generally hardworking, which promotes economic self-sufficiency. They also have a great ability to adapt to different situations, which facilitates acculturation. Filipinos have been likened to bamboo; they are flexible and adaptable, strong and resilient. They have an innate drive to go on and to be successful, and are extremely tolerant in enduring difficulties. Moreover, Filipinos use humor to cope with difficulties and to express frustration and anger in an acceptable way.

Filipino American clients' traits of resiliency can be an asset in the helping process. In the beginning phase of assessment and initial engagement, these traits serve to motivate clients to find solutions to problems. Their creativity and ability to generate resources can be utilized in planning interventions. The professional needs to tap their potential in mobilizing community services in response to their needs.

INDIGENOUS STRATEGIES AND WESTERN INTERVENTIONS

The aim of empowerment practice in social work is to increase the actual power of the clients or community, so that they themselves can take action and prevent the problems they are facing. Utilization of indigenous strategies in working with clients effectively builds on their strengths and problem-solving capacities. Rooted in their value system, these methods have worked in the past and are familiar to clients. They are then more inclined to use such strategies, thus increasing the likelihood of success.

In Filipino culture, mutual support networks are formed, members of which assist each other during times of difficulty. These networks encompass the nuclear family, the extended kinship system, close friends, and neighbors.

In the Philippines, community members practice *bayanihan*, which means "mutual help." Individuals and families help each other, such as preparing food for a wedding, hosting a funeral wake, raising funds for a town *fiesta* (religious celebration), and dealing with a community issue. In the smaller neighborhood system, neighbors might assist each other by babysitting, lending tools or food ingredients, and protecting each other's houses against thieves. In the process, intimate relationships and trust are formed. The practice of *damayan* is established, which means "helping those in need" in times of crisis.

Informal neighborhood chat groups, friendship groups, family dialogues, and family reunions provide a venue for talking about problems, venting feelings, seeking advice, and receiving emotional support and practical help. According to Lourdes Lapuz (1977), relatives, friends, and neighbors serve as an informal marriage counseling service in the Philippines. This is successful in partially relieving marital tension when relational problems are not too severe. The couple, however, risks the possibility of being judged or blamed, or being subjected to gossip, plain meddling, or even dubious gratification over another person's misery.

Indirect methods, rather than open confrontation and other direct approaches, are used in resolving conflict. Outside the boundaries of the nuclear family, *tsismis* (gossip) becomes a tool for changing behavior. Persons are criticized without open conflict, and this can motivate them to change when they become aware of the criticism (Cimmarusti, 1996). Gossip, or the fear of it, is a means of social control that keeps people from deviating from the norm (Jocano, 1975). In another conflict resolution method, triangulation, an individual relays concerns about another to a third person, who in turn communicates the complaints in an appropriate manner. The mediator has to have a high or respected position in the clan for the recipient of the complaint to react positively (Cimmarusti, 1996).

Filipino American families do not have the same network of support as families in the Philippines. They tend to deal with problems within the extended family system or support network and discourage soliciting external help. Assistance is mobilized by one's support system. When conflict such as that between spouses or between parent and child is unresolved, a mediator or go-between may be used (Agbayani-Siewert, 1994). Help might be sought from an elder or respected member of the support network, or at times, a religious person. External help, such as from a counselor, is sought only when the problem escalates or reaches an acute stage (Tompar-Tiu & Sustento-Seneriches, 1995).

Illness and behavioral and emotional disturbances are commonly attributed to spiritual factors; hence, interventions beyond the physical are used (Anderson, 1983; Tompar-Tiu & Sustento-Seneriches, 1995). Prayer is a popular help-seeking behavior and a source of comfort. Acts are performed to right the wrong that might have caused the problem, such as penance, sacrifices, and religious devotions. The guidance and blessing of religious clergy are sought. Traditional healers may be involved, and herbal remedies may be used to treat a disorder. Even in the United States, the services of indigenous interventionists are utilized, and traditional healing methods are applied, often in conjunction with Western interventions (Tompar-Tiu & Sustento-Seneriches, 1995).

In many instances, however, indigenous interventions prove inadequate in addressing issues faced by Filipino Americans. When traditional help mechanisms fail, what interventions appropriate to Filipino American families are sensitive to their culture and value system? The use of family therapy is supported by cultural values that encourage and facilitate collective problem solving and conflict resolution among family members. These values include harmony, reciprocity of benevolence, importance of the family, and respect for authority. The therapist can focus the family on the need for cooperation, communication, and negotiation to preserve family harmony and integrity.

To be more effective, the therapist may consider joining with the family while holding on to the use of his or her authority. This could facilitate engagement of clients in the therapeutic relationship rather than maintenance of a distant, professional stance. In the Philippines, interventionists frequently meet with families in their homes, and the main session is often preceded by informal chats and snacks offered by the family. Such gestures from professionals convey a sincere desire to help the family and are most often received with warmth, break down of defenses and guardedness, and reciprocity, with clients becoming more responsive to services. Especially for resistant clients, home visitation and even counseling sessions conducted in the home should be considered.

Because Filipinos regard professionals highly, the therapist can use his or her authority and influence as an agent of change in the family. He or she can adopt an educational role. Therapy should educate both parents and children "about the tensions between the two cultures, generations, value systems and behavioral styles to provide both parents and children with a better understanding of their own conflicts and ways to cope with them" (Agbayani-Siewert, 1994, p. 436).

Some techniques that might be especially applicable are meaning-oriented techniques such as reframing and circular questioning, which may be less threatening and more useful than action-oriented techniques such as enactment and role play (Cimmarusti, 1996). Agbayani-Siewert (1994) suggested the use of vignettes as a problem-solving tool and nonthreatening way to discuss a sensitive topic. Assigning tasks that involve acts of kindness utilize the value of indebtedness, thus setting into motion reciprocal exchanges between family members (Cimmarusti, 1996).

With the consent of the family, members of their support network can become involved in the intervention process. Sessions that include these people might be held to mobilize their participation in treatment planning and implementation. The use of traditional conflict resolution mechanisms, such as use of mediators and involvement of a spiritual mentor, might be integrated into family therapy or marital counseling.

Because of the collectivist nature of Filipino culture, group therapy can be a productive tool for the therapist. On the one hand, due to fear of shame and loss of face, there may be initial resistance to disclosure in a group setting. As trust is developed and relationships are established among members, however, the support group can be an important source of help. It can become a venue where collectivistic values and practices are applied and utilized. Because Filipinos are fond of social activities that involve eating, singing, and dancing, these could be combined with the therapeutic process to maintain the clients' interest.

To further facilitate the *bayanihan* and *damayan* system, the helping professional needs to connect the family with resources in the community and create or widen the support system of the family. Churches and Filipino organizations are popular places for getting together, developing relationships, and accessing information and support. Youth can benefit from community resources (e.g., mentorship and afterschool programs), because many parents work full-time or have multiple jobs, and children might be left without supervision. In reaching out to members of the mentally ill population and their families, aggressive outreach and creative approaches are needed to counteract the stigma around help seeking (Tompar-Tiu & Sustento-Seneriches, 1995).

PRINCIPLES OF CULTURALLY APPROPRIATE PRACTICE

Recognize the Multiple Stressors of Immigrants

Be aware that Filipino immigrant families experience tremendous stress associated with the immigration and acculturation process. Explore how this interacts with their experience of a particular problem or situation to have a more comprehensive and accurate view of the person-in-situation dynamics.

Acknowledge Individual Differences

There are wide variations among Filipino families, and they differ in level of adherence to cultural values and practices. Some factors that determine this level of adherence and need to be assessed include the family's length of stay in the United States, level of acculturation, generational level, and background in the Philippines (including subethnic and urban–rural origin, socioeconomic status, educational attainment, and professional level).

Assess Culture-Bound Perceptions of the Problem and Solutions

Examine the client and the family's perspectives on the problem, its causes, and solution. Explore the relevance of faith, spiritual beliefs, and cultural interpretations, and how these affect their receptiveness and participation in the helping process. Determine the types of interventions being utilized, including indigenous methods. Educate them about their options, but respect their adherence to traditional views and practices, and their right to self-determination.

Note Inaccurate Presentation of Symptoms

The client's affect might be incongruent with mood and concerns. For example, a client might smile while talking about sad events or negative feelings. Possible explanations include shyness in talking about feelings, socialization in restraint of feelings, and fear of rejection. Congruence between affect and mood increases as trust is developed. Additionally, Filipino American clients tend to present somatic symptoms or environmental stressors first, while denying or minimizing emotional and mental problems.

Recognize the Important Role of the Family

Because of the immense role the family plays in the life of the Filipino American, treatment goals and interventions should be directed at the entire family system. It is important to assess the family's part in the problem situation. In assessment, observe family interaction and decision-making patterns. Observe the couple's relationship, whether egalitarian, patriarchal, or matriarchal in structure. Know who is part of the family, taking into consideration the extended kin, the *compadre/comadre* system, and the involvement of religious people.

Engage family members actively in assessment, treatment planning, and implementation, involving them in the decision-making processes, if in keeping with treatment goals. Determine who plays an important role in family affairs, and assess their willingness to be part of the helping process. Their participation may prove to be a significant contributing factor in the success of the intervention. According to McLaughlin and Braun (1998), their personal experience working with Filipino American clients in Honolulu suggests that patients may not be compliant if a health care worker disregards other family members' opinions.

Work Initially with the Existing Hierarchy of Power

Be aware of the power structure and who is held in authority and address these persons with respect. It is often best to work with the existing hierarchy of power, especially in the initial stage of treatment. If in keeping with service goals, aligning with those in authority could be beneficial. If an important family member is not given due consideration, he or she might dissuade the client from participation. At the same time, be aware of the feelings of other family members toward the family authority and treat the other members with importance. Also, convey respect to senior members.

Avoid Open Criticism and Confrontation

Open criticism and confrontation might be offensive and lead clients to drop out of treatment prematurely. Indirect communication might be more effective at the start. Humor can be very effective in getting the message across in a nonthreatening way. As rapport and relationship are developed, clients will have increased openness in accepting feedback. In doing so, clarify your intent, and be sensitive to *hiya* (shame) and *amor propio* (self-regard).

Develop a Relationship

Relationship is highly valued by Filipinos. They tend to work best with people with whom they feel comfortable and have an established relationship. They may ask personal questions to build rapport with the helping professional. For example, a client might ask a Filipino professional about his or her area of origin in the Philippines, and length of stay in the United States. Some personal information may be essential in building a working relationship. A sense of indebtedness to the professional may develop because of the relationship and help extended, and this encourages treatment continuity and cooperation.

Utilize Respect for Authority

Because Filipinos put a high value on education, they ascribe high status to professionals and regard them as authorities, sometimes addressing them as ma'am, sir, or doctor. This can be a positive factor in engagement of clients in the therapeutic process and can promote treatment compliance. On the other hand, clients may keep their true feelings and thoughts from the professional, or refrain from clarifying or asking questions because of the difference in status. Balancing efforts to establish a personal relationship and maintain professional distance is essential. Imposing a distance and failing to connect on a more personal level with the client may weaken the therapeutic relationship. Assure clients that they can respond to, question, or challenge input or feedback.

Be Sensitive to an Indirect Communication Style

Clients may agree to a plan because of the desire to please and maintain a good relationship with the therapist. "Yes" does not always mean *yes*; indecisiveness could mean "no". "I might" or "I am not sure" is often said instead of "no". Be sensitive to verbal and nonverbal cues. Take note of the possibility that clients are withholding their feelings and thoughts to maintain peace. Disagreement may be expressed in indirect ways, such as by missing appointments or nonperformance of assigned tasks. Explore ambiguous responses and unfinished sentences. As clients develop a relationship with the professional, a more direct communication style will likely develop.

Be Aware of Communication Barriers

Be aware of Filipinos' idiosyncratic use of English, confusion with pronouns, limited words in describing feelings, and other language difficulties. Filipino Americans might deny language problems, because facility with the English language is a status symbol. As Filipinos typically learn English, starting from kindergarten in the Philippines, possession of English-language skills should not be equated with a high level of acculturation. Always give clients the opportunity to clarify and ask questions.

Deal Sensitively and Politely with Gifts

Filipino American clients may offer food or gifts as a gesture of reciprocity, as appreciation for help extended to them. In keeping with Filipino hospitality, it is typical for families to serve food to guests in their homes. When food is offered during home visits, it is often polite to accept it. One has to be sensitive, however, to the possibility that the offer is a mere gesture of politeness. If forms of hospitality have to be refused, this should be done in a courteous and sensitive manner.

Be Cognizant of Intergenerational Tension

First-generation immigrant parents may base their expectations of their children on how they were socialized in their country of origin. Second-generation immigrant children tend to adhere to the value system of American society. The practitioner needs to be aware of this tension and recognize the struggles of both parents and children while educating them about the conflict. One might take the role of mediator, facilitating open dialogues, with observance of mutual respect. Both parties need to engage in open communication and may have to compromise to achieve treatment goals. While advocating for the child, the practitioner has to be mindful of the cultural importance of the family unit (Agbayani-Siewert, 1994).

Parents need to be educated about children's developmental processes and needs in the American context, value conflicts experienced by immigrant youth, struggles in mediating between two cultures, and pressure exerted on children by unrealistic parental expectations. Encourage loosening of family boundaries to utilize external help such as counseling, when appropriate, reframing this as a means of strengthening family relationships rather than as a threat to family solidarity. Likewise, encourage exposure and connection of children to Filipino culture to promote a stronger sense of ethnic identity. Development of children's appreciation of the culture promotes a better understanding of their parents' values, traditions, and perspective, and contributes to bridging of generations.

CASE VIGNETTE

Tim, a 15-year-old Filipino American male, was referred to the counselor by his 10th-grade teacher. He had been cutting classes frequently, and his grades were failing. This was a drastic change from his previous academic performance; Tim had always excelled in class in previous grades.

In the first session, Tim was brought in by his father, Ben, a 45-year-old Filipino immigrant who migrated to the United States 18 years earlier to marry his Filipino fiancée Nelia. She had come to the United States 5 years earlier as a nurse. Shortly after marriage, they had one child, Tim. Four years ago, Nelia died unexpectedly. Ben did not pursue a relationship after her death.

Ben expressed concern about Tim's behavior. He could not understand what happened with his son, who used to be a serious student. In the past, it was never a problem getting him to do chores and follow house rules. This last year, however, Tim had been increasingly rebellious, refusing to do homework, failing to do chores, and coming home past curfew time. Lately, he had been associating with peers who smoked and drank beer.

Also, Ben mentioned that Tim had not come home one night the previous week. Late in the evening, Ben's brother Lucio called and informed him that Tim had come to their house and had refused to return home. In the morning, Lucio brought Tim back. Ben said he was at a loss on what to do. Throughout the session, Tim remained very quiet, gave monolingual responses, and appeared tense.

The culturally competent counselor recognized that she needed to get more information from Tim, as well as build rapport and engage him in therapy. She wondered whether Lucio served as a mediator between father and son, in which case, he could have a vital role in the therapeutic process. The counselor asked Ben's permission to have Lucio bring Tim to the next session. Ben agreed.

Tim and Lucio arrived at the next session. Tim appeared relaxed. With the counselor's probing and Lucio's gentle prodding, Tim was able to verbalize his feelings toward his father and about the situation. He felt that his father was very controlling, imposing his own standards and desires on him. His father always compared Tim to himself as a youth in the Philippines, where he was an obedient, hardworking child. Tim felt that his father did not understand him. At the same time, he was worried about his father, and believed he had not gotten over his mother's death. Tim thought his father had become stricter after his mother's death, imposing unreasonable restrictions on his behavior.

Lucio agreed that Ben continued to grieve about Nelia's death. He worried about him too, because he seemed to be isolating himself, often missing family events. Tim verbalized how he wanted family relationships to be harmonious again, like when his mother was around. The counselor assured him that she believed this was a common desire between father and son.

In the next session, the counselor met with Ben and Lucio. The latter helped her communicate to Ben their concerns. Ben admitted continued grief about his wife's death. He felt unable to provide the nurturing his wife had provided to Tim. He felt pressure that, as a single parent, he had to take charge over his son's behavior. He verbalized feeling overwhelmed by the responsibilities of single parenting. Nelia had played an active role in child rearing and discipline. Although Ben wondered whether he might be imposing excessive control over his son, he also talked about how, as a youth in the Philippines, he was always obedient and respectful to his parents.

The counselor educated Ben about normal adolescent needs in the United States and value conflicts experienced by Filipino immigrant youth. Ben agreed that it was fine for Tim to talk with Lucio and have him intervene if, for some reason, Tim did not feel comfortable approaching Ben.

In the next sessions with Ben and Tim, the counselor facilitated open dialogues, while setting ground rules of mutual respect and harmonious interaction. She assigned kind acts for Tim and Ben to do for each other, fueling patterns of reciprocity. At her suggestion, Ben began attending family get-togethers again and went on fishing trips with Tim. The counselor connected Ben with a Filipino organization, through which he got in contact with other Filipino American single parents and established some friendships. Tim was referred to a youth center, where he got involved with cultural programs that increased his knowledge and appreciation of Filipino culture, and was steered away from unwholesome peers.

Ben had reservations about going to another therapist to deal with grief and loss issues. He had a good relationship with a Filipino priest, however, and began meeting with him. He agreed to seek out a counselor if religious intervention proved inadequate.

As a result of the social worker's interventions and cultural sensitivity, positive changes were introduced into the family system, and the family unit was stabilized. She mediated between father and son and facilitated communication between them, utilizing the help of extended kin as go-betweens. To decrease the parent–child gap, the father was educated about generational and cultural differences between him and his son, and the son was linked with community programs that promoted appreciation of and connection with his ethnicity. Among the cultural values that were beneficial to the change process were reciprocity and family orientation. Community resources that were utilized integrated the family with their cultural and spiritual community, thus increasing support and decreasing isolation.

CONCLUSIONS

Filipino immigrants experience major transitions, including loss of occupational status, decrease of social support, economic pressures, and adjustment difficulties. Problems arise in the husband–wife and parent–child systems. In adoption of the strengths perspective in social work assessment and practice, Filipino cultural values are recognized as strengths that help Filipino Americans cope with the stress of immigration and adaptation. Their cultural value system is based on collectivism, family orientation, spirituality, and resiliency.

Utilization of indigenous strategies in working with clients builds on their strengths and empowers them to solve their own problems. Some of these strategies include *bayanihan* and *damayan*, seeking advice from one's support network or a religious person, use of mediation, and religious acts. Western interventions can also be beneficial when adapted to Filipino cultural values and ways. In working with Filipino American children and families, observance of culturally appropriate principles is necessary for an effective helping process.

REFERENCES

Aesquivel, C. (1990). Babies making babies: Teen pregnancies rise in the Asian Pacific community. *Pacific Ties*, 7(3), 3.

Agbayani-Siewert, P. (1988). *Social service utilization of Filipino Americans in Los Angeles*. Unpublished manuscript, School of Social Welfare, University of California, Los Angeles.

Agbayani-Siewert, P. (1994). Filipino American culture and family: Guidelines for practitioners. *Families in Society: The Journal of Contemporary Human Services*, 75(7), 429–438.

Almirol, E. (1986). Exclusion and institutional barriers in the university system: The Filipino experience. In G. Okihiro, S. Hune, A. Hansen, & J. Liu (Eds.), *Reflections on shattered windows: Promises and prospects for Asian American studies* (pp. 59–67). Pullman: Washington State University.

Anderson, J. (1983). Health and illness in Pilipino immigrants. *Western Journal of Medicine*, 139, 811–819.

Azores, T. (1986-87). Educational attainment and upward mobility: Prospects for Filipino Americans. *Amerasia Journal*, 13, 73–84.

Baysa, E., Cabrera, E., Camilon, F., & Torres, M. (1980). The Filipinos. In N. Palafox & A. Warren (Eds.), *Cross-cultural caring: A handbook for health care professionals in Hawaii* (pp. 197–231). Honolulu: Transcultural Health Care Forum.

Braun, K. L., & Browne, C. V. (1998). Perceptions of dementia, caregiving, and helpseeking among Asian and Pacific Islander Americans. *Health and Social Work*, 23(4), 262–273.

Cabezas, A., Shinagawa, L. H., & Kawaguchi, G. (1986). New inquiries into the socioeconomic status of Pilipino Americans in California. *Amerasia*, 13, 1–21.

Carandang, L. A. (1979). The Pilipino child in the family: A developmental–clinical approach. *Philippine Studies*, 27, 469–482.

Chan, S. (1998). Families with Pilipino roots. In E. W. Lynch & M. J. Hanson (Eds.), *Developing cross-cultural competence: A guide for working with children and their families* (2nd ed., pp. 259–300). Baltimore: Brookes.

Cimmarusti, R. A. (1996). Exploring aspects of Filipino-American families. *Journal of Marital and Family Therapy*, 22(2), 205–217.

Domingo, K., & Wong, R. (1990). Asian gangs in LA. *Pacific Ties*, 7(3), 12–13.

Enriquez, V. (1993). Developing a Filipino psychology. In U. Kim & J. W. Berry (Eds.), *Indigenous psychologies: Research and experience in cultural context* (pp. 152–169). Newbury Park, CA: Sage.

Espiritu, Y. L. (1994). The intersection of race, ethnicity, and class: The multiple identities of second-generation Filipinos. *Identities*, 1(2–3), 249–273.

Guthrie, G., & Jacobs, P. (1966). *Child-rearing and personality development in the Philippines*. University Park: Pennsylvania State University Press.

Heras, P., & Revilla, L. A. (1994). Acculturation, generational status, and family environment of Pilipino Americans: A study in cultural adaptation. *Family Therapy,* *21*(2), 129–138.

Jocano, F. L. (1997). *Filipino value system: A cultural definition.* Quezon City, Philippines: PUNLAD Research House.

Jocano, F. L. (1975). *Slum as a way of life.* Quezon City, Philippines: New Day.

Kao, G. (1995). Asian Americans as model minorities?: A look at the academic performance of immigrant youth. *Social Science Quarterly, 76,* 1–19.

Lapuz, L. V. (1977). *Filipino marriages in crisis.* Quezon City, Philippines: New Day.

McLaughlin, L. A., & Braun, K. L. (1998). Asian and Pacific Islander cultural values: Considerations for health care decision making. *Health and Social Work, 23*(2), 116–126.

Okamura, J. Y., & Agbayani, A. (1991). Filipino Americans. In N. Mokuau (Ed.), *Handbook of social services for Asians and Pacific Islanders* (pp. 97–115). Westport, CT: Greenwood Press.

Oliver, J. E., Grey, F., Stiles, J., & Brady, H. (1995). *Pacific rim states Asian demographic data book.* Oakland: University of California, Office of the President.

Padilla, A., Wagatsuma, Y., & Lindholm, K. (1985). Acculturation and personality as predictors of stress in Japanese and Japanese Americans. *Journal of Social Psychology, 125,* 295–305.

Ponce, D. E. (1980). The Filipinos. In J. McDermott, W. S. Teng, & T. Maretzki (Eds.), *People and cultures of Hawaii: A psychocultural profile* (pp. 155–163). Honolulu: University of Hawaii Press.

Pulido, M. (1990). Conflict in Cerritos. *Pacific Ties, 7*(3), 10, 15.

Roces, A., & Roces, G. (1985). *Culture shock.* Singapore: Times Books International.

Rumbaut, R. G. (1995). The new Californians: Comparative research findings on the educational progress of immigrant children. In R. G. Rumbaut & W. A. Cornelius (Eds.), *California's immigrant children* (pp. 17–70). La Jolla: Center for United States–Mexican Studies, University of California, San Diego.

Rumbaut, R. G. (1996). The crucible within: Ethnic identity, self-esteem, and segmented assimilation among children of immigrants. In A. Portes (Ed.), *The new second generation* (pp. 119–170). New York: Russell Sage Foundation.

Santos, R. A. (1983). The social and emotional development of Filipino-American children. In G. J. Powell (Ed.), *The psychosocial development of minority group children* (pp. 131–146). New York: Brunner/Mazel.

Takaki, R. (1989). *Strangers from a different shore: A history of Asian Americans.* Boston: Little, Brown.

Tompar-Tiu, A., & Sustento-Seneriches, J. (1995). *Depression and other mental health issues.* San Francisco: Jossey-Bass.

U.S. Bureau of the Census (1991). *Statistical abstract of the United States: 1991* (111th ed.). Washington, DC: U.S. Government Printing Office.

U.S. Bureau of the Census (2000). *Statistical abstract of the United States: 2000* (120th ed.). Washington, DC: U.S. Government Printing Office.

Wolf, D. L. (1997). Family secrets: Transnational struggles among children of Filipino immigrants. *Sociological Perspectives, 40*(3), 457–482.

Ying, Y., & Hu, L. (1994). Public outpatient mental health services: Use and outcome among Asian Americans. *American Journal of Orthopsychiatry, 64*(3), 448–455.

CHAPTER 5

Korean Children and Families

SUNG SIL LEE SOHNG
KUI-HEE SONG

Of the over 1 million Korean Americans living in the United States today (U.S. Bureau of the Census, 2001), some are descendants of the first wave of labor immigrants who arrived in Hawaii at the turn of the century. The second wave came to the United States during and after the Korean War (1950–1953) as wives of American servicemen, war orphans, and students. Most Korean Americans, however, have come to the United States since 1965, both as new immigrants and as relatives of those who came earlier.

Coming from a monocultural, monoracial environment, Korean immigrants had to learn a new language, new customs, and new ways of living in a multilingual, multicultural, and multiracial society. As a racial/ethnic minority, they were subjected to overt and covert forms of prejudice, stereotype, and discrimination. Slowly but steadily, they have made progress. They settled in run-down sections of inner cities and turned them into booming commercial districts. They built Koreatowns, established churches and temples, started businesses, bought homes, and put their children through college. Their work ethic and faith in their adopted country as a land of opportunity helped them to move ahead. What often goes unreported beyond this "model minority" is that many Korean immigrant families, like many other Asian immigrants, struggle with conflicting pressures: to preserve cultural heritage and traditional values, and to adapt to social changes for survival and mastery of a new sociocultural environment.

In this chapter, we explore a brief history of Korean immigrants and examine the interplay between Korean and American cultures, and how the related elements of culture and power affect Korean immigrants' lives. We believe that a dialectical view of culture and its link to social power is essential to understand the social dynamics that support the various forms of dominant and subordinate power relations in the United States.

Much has been said about Korean Americans today being positioned on the *in-between*—on the cusp, at the interstice, in the buffer zone—between Korea and America, between black and white, between mainstreamed and marginalized (Kim, 1997). The *in-between* is a precarious and dangerous position to occupy for those who are not fully aware of where they are and what their position means in the larger picture. The "middleman minority" is the term used to explain the phenomenon of an alien or immigrant group's concentration in small business (Rinder, 1959). We discuss the similarity of the role of Korean immigrants (especially entrepreneurs) in the traditional middleman minority role. Our analysis provides a political–economic context for today's changing Korean immigrant families to identify culturally appropriate and empowering practice principles in Korean immigrant child and family groups.

KOREAN IMMIGRATION HISTORY
FROM A GLOBAL PERSPECTIVE

U.S. policy makers and the public alike believe the causes of immigration are self-evident: People who migrate to the United States are driven by poverty, economic stagnation, and overpopulation in their home countries. It is assumed that immigration is unrelated to U.S. economic needs or broader international economic conditions. In this context, the decision to permit immigration becomes a humanitarian matter; we admit immigrants by choice and out of generosity, not because we have any economic motive or political responsibility to do so (Sassen, 1998). We counter this widely held perspective and examine how political, military, and economic conditions in the United States and Korea have shaped the history of Korean immigration.

The First Wave

The first Korean Americans were laborers recruited to work in the sugar plantations of Hawaii. About 7,000 men, mostly unmarried, arrived between 1903 and 1907. They were brought in to offset the labor shortage created when the Chinese exclusion acts passed by Congress became applicable to Hawaii in 1898, and waves of anti-Japanese sentiment discouraged Japanese immigration. Before the 1924 immigration law revision that completely prohibited immigration from Asia, the Korean laborers in Hawaii had managed to bring in approximately 1,100 Korean picture brides

(Patterson, 1988). These women were often better educated than their men, and they energized the small Korean American community. They led their families from the farms of Hawaii into the city of Honolulu, and then to California, participating in church activities and contributing to the independence movement aimed at freeing their homeland from Japanese colonial rule from 1910 to 1945 (Yu, 1993).

A few Korean students then came to the United States between 1899 and 1909, followed by 541 political exiles, who came by way of China or Europe without passports between 1910 and 1924, after Japan annexed Korea. Between 1921 and 1940, 289 additional Korean students came to the United States on Japanese passports. Many of these exiles and students found ways to stay in the United States and became leaders of the pre–World War II Korean American community (Choy, 1979; Hurh & Kim, 1984).

The early Korean immigrants were forced to live with open discrimination. A powerful coalition of Americans—members of labor unions, radicals on both ends of the political spectrum, and intellectuals—opposed Asian immigration. The lives of the early Korean Americans were limited not only by immigration laws, which separated them from their families, but also by explicitly anti-Asian laws such as California's Anti-Miscegenation Law (1901), which prohibited their intermarriage with whites, and its Alien Land law (1913), which prevented them from owning land. These social conditions posed serious obstacles to the socioeconomic mobility of Asian immigrants. Some Koreans settled on the fringes of Chinatowns or Japantowns. Many lived as migrant farm workers. Because of antimiscegenation laws and the male–female ratio of 10 to 1, many of the original Korean immigrants remained single throughout their lives, which resulted in minimal growth in the Korean American population (Yu, 1993).

The Second Wave

American intervention in the Korean War triggered the second wave of Korean immigration: wives of American servicemen, war orphans, and students. Between 1951 and 1964, approximately 6,500 brides, 6,300 adopted children, and 6,000 students came to this country (Hurh & Kim, 1984). These three groups have continued to be significant components of Korean immigration to the United States.

In the period following the Korean War, the United States actively sought to promote economic development in Korea and Southeast Asia as a way of politically stabilizing the region. In addition, U.S. troops were stationed in Korea, the Philippines, and Indochina. Together, U.S. business and military interests created a vast array linking Korea and Southeast Asian countries that would later produce large migration flows to the United States.

The Third Wave

The third wave of Korean immigration began with the passage of the Immigration Act of 1965, which had the most significant effect on the Korean American community. Although the immigration of Koreans to the United States is a century old, the Korean American community before 1965 was insignificant in terms of population size. The rate of immigration accelerated from 70,000 in 1970s to 355,000 in 1980, and to 800,000 in 1990, according to statistics from the 1990 U.S. Bureau of the Census, putting Korea among the top five countries of origin of immigrants to the United States.

In the 1960s and 1970s, the United States played a crucial role in the development of today's global economic system. It was a key exporter of capital, promoted the development of export–manufacturing enclaves in many Third World countries, and passed legislation aimed at opening its own and other countries' flow of capital, goods, services, and information. The emergence of global economy and the economic role played by the United States in this process contributed both to the creation abroad of pools of potential emigrants and to the formation of linkages between industrialized and developing countries that subsequently were to serve as bridges for international migration. The massive increase in foreign investment during this period, particularly in South Korea, Taiwan, and the Philippines, along with the establishment of political, military, and economic linkages with the United States have been instrumental in creating conditions that allowed the emergence of large-scale emigration (Sassen, 1998).

Although the structural linkages between the United States and South Korea were an important factor in the massive migration of the post-1965 Korean immigrants, many new Korean immigrants were attracted by a perceived economic mobility. Whereas better economic opportunity in the United States is a pull factor for new Korean immigration, political problems, social insecurity, and fear of another war in Korea are push factors.

THE MIDDLEMAN MINORITY AS AN ECOLOGICAL ADAPTATION

The new wave of Korean immigrants began landing at Los Angeles, New York, and other major international airports in the late 1960s, a time when Jewish stores and corporate chains were withdrawing from inner cities. Korean immigrants filled the vacuum. They leased stores and bought markets, unaware of the events that had led to the vacuum or that they were placing themselves between two starkly contrasting and often hostile worlds: the poverty-stricken inner city and the affluent suburbs. A typical pattern in the 1970s was for a newly arrived family to start a small business after a few years of work on assembly lines or with maintenance companies. Because of the heavy reliance on ethnic networking, an ethnic Korean concentration developed, for example, in labor-intensive, small grocery, dry cleaning, liquor, and fast-food businesses.

Many Korean immigrants who support themselves by running small businesses thus have gained the reputation as a trading minority. Survey studies lend statistical support to the visibility of Korean immigrant entrepreneurship. According to a survey conducted in 1973, 25% of Korean heads of household in Los Angeles were engaged in small business (Bonacich, Light, & Wong, 1976). The self-employment rate in the Los Angeles Korean community increased to 40% in 1977 (Yu, 1982), then to over 50% in 1986 (Min, 1989). The New York Korean community exhibited an even higher self-employment rate, 52%, of Korean workers (Min, 1991). Overall, more than 40% of Korean immigrants in the United States seem to be self-employed.

A significant effect of the 1965 Immigration and Naturalization Act on immigration patterns was a dramatic change in the socioeconomic background of immigrants. Whereas the earlier immigrants consisted largely of farmers and unskilled workers, the post-1965 immigrants were mainly recruited from the urban, middle-class strata of each source country. Upon their arrival, however, the majority of Korean immigrants faced unfavorable labor market conditions. It is well documented that many college-educated Korean immigrants hold blue-collar jobs, and many professionals are either unemployed, underemployed, or turn to nonprofessional jobs, primarily because of language and cultural barriers, racial discrimination in hiring and promotion, low wages in the general labor market, and lack of transferability of work experience, education, and skills acquired in Korea (Chang & Moon, 1998).

Min (1991) argues that Korean immigrants turn to small business to make a living mainly because of their *disadvantages* in nonbusiness occupations, not because of their advantages in small business. The majority of Korean businesses are located in crime-ridden, low-income residential and downtown commercial areas that are not attractive to white merchants (Light & Bonacich, 1988; Min, 1989).

Other ethnic and immigrant groups, such as Jews in Medieval Europe, Chinese in Southeast Asia, and Indians in East Africa, specialized in small businesses. The term used to explain the phenomenon of an alien immigrant group's concentration in small business is the "middleman minority" (Rinder, 1959). In many African and Southeast Asian countries, the white colonial power promoted outsiders as entrepreneurs to prevent trade from falling into the hands of a potentially powerful indigenous group (Skinner, 1963; Yambert, 1981). Thus, Jiang (1978) has indicated that alien merchant groups possessed revenues and resources disproportionately and were relegated to positions of low status, low power, and few noncommercial privileges.

Korean immigrant entrepreneurs in the United States take on a role similar to that of the traditional middleman minority (Bonacich, 1988; Min, 1989; Portes & Manning, 1986). U.S. structural forces encouraged Korean small businesses in minority areas. Residential succession is the process by which minority members are slowly replacing whites in certain areas (Aldrich, 1975). As Aldrich demonstrated, blacks and other minority groups in the United States are slow in taking over white-owned businesses or establishing new businesses in racially changing areas because of their low levels of capital and business experience. As a result, residential succession increases the number of vacant sites for businesses in inner cities and newly established black residential areas, which provides new immigrants with business opportunities. No doubt, this residential succession process has encouraged Korean immigrant entrepreneurship in transitional areas. Another structural force encouraging Korean immigrant entrepreneurship in minority ghetto areas is that large corporations are unwilling to maintain or establish business in these areas largely because of high crime rates and low profit margins.

Korean store owners operating businesses in black areas, like middleman minorities in other societies, have faced a high level of hostility and violent reactions from African American customers. The Korean–African American conflicts have increased over the years in New York, Chicago, Atlanta, and Philadelphia, rapidly escalating after a series of organized boycotts in these cities in 1990. The Los Angeles riot in spring 1992, following the verdict in Rodney King's trial, destroyed many Korean-owned businesses. The conflict is further aggravated by Korean immigrant entrepreneurs' high visibility (because of racial, cultural, and class differences from the local residents), and by their vulnerability (because they are politically and culturally disadvantaged as a result of limited English proficiency and unfamiliarity with African American culture). These race, culture, and language gaps reinforce the perception of adversarial positions between the two groups.

When Korean immigrants operate small businesses in communities of color, they are structurally placed in the position of middleman. They obtain supplies from white-dominated American and international corporations, then sell the supplies to the residents of local communities. Through these business transactions, Korean entrepreneurs share profits with those who control the corporations. But as the local retailers in African American communities, Korean entrepreneurs alone are marked as a convenient scapegoat for hostility and resentment toward the establishment. In short, Korean small business owners illustrate a classical case of middleman minority. This interminority group conflict reflects each group's respective position in the white-dominated American economic system.

The Los Angeles riot in 1992 demonstrated that Korean Americans must build healthy relationships with other minority communities, organize themselves politically, and fight racism—their own, as well as that of others. In this respect, the riots were a "wake-up call," and Korean Americans are rebuilding Korean communities that will be an integral part of the total community, benefiting not only Koreans but also their non-Korean neighbors.

CONTEXTUALIZING THE KOREAN AMERICAN COMMUNITY TODAY

The Korean American community can be broken down into three generational categories. The first is the *il-se* (first generation), composed of those who came to the United States as adults. The second is the *il-jom-o-se* (the one-and-a-half generation, born in Korea but raised in the United States), and the third is the e-se (the American-born second generation). The *il-se* speak Korean and tend to think and behave like Koreans. The *il-jom-o-se* and *e-se* speak mostly English and tend to think and behave like Americans, which distances them from their elders. All Korean churches and community organizations are defined on the basis of the language they use, for the Korean-speaking adults and their English-speaking children lead separate lives and socialize in different orbits (Yu, 1993).

Korean immigrant parents and their children approach life in the United States in different ways. The parents already have a strong, positive Korean identity, because their own upbringing was in Korea, where they were part of an established culture. They have the courage and self-esteem necessary to venture into new territory despite their cultural and linguistic disadvantages.

Younger Koreans, however, are growing up in a minority culture. Second-generation Korean Americans generally lack the feeling of mastery over their environment that their parents possess. Under the circumstances, they have difficulty developing pride and confidence in their ethnic heritage and struggle constantly to discover and define themselves. They often feel alienated in Koreatown, Korean churches, and Korean community organizations, and they are assimilated into the mainstream society with difficulty. The resulting lack of a "positive self-identity" is one of the most serious problems younger generation Koreans face in this country, and it can lead to a sense of alienation, helplessness, and despair.

Korean parents make enormous sacrifices to provide their children with a good education, and most Korean children understand their parents' plight and try to live up to their expectations. As a result, many Korean children excel in school. For Korean American families, like other Asian American families, educational success is not only an individual matter but, it also becomes a serious family concern. Recently, however, a few researchers (Liu, Yu, Chang, & Fernandez, 1990; Pang, 1991; Schneider & Lee, 1990) have discussed the manifest problems of low self-esteem, high achievement anxiety, and low social skills in relation to parental pressure found among some high-achieving Asian American students. These studies report on the increasing rate of high school dropouts, substance abuse, teen pregnancy, and gang activity among Korean and Asian American youth. They point out that cultural–parental pressure to succeed can be a stress factor that may lead young Asian Americans in general, and Korean Americans in particular, to the development of mental as well as behavioral problems.

The language and culture gap between generations plague the Korean American family. Language use is the most conspicuous difference. School-age children quickly realize that they are different from others. Therefore, they begin the difficult and painful process of redefining their ethnic, cultural, and individual identity. As they grow, the children often turn against their Korean ethnicity, hating their own looks and other markers of their cultural identity. The process of devaluation of their Koreanness, self-redefinition, and eventual self-acceptance is long and convoluted, and some children inevitably fall through the cracks into a delinquent subculture. Because of this process of rejection and redefinition, Korean American children begin to lose their Korean-language proficiency rapidly after they start school. Without English skills, however, parents lose their primary means of communication with their children. Many immigrant families are forced to live without effective parent–child communication, a vital part of stable emotional and intellectual development.

As discussed in the previous section, an estimated one-third of adult Korean immigrants own and operate small businesses, working an average of 60 hours per week, leaving little time for formal learning of the language and the systems of their new society, whereas their younger children adapt more quickly to their new environment, learning English and a different code of ethics and behaviors. Generational differences, highlighted by cultural and linguistic gaps, can and do create damaging barriers within all arenas of family life.

Another important difference between adult and younger Koreans is the degree of hierarchy and male dominance in the lifestyle and value system. Adult Koreans tend to have hierarchical, authoritarian, and patriarchal relationships, characterized by rigid gender and age distinction in the family relationship. Parents are traditionally accorded unquestioning respect and function as the highest authority in the home. Family obligation is a primary role for parents to bring up children well. Authoritarian control and subsequent poor communication, on top of language barriers between parents and children, are a primary source of conflict in the Korean American family.

Changing gender roles also affect the traditional lines of authority, especially Korean male dominance. The 1990 Census indicated that 56% of Korean American women 16 years or older worked outside the home (U.S.

Bureau of the Census, 1994). Also, Min (1992) found that 70% of Korean married women in New York City worked outside the home. A number of studies of Korean entrepreneurship found that the women are crucial to starting and maintaining small family businesses; their availability and willingness to work long hours are major factors in achieving economic success (Hurh & Kim, 1984; Min, 1992).

Several studies (Min, 1992; Song & Moon, 1998; Yu, 1993) show first-generation men continue to insist on patriarchal authority within the family and relegate household tasks to the women in the family regardless of whether they also work outside the home. As Korean American women have increased both their economic power and their feminist consciousness, they have begun to challenge the traditional male order. Some resort to divorce, others marry out of the Korean American community, and still others stay single to pursue professional careers.

Korean immigrant men, on the other hand, already feel beleaguered by their circumstances. They face the language barrier and discrimination outside the home, and are frustrated by the underutilization of their education and occupational skills. The erosion of their traditional authority over children and spouses makes them feel even more helpless, and the accumulated anger often explodes in the context of their relationships with their wives and children. The traditional authoritarian and male-dominant values of Korea and the egalitarian ideals of U.S. society have not yet been constructively synthesized within the Korean American family.

In summary, Korean immigrant families and children have been exposed to conflicting dual socialization processes, with often mixed, contested, and ambiguous cultural values. Yet despite the different language-use patterns and levels of assimilation, in many respects, the Korean American community holds together across generational and gender lines. The sense of belonging created by family ties, cultural values, and common ethnic identity is a powerful force for social cohesion. Perhaps the cultural attachment to Korean customs and values is not only an obstacle to functioning in U.S. society but also an aid in coping with and a buffer against harsh environments.

INDIGENOUS KOREAN *HAAN* TRANSFORMATION PROCESSES AS A CULTURALLY COMPETENT PRACTICE APPROACH

We argue that the culturally competent practice with immigrant families entails assisting them in their ongoing cultural negotiation in which multiple, often opposing, ideas and ways of being are addressed, appropriated, and negotiated. This practice goal works within, rather than against, the grain of the cultural understandings. Such practice inevitably entails a redefinition and renegotiation of the needs and goals inherent in any socially and culturally constituted relationship of relevance. From this orientation, we propose that Korean *haan* (Kim, L., 1992; Kim U. & Choi. S., 1995) transformation processes exemplify the use of cultural values as strengths, culturally competent assessment, and intervention methods pertinent to immigrant Korean children and families.

"Although the exact translation and interpretation of the meaning of *haan* into the word in English is not easy, it denotes the long-held entangled emotions of suffering that are developed over time by tragic life events and oppressing environments" (Song, 1999, p. 174). A unique Korean folk term for feelings of suppressed anger and resentment due to such circumstances is called *haan*. The concept of *haan* is essential in understanding Korean women who have been oppressed individually and collectively in a male-dominant society. For example, brutal treatment by husbands or in-laws is often mentioned by *haan*-burdened women. Many Korean women's beautiful but painful poems, songs, and novels are rich in the expression and reflection of feelings of *haan*. Feelings of personal *haan* and feelings of victimization are very important issues to be explored in working with Korean immigrant mothers and women. To understand them, one has to understand their *haan*.

Throughout history, Korean women have untangled the complex webs of *haan* through their survival wisdom and endurance. *Haan* reflects a deep intrapsychic process associated with interaction with the external historical–social–cultural environment. *Haan* is also deeply imprinted in the collective subconscious of Koreans, who have suffered much and endured oppression and pain in their history. *Haan* is, however, not a passive process of suffering with acceptance and resignation, but an active process of suffering with a will to endure pain, to overcome, and to triumph someday. For this reason, *haan* involves very complex and comprehensive mental processes and has a transforming power that has not yet been recognized in Western culture.

THE FOUR PHASES OF *HAAN*

Generally speaking, there are four experiential phases of *haan*: from the stage of fermenting one's entangled emotions of suffering, through the stages of reflecting and disentangling, to the transformation in emptying one's mind (Choi, 1994; Kim & Choi, 1995; Song, 1999). We conceptualize the *haan* transformation processes as a generative process in which new meanings emerge and are mutually constructed between client and practitioner through therapeutic dialogue. This conceptual framework is based on the premises that (1) narrative is a way we use language to relate to others; (2) we live in and through the narrative identities that we develop in dialogue with one another; (3) narrative is a discursive schema with culturally driven rules and conventions that provide structure and coherence to the fragments of our life events and experiences; (4) we organize, account for, and make sense of experience through narratives or stories; (5) therefore, the dialogical basis of the narratives is always changing and evolving.

The transformative power of *haan* shares similar premises developed by the clinical theory of dialogical conversation (Anderson & Goolishian, 1992; Seikkula, 1995; Song, 1999). In these therapeutic processes, the role of the practitioner is that of a dialogical artist whose expertise is in the arena of creating a space for and facilitating a dialogue as a participant–observer and a participant–facilitator. The practitioner exercises this art through therapeutic questions. The therapeutic question is the primary instrument to facilitate the development of conversational space and the dialogical process from *a position of not knowing*. A practitioner participates with a client in the telling, retelling, hearing, and creating of the client's well-being and problem narratives. The aim of dialogical engagement is to connect, collaborate, and construct mutually acceptable reality with the client in the creation of a new narrative and the creation of opportunity for new agency. Culturally competent practice is simply the expertise required to participate in this process.

CASE ANALYSIS FROM A KOREAN *HAAN* CULTURAL PERSPECTIVE

The *haan* transformation processes suggest that there is a generic set of developmental stages or domains. Each domain is a "stage" only in the sense that, with some predictability, one set of attitudinal clusters precedes the next set for most Korean people. We present the stages, for the purpose of conceptual clarity, as if a person moves neatly from one stage to the next. In reality, most people experience several stages simultaneously, living a mixture of overlapping multiple stages.

The Kim family, a Korean first-generation immigrant family, is composed of a maternal grandmother, her 38-year-old daughter, 42-year-old son-in-law, and three grandchildren: Lisa, age 13, Christina, age 7, and 6-month-old David. All three children were born in the United States. The family owns a grocery store, where Mrs. Kim works 7 days a week, with long hours. Recently, the family moved from a large metropolitan area to a suburban area with a good school district. The Kim family was referred for family counseling by a school counselor about alleged child physical abuse. One of the authors (Song) worked with the Kim family for 4 months. The mother was the primary client in unraveling her *haan* transformation experiences through the dialogical processes.

The first phase of *fermenting* involves internalizing the tragic and oppressive suffering significant to a Korean immigrant family. In the analysis of the first stage experience of fermenting, Mrs. Kim realized her multiple, helpless predicaments. The complex tragic events and situations of her story are as follows: She was born and lived in poverty in her early days. Mrs. Kim also made an irrevocable mistake that produced tragic consequences in her life. In a way, her decision to get married was to escape from adversity. Her husband's mental illness was a devastating turning point in her marital life. Moreover, as a daughter-in-law and wife, she was powerless to confront her authoritarian parents-in-law and her husband. Because she was powerless to change her situation, she had to accept her fate and live with it. Experiences of oppressive events and situations provoked raw emotions of anger, fury, frustration, vengeance, and outrage. Yet she was culturally asked to ferment these raw emotions and transform them into socially acceptable emotions.

In this stage, it is critical that the practitioner listen patiently without interrupting the long-lasting storytelling and maintain coherence with client's subjective story. He or she works within the client's reality—her language, vocabulary, and metaphor—about the child abuse problem and its imagined solutions. The practitioner allows room for the client's familiar experiences and descriptions, so that the client's energy is not spent convincing the practitioner of her view. It also helps lessen the chance that the practitioner's voice might dominate and shape the story to be told, thus precluding the client's version; the practitioner guides the development of future versions with helpful nuances. Toward this end, the practitioner must create and safeguard room for the client's first-person narrative (Anderson, 1997).

The second stage mainly involves *reflecting* on the Kim family's voice and experience, and its influences on Mrs. Kim's paralyzed mind in several ways. She began to protest against her fate by saying:

> "Because my life was so much difficult, I want to escape from the situation. Because it was so hard for my family to make a living, . . . I wanted to get away from the situation . . . from my family's poverty."

She refused to accept the cruel fact that she alone must bear the burden of her tragedy. During session 1, when reflecting on her difficult relationship with husband, she said: "I couldn't put up with him, [husband] . . . and also I couldn't live with mother-in-law together any more.

Then, Mrs. Kim was able to transform the emotional venom of grudge into detached tears of *haan* with both cries and laughs. During session 2, she expressed:

> "I don't need to . . . talk about all the stories that I have lived until now, do I? While being pregnant . . . well [smiling in a way of lamenting], I believed God. I had thought constantly that my husband was a miserable man [tears in eyes]. And I began to think that if I had turned back

from and left him, what would have happened to this man? For I had kept thinking this kind of thought in my mind, I could hardly have left him [laughing and crying]."

The third stage of *disentangling* is manifested when the client demonstrates a release of tangled emotions in several ways: (1) The client's personal entangled feelings of *haan* become public, communicated, shared, and accepted; (2) he or she has companions to provide consolation and to help enhance self-dignity; (3) he or she is bound up with all participants in full affection; and (4) he or she develops strong optimistic themes in the experience of *haan*. The client is able to easily relate to other's suffering and forgive the mistakes of the others. For example, to release unspoken mental anguish or grief from her self-imposed prison by letting it evaporate, Mrs. Kim read her letter to her mother in the presence of family members in a reflective–retrospective manner.

By session 6, when addressing her strong sense of self-responsibility and hardworking style, she stated:

> "I guess the motivation came from my childhood in the course of growing up. I saw the hardship of my mom while she was young and lived with my father. Because my father lived as he pleased and didn't take care of the family, the children became the final victim. Of course, so was the mom."

By session 12, Mrs. Kim was able to relate easily to others' suffering and forgive their mistakes:

> "I was really surprised to hear what Christina said, because I didn't know what she thought about. Although I always tell her to clean up and read books, I had no idea about whether she really thinks it important or she really thinks that she wants to do it or not. But when she told me that, I feel reassured. . . I hated my father so much. I really was so angry with my father that I couldn't forgive him. Now when I think of him, I really thank my father so much just only for his living a healthy life."

For the practitioner, asking questions and probing are most helpful to the client, because emphasis is on openness to new narratives. He or she questions from the position of not knowing within the conversation, helping the client tell, clarify, and expand on a story, thus opening up new avenues and exploring what is not yet known. It is in this local and continuing process of question and answer that a particular understanding or a particular narrative becomes a starting point for the new and "not-yet-said" (Anderson & Goolishian, 1992).

The last stage, the *mind emptying*, is a leap from the reflecting phase.

At this phase, Mrs. Kim appears to embrace both positive and negative aspects of life as it was, to realize the meaning of her suffering, to put life into a universal perspective such as human dignity/rights of women/children and compassion/love, and to find peace and harmony in her life with the others.

In session 6, looking back on her suffering experience in the early childhood due to poverty, she stated:

> "I don't have to blame anyone else, and I was made that way like mannish, like an untamed pony galloping everywhere. I believe that I have to do what I can do, and I was able to do anything when I did my best. I have a feeling of accomplishment in the process rather than difficulty. I enjoyed it. I was really active when I was young. Active . . . anyway, I think that bright and gloomy side of people's life always existed side by side."

When the therapist asked about how her mother did spank her when she had to, Mrs. Kim immediately replied by retelling her mother's negative and positive aspects:

> " I felt really happy to see my parents get along well together at my wedding. Of course, my father gave my mother very hard time, but seeing both of my parents living along . . . I felt really happy."

In another dialogue, Mrs. Kim realized the meaning of her suffering.

> "What I often told my mother . . . sometimes my mother still laments her life and so how I always comfort her is saying, 'Mother, your life is truly . . . worthy.' I always said that."

By session 12, in a letter to her loving mother that she read before the family and therapist:

> "Mother! It seems like a very old story but I think that it was so painful and difficult childhood for me . . . And yet I image how I would have been different if I had been born in a very rich family. There is an old saying that people need to go through adversity at early ages. Now I am so thankful to the hardship, although it had given to me against my will. Because of the sheer strength, at present time, I am doing my best while thinking back on the tough days. . . . And also I always appreciate your love deep in my heart."

An indigenous Korean cultural perspective of *haan* represents cultural significance of dialogue as a way of understanding therapeutic narrative changes in multiple communicative relationship meanings and actions. Mrs. Kim entered the therapy with monologue-fixed and single-voiced narratives about her relationship with her husband, children, parents-in-law, and her family of origin. Her speech had three interwoven aspects: (1) negative and self-accusing voices about self and other, (2) talk about the already spoken-about and seen world for the purpose of solving problems and conflicts, and (3) fixed and constricting narratives.

> "I had to do it all alone; no one helped me. My husband is so dependent on me; like my husband, Christina, my second child, is very much like her father in character and so she relies on others. She is so lazy that she got beaten. She deserves to get beaten."

Following the *fermenting* monologue with the therapist, Mrs. Kim constructed a dialogue between herself as unloved child/daughter-in-law/wife and her imagined voice of love, such as the God and the mother. In *reflecting* and *disentangling* stages, several new narratives emerged: leaving home to make a better living, her parents' reconciliation at her brother's wedding, and a very shaky new idea of herself as both a victim of parental failure and a possible resource to her husband, children, and parents-in-law. The reflecting therapist commented on the story, adding another voice, and offered an idea for another story. Internal dialogue between Mrs. Kim's self as an abusing mother and an abused child emerged. With the aid of the therapist, Mrs. Kim and Christina wrote letters to each other, adding more voices, and a new narrative potential emerged. The letters acted as representatives of their inner dialogues, and when they were heard, witnessed by relevant others, the emotional life of all participants changed. As Christina, the abused daughter, wrote and spoke aloud about her experiences, the mother's and father's understanding of their daughter and of each other changed. This dialogical interaction created an emotional charge that changed the whole family's stereotypical ideas about mother–daughter relationships. These relationships could include longing, vulnerability, and tenderness, as well as rage and disappointment. Reading the letters aloud holds these voices and ideas in tension, which increases possibilities for new narratives in the family.

PRINCIPLES OF CULTURALLY APPROPRIATE PRACTICE

From the foregoing case example, we can find out the major culturally competent practice principles. A key principle of the *haan* transformation process is that once the Korean immigrant client ensures the emotional security of affectionate relationship with the social worker, he or she can then participate more in the dialogical conversation process, which helps to release entangled emotional sufferings and agonies, and then move toward a constructive, caring action. Based on the principle of emotional security of affectionate relationships, the social worker is never critical of what the client is saying or feeling. The aim of dialogue in *haan* processes is to connect, collaborate, and construct mutually acceptable reality with the client in creating a new narrative and opening an opportunity for new therapeutic action.

Another principle of *haan* transformation in the therapeutic action is that when the practitioner maintains coherence with Korean clients' subjective stories about what they experience in life, they can perceive themselves more positively and decrease destructive relationship in the family. From the principle of maintaining coherence with clients' subjective stories, there should never be added pressure on clients to cover content surrounding the life events precipitating the child abuse problem. The social worker helps clients have self-images of being listened to and respected; and becoming a dignified human being in the presence of self-consciousness. Based on the principle of maintaining coherence with clients' subjective stories, the social worker needs to be cautious about the fact that Korean immigrant family clients describe child abuse problems not so much in simple action or behavior as in an encompassing pattern. The natural process of description of child abuse problems is not significantly related to independent individual members (e.g., I, you, he or she); she rather, it describes interlocking relationships between family members (e.g., grandparents–parents and child, parents-in-law–daughter-in-law, daughter and son, sister and sister). This reflects how the Korean immigrant client has a more relational self-view or interdependent self-construal than an individualistic self-view. This argument is also supported by Keeney's (1987) view that treating child abuse as a problem involves addressing multiple descriptive and semantic frames, called "recursive dialectic of semantics."

The final principle in the *haan* transformation process is that the social worker's conversational questions allow clients to tell, clarify, and expand on a story about lived experience, and provide structure and coherence to the fragments of their life events and experiences. These questions is the primary instrument for the social worker in facilitating the development of conversational space and the dialogical process. Each question leads to an elaboration of description and explanation, and another question. This principle emphasizes the importance of becoming as interested and open as we can, actively utilizing our curiosity about the client's story. Based on this principle, questions are always asked from the position of not knowing rather than imposing the social worker's ideas. Questions from this position are more likely to come from inside rather than outside the interactive conversation (Anderson, 1997).

The foregoing major principles illustrate empowerment based in culturally competent practice with Korean immigrant families and children to help disentangle the entangled relation between the client and others. By telling a story in a situation of affection and emotional security, the Korean clients engage in the creation of multiple meanings in ways that are consistent and coherent, with long-lasting cultural strengths, such as interdependent living in harmony and peace with self and others.

CONCLUSIONS

We argue that the indigenous Korean *haan* transformation processes addresses culturally relevant assessment and intervention strategies, and add to an integrative way of balancing the Western dialogical and an indigenous Korean *haan* perspective. As a result, this process may contribute to maximizing the manifestation of clients' own voices and stories, while minimizing the risk of bias from a point of view of predominant cultural meaning and interpretation, in the information practitioners gain through dialogical conversation.

From this perspective, the current child protective service delivery system needs to be examined critically for its countertherapeutic effect among court-mandated cases of diverse cultural background. The current therapeutic culture involves multiple service delivery systems, with an emphasis on pathologizing, victimizing, and authoritative intervention.

Thus, there has been an ongoing need for an alternative conceptual framework for culturally competent practice that reflects a move from a hierarchical to a horizontal, egalitarian, and collaborative effort. Such an approach permits and frees the practitioner from the position of expert and makes him or her coparticipant in the co-creation of a new therapeutic reality. It has become possible within this orientation to move from a therapy that is interventionist toward therapy that relies on the expertise and integrity of the clients.

REFERENCES

Aldrich, H. (1975). Ecological succession in racially changing neighborhoods: A review of the literature. *Urban Affairs Quarterly, 10*, 32–48.

Anderson, H. (1997). *Conversation, language, and possibilities: A postmodern approach to therapy.* New York: Basic Books.

Anderson, H., & Goolishian, H. (1992). The client is the expert: A not-knowing approach to therapy. In S. McNamee & K. J. Gergen (Eds.), *Therapy as social construction* (pp. 25–39). Newbury Park, CA: Sage.

Bonacich, E. (1988). The social costs of immigration enterpreneurship. *Amerasia Journal, 9*(2), 127–135.

Bonacich, E., Light, I., & Wong, C. (1976). Small business among Koreans in Los Angeles. In E. Gee (Ed.), *Counterpoint: Perspectives on Asian America* (pp. 437–

449). Los Angeles: Asian American Studies Center, University of California, Los Angeles.

Chang, H. K., & Moon, A. (1998). Work studies, conjugal power relations, and marital satisfaction among Korean immigrant married women. In Y. I. Song & A. Moon (Eds.), *Korean American women: From tradition to modern feminism* (pp. 75–87). Westport, CT: Praeger.

Choy, B. Y. (1979). *Koreans in America*. Chicago: Nelson-Hall.

Hurh, W. M., & Kim, K. C. (1984). *Korean immigrants in America: A structural analysis of ethnic confinement and adhesive adaptation*. Rutherford, NJ: Fairleigh Dickinson University Press.

Jiang, J. (1978). Toward a theory of Pariah enterpreneurship. In G. Wejeyewardene (Ed.), *Leadership and authority: A symposium* (pp. 146–162). Singapore: University of Malay Press.

Keeney, B. P. (1987). Ecosystemic epistemology: An alternative paradigm for diagnosis. *Family Process, 18*, 117–129.

Kim, E. (1997). Korean Americans in U.S. race relations: Some considerations about Korean American work in coalition with other people of color in the 1990s. *Korean American Historical Society Occasional Papers, 3*, 75–84.

Kim, L. (1992). Psychiatric care of Korean Americans. In A. Gaw (Ed.), *Culture, ethnicity and mental illness* (pp. 347–375). Washington, DC: American Psychiatric Press.

Kim, U., & Choi, S.-C. (1995). Indigenous form of lamentation (*han*): Conceptual and philosophical analysis. In H.-Y. Kwon (Ed.), *Korean cultural roots: Religion and social thoughts* (pp. 245–266). Chicago: North Park College and Theological Seminary.

Light, I., & Bonacich, E. (1988). *Immigrant entrepreneurs: Koreans in Los Angeles, 1965–1982*. Berkeley: University of California Press.

Liu, W. T., Yu, E., Chang, C., & Fernandez, M. (1990). The mental health of Asian American teenagers: A research challenge. In A. Stiffman & L. E. Davis (Eds.), *Ethnic issues in adolescent mental health* (pp. 92–112). Newbury Park, CA: Sage.

Min, P. G. (1989). *Some positive functions of ethnic business for an immigrant community: Koreans in Los Angeles*. Final Report submitted to the National Science Foundation, Seoul, Korea.

Min, P. G. (1991). Korean immigrants' small business activities and Korean-black interracial conflicts. In T.-H. Kwak & S. H. Lee (Eds.), *The Korean-American community: Present and future* (pp. 13–28). Pusan, Korea: Kyung Nam University Press.

Min, P. G. (1992). Korean immigrant wives overwork. *Korean Journal of Population and Development, 91*, 557–592.

Pang, V. O. (1991). The relationship of test anxiety and math achievement to parental values in Asian-American and European-American middle school students. *Journal of Research and Development in Education, 24*(4), 1–10.

Patterson, W. (1988). *The Korean frontier in America: Immigration to Hawaii, 1986–1910*. Honolulu: University of Hawaii Press.

Portes, A., & Manning, R. (1986). The immigrant enclaves: Theory and empirical examples. In J. Nagel & S. Olzak (Eds.), *Competitive ethnic relations* (pp. 47–68). New York: Academic Press.

Rinder, I. (1959). Strangers in the land: Social relations in the status gap. *Social Problems*, 6, 253–260.

Sassen, S. (1998). *Globalization and its discontents*. New York: New Press.

Schneider, B., & Lee, Y. (1990). A model for academic success: The school and home environment of East Asian students. *Anthropology and Education Quarterly*, 21, 358–377.

Seikkula, J. (1995). From monologue to dialogue in consultation within larger systems: Human systems. *Journal of Systemic Consultation and Management*, 6, 21–42.

Song, K.-H. (1999). *Helping Korean immigrant families to change child abuse problem: A postmodern multicultural language systems perspective*. Unpublished doctoral dissertation, Loyola University, Chicago.

Song, Y., & Moon, A. (1998). The domestic violence against women in Korean immigrant families: Cultural, psychological, and socioeconomic perspectives. In Y. Song & A. Moon (Eds.), *Korean American women: From tradition to modern feminism* (pp. 161–173). Westport, CT: Praeger.

Skinner, E. P. (1963). Strangers in West African societies. *Africa*, 33, 307–320.

U.S. Bureau of the Census. (1994). Characteristics of the Asian and Pacific Islander population in the U.S. *1990 census of population and housing subject summary tape file (SSTF5)*. Washington, DC: U.S. Government Printing Office.

U.S. Bureau of the Census.(2001). Profile of general demographic characteristics for the U.S.: 2000. Table DP-1. *U.S. Dept of Commerce News*. Retrieved from *http://factfinder.census/gov/servlet/QTTable?_ts=71761469080*. Data Set: Census 2000 Summer file 1 (SF1) 100 percent geographic—United States.

Yambert, K. A. (1981). Alien traders and ruling elites: The overseas Chinese in Southeast Asia and the Indians in East Africa. *Ethnic Groups*, 3, 173–198.

Yu, E. Y. (1982). Occupations and work patterns of Korean immigrants. In E.-Y. Yu, E. Phillips, & E. S. Yang (Eds.), *Koreans in Los Angeles: Prospects and promises*. Los Angeles: Center for Korean and Korean-American Studies, California State University.

Yu, E. Y. (1993). The Korean American community. In D. N. Clark (Ed.), *Korea briefing, 1993* (pp. 35–42). Boulder, CO: Westview Press.

CHAPTER 6

Lao Children and Families

ALFRED S. BEDNORZ
KATHY CALDWELL

The Lao are some of the most humble and ingratiating Southeast Asians one will meet. Their history as a people bespeaks a similar attitude. Laos is a small, landlocked country in Southeast Asia, between Vietnam to the east, Cambodia to the south, Thailand and Burma to the west, and China to the north. The Lao economy is based largely on agriculture, with rice being the most important crop. In the aftermath of the Fall of South Vietnam and Cambodia, Laos ceased to be a constitutional monarchy when, on December 2, 1975, the Lao People's Democratic Republic was established. Soon after this declaration, people left Laos in waves because of fear and the repressive measures of the new government (measures such as incarcerating individuals allied with the past government or the United States in "reeducation camps" and forcing collectivization of farming). Over 250,000 Lao came to the United States from 1975 to 1996 when Lao resettlement formally ended. Most of the resettlement in the United States occurred primarily in California, Iowa, Minnesota, Texas, and Washington (Keovilay & Kemp, 2000).

This chapter reviews the history and the adaptations of the Lao refugees to the United States. Problems and issues regarding Lao refugee children and families, and cultural values, as strengths in assessment are also discussed. Finally, indigenous strategies and Western interventions, as well as culturally competent practice principles with a case example, are offered.

HISTORICAL BACKGROUND

The Lao, an ancient people, moved from the Yunnan area of China, settling in the northern part of the country, in approximately 600 A.D. Their history is one of ancient kingdoms, dominating and being dominated by neighbors—the Thai, the Chinese, and the Vietnamese. Their primary influence seems to be from Thailand (the old Kingdom of Siam). By the early 1700's, there were three major kingdoms in Laos: the kingdoms of Luang Prabang in the north, Vientiane in the center, and Champassak in the south. In fact, the Lao national symbol is of a three-headed elephant, with a white parasol, on a five-step platform. The elephants symbolize the three kingdoms, the parasol is a symbol of royalty and the five steps symbolize the five commandments of Buddhism; prohibiting killing, stealing, lying, adultery, and abuse of alcohol (Center for Applied Linguistics, 1981).

The Lao people comprise many ethnic groups. The Lowland Lao, who live along the rivers, are the politically and culturally dominant group, making up almost two-thirds of the population and speaking a language closely akin to Thai. The people of the Highland, known collectively as Lao Sung (predominately Hmong and Mien), are the original settlers of Laos from south China. In the central and southern mountains, Mon-Khamer tribes, known as Lao Theung, or Midslope Lao, predominate. Large pockets of Vietnamese and Chinese also live in Laos, particularly in towns and cities.

The Lao link with the Thai people may have in many ways led to their downfall. When the French colonized the area in the mid 1880's, they attempted to sever the cultural ties with Siam (under the influence of the British) and replace them with ties to Vietnam, in the French sphere of influence. This restructuring of political influence would spell disaster for Laos in the 20th century. With the fall of French domination in South East Asia, also know as French Indochina, Laos gained freedom and autonomy as a country but was found to be in an influence vacuum, because ties with Thailand had been severed by French domination, and the France had been forced out of the area by the Vietnamese.

The Geneva Accords of 1954, which proclaimed the sovereignty of Laos, also created a government with three major parties that worked against each other attempting to gain primary power. The country tottered precariously throughout the 1950s, 1960s, and early 1970s under a U.S.-backed monarchy, until the American government pulled all of its troops out of South Vietnam. Although Laos was officially neutral, a growing American and North Vietnamese military presence in the country drew Laos increasingly into the "Vietnam War." For over a decade, Laos was subjected to the heaviest bombing in the history of warfare as the United States sought to destroy the Ho Chi Minh Trail that passed through eastern Laos (U.S. Department of State, 2000).

In the mid-1970s, the Pathet Lao, a political party allied with North Vietnam and originally a resistance organization connected to the communist struggle against colonialism, swept out the two remaining political parties and proclaimed an end to the monarchy, and a the beginning of the People's Democratic Republic of Laos. Thousands who had been in the Royal army, allied with the United States, or had any ties with the old Lao government, fled the country, or were apprehended and placed in "reeducation camps." The camps were basically prison camps in which the "inmates" were continuously reminded of the error of their political beliefs. When the "inmates" were not being "reeducated" they were forced to work, constantly under the threat of interrogation and, even worse, death.

The newly powerful communist government of Laos, with the help of the North Vietnamese army, attempted to reorganize the country under standard communist ideologies by collectivizing farming in Laos and centralizing power. This led to massive economic problems that increased the flow of refugees out of the country and into neighboring states, primarily Thailand.

As this was occurring in southern and central Laos, the people of northern Laos (primarily comprised of the Hmong and the Mien) faced systematic annihilation as a reward for their faithful service to the government of the United States. Most Hmong men from 12 to 55 years of age were recruited by the U.S. Central Intelligence Agency to fight the North Vietnamese and Lao communists (Center for Applied Linguistics, 1981). When the Royal Lao government fell, they were forced to flee or be slaughtered. Estimates are that more than 300,000 persons had fled the country by the mid 1980's (U.S. Department of State, 2000).

Life in the refugee camps in Thailand, though far from pleasant, seemed better than the options in existence at home. The Lao (men, women, and children) were not particularly welcome in Thailand, but with the assistance of Western countries (the United States and Europe, especially France) and Japan, they were allowed to remain. For those lucky enough to have ties to the United States, processing proceeded, and the Lao eventually were allowed to enter the United States as refugees. Prior to the Refugee Act of 1980, the definition of a refugee was somewhat nebulous, although the United States accepted the definition used by the United Nations 1951 Convention Relating to the Status of Refugees, which defined a refugee as

> a person who, owing to a well-founded fear of being persecuted for reasons of race, religion, nationality, membership in a particular social group, or political opinion, is outside the country of his nationality, and is unable to or, owing to such fear, is unwilling to avail himself of the protection of that country. (United Nations High Commissioner for Refugees, 2001)

The United States accepted this definition but placed many qualifiers to it, the most significant being that the "refugee" must be of compelling interest to the United States. This most often meant that the person had to have been a member of the ousted government or its armies, or an individual who had worked closely with the military of the United States or for the government of the United States (e.g., embassy workers), or for companies in the United States or charitable groups from the United States (e.g., the Salvation Army).

The United States Congress passed into law the Refugee Act of 1980, which standardized the definition of a refugee as

> any person who is outside any country of such person's nationality or, in the case of a person having no nationality, is outside any country in which such person last habitually resided, and who is unable or unwilling to return to, and is unable or unwilling to avail himself or herself of the protection of, that country because of persecution or a well-founded fear of persecution on account of race, religion, nationality, membership in a particular social group, or political opinion. (U.S. Code: Title 8, Section 1101)

Other Western countries opened their arms to the refugees, and most were eventually resettled in Western countries. Those who were not accepted for resettlement in other countries were eventually repatriated to Laos. For the Lao men, women, and children, who entered the United States, life was very different from what they had experienced in their home country.

ADAPTATION TO THE UNITED STATES

The Lao had to readily adapt to numerous situations when they entered the United States. The first and perhaps most important adaptation was being placed in an alien land, the United States, with its strange customs and practices, where few people spoke their language.

Weather

One major adaptation was a need to understand the weather and how very different it was from Laos. Many areas of the United States experience rapid temperature changes in the fall and winter. The Lao who resettled in such areas may have never seen snow, sleet, or icy conditions. It was a source of wonder for Lao children when the first snowfall occurred. One could go out into the Lao community and see adults and children outside in the snow, staring up with faces filled with wonder and amazement. Parents had to be instructed to dress their children and themselves appropriately for winter. Although this may seem an insignificant thing, it only takes one or two cases of frostbite for the importance of the matter to sink in.

Time

The matter of time, and the importance of it, was also a source of adaptational angst for most Lao and their caseworkers. The Lao concept of time is much more fluid than that of most Americans. When a caseworker told a family that they would pick them up at 3:00 P.M., the caseworker meant just that. Very often, the Lao family would finally gather to be met by the caseworker by 3:30 or 3:45. One of the earliest lessons that both caseworkers and refugee families had to learn was that if an appointment was to be kept, the family really did have to gather and be ready to be picked up at the assigned time. The caseworker, many times, had to learn to tell families to gather together earlier than required, to make certain that they would be ready and "on time" for their appointment. As Lao refugees had to learn to deal with American caseworker time, so, too, did caseworkers have to learn to deal with "Lao time." When the refugees had a function, such as a wedding, caseworkers soon learned to arrive less punctually, or they would be the first ones to arrive. Lao refugees had to learn to be punctual for job shifts, or they would soon lose their jobs. All in all, the Lao had to learn to be clock conscious and "on time" for all things American.

Housing

Housing was also an area of adaptation for the Lao refugees. Few homes, and no apartments, can accommodate a large refugee family. Although apartment complexes and landlords, in general, were amenable to renting to refugee families, the number of people in a family quite often created a problem. Many cities also have codes that regulate the number of people that can live in an apartment. Families certainly did not want to be separated, nor did resettlement agencies want to separate them. So in many instances, the resettlement staff were able to rent multiple apartments next door to each other for a large family. For many of the families, an apartment was designated for the parents, and cooking and eating, and another apartment was designated for sleeping and living space for married sons and their families. The plumbing in each apartment, duplex, or home was to many a source of wonderment. The first wave of Lao refugees resettled was former military that did not necessarily have indoor plumbing in their native country. For those who came from the few cities, simple things such as our commodes were very different from the ones in their homeland. Each caseworker had to teach refugee families how to use the accommodations in the bathrooms and the kitchens.

One problem that soon arose as Lao resettled in the United States was the rice in the kitchen sink. Families consumed large quantities of rice, and the women had to be taught to not let uncooked rice go down the drain, because sinks soon clogged up. Many landlords had to impose fines for cleaning out kitchen sink drains filled with rice.

PROBLEMS FOR CHILDREN AND FAMILIES

Numerous problems existed for the Lao resettling in the United States. All members of the family system were affected, and many cities in which the Lao were resettled had a difficult time adjusting to the Lao. Amarillo has a population of approximately 190,000 individuals, and about 79% are Caucasian. Hispanics make up approximately 13%, blacks approximately 5%, 1% are other, and, currently, 2% are Asian. The residents had mixed reactions to the quick influx of Southeast Asians. Initially, the response was negative, particularly regarding those who arrived soon after the end of the Vietnam War. With time, however, the Asians were much more accepted, but this is most likely due to the cultural values, perceived as strengths by Americans, of humility, an excellent work ethic, and the Lao personality, which is considered reserved. A myth exists that the Lao are "passive," but in reality they are hardworking and humble. The refugees are empowered by their ability to establish jobs through niche building and their ultimate successes in the United States. They are not likely to speak out publicly or cause problems that reflect poorly on their families.

The most significant issue for the adults was their loss of status and economic class after arriving in the United States. The first wave of Lao refugees consisted of military officers, and government workers, who were more highly educated than the later wave of farmers and laborer refugees. A highly respected dentist in Laos could not practice dentistry in the United States. Certifications and licenses are not reciprocal, and in order for the Lao to work in their professions, they would have to start all over again. The latter wave of refugees who worked primarily in agriculture was less educated. In Laos, public school was not compulsory until 1975. The refugees who came to the United States were older and had not acquired a great deal of schooling. Most were educated enough to read and write, the men more so than the women. The more highly educated refugees have, and continue to experience, feelings of great loss of the status and identity they worked so hard to achieve in Laos.

The refugees usually arrived by plane late at night, so they were taken to their apartments and shown how to use the basic facilities with which they were unfamiliar. The very next morning, the entire family would have an intake completed at the resettlement office and would have to be "oriented" to U.S. expectations and customs, and sign a number of agreements included in the resettlement paperwork. They arrived with the clothes on their backs and perhaps a small duffel bag—their entire possessions to begin a new life in the United States.

Within the first 30 days, the Lao were exposed to Western medicine requiring tests to determine overall health, parasitic infection, and diseases from their country of origin. One major cultural discrepancy was that the resettlement agency staff had difficulty explaining to the refugees that stool samples were needed, which necessitated the refugee filling a bottle with a stool sample. The Lao eat with their fingers, not utensils, and they were extremely hesitant to do anything unclean with their hands.

The refugees were required to obtain employment very soon after their arrival in Texas. Trips to the Texas Department of Human Services offices were required to apply for Medicaid and Refugee Cash Assistance (RCA), and to the Social Security office to obtain social security numbers.

Fortunately, former refugees had been hired at the resettlement agency to act as interpreters and case managers for the new arrivals. These case managers were responsible to provide all of the family's transportation to medical appointments and job interviews, and for conducting frequent home visits to resolve refugees' questions and concerns. The case managers conducted all the translating for every visit the family made to obtain services. They were also on call 7 days a week to translate for the police department, local hospitals and clinics, and any other resource with which the family came into contact. As children attended school, their ability to speak English increased quickly. Sometimes children had to interpret for their parents, if a translator was unavailable from the resettlement agency. This created problems, because it clashed with the Lao hierarchy. Children could not ask personal questions of their parents out of respect for their elders. Children were not allowed to translate for their parents; thus, service providers and medical personnel often obtained very sketchy information.

The hiring of former refugees as case managers was highly effective in empowering new arrivals by easing the initial culture shock. However, things were not problem-free. Because the case managers were former refugees and of the Lao culture, their ability to ask very personal questions of the new arrivals, particularly to the women, was inhibited because of cultural mores. It was difficult for male case managers to ask for any medical information from female family members. Additionally, the heads of household were generally older than the case managers, and utmost respect for those individuals who are older is of great significance in the Lao culture. The case managers had difficulty instructing the elders on matters of hygiene and the need to obtain employment that was beneath their status. When conflicts arose, the case managers had to learn to get involved in the family's "business" to resolve situations. This contradicted Lao culture, because families problem-solve only within the extended family. Because everything was new to the refugees, the case managers were forced to intervene, which made both parties uncomfortable.

After the first 30 days, when all of these tasks were completed, the refugees were taken to job interviews in the hope of gaining employment before the 90-day government assistance ended. At this point, refugees experienced the humiliation of going to work at the local beef packing plant that for many of the earlier, more educated arrivals, was beneath them. The laborers and farmers adapted more easily, because they were used to manual labor. The packing plant began hiring Southeast Asian refugees, because English was not a necessity to learn their jobs, which consisted mainly of butchering cattle on the kill floor or repetitive cutting of particular cuts of beef. In other words, one employee was responsible for making the same cut of beef (e.g., a sirloin steak) on each section of cow that passed on a conveyer belt, while another cut only rump roasts.

Over time, this work has resulted in high rates of carpal tunnel syndrome (a painful condition of the wrist and hand caused by repetitive motions) and injuries with knives. Additionally, the conditions are bleak, because the factory has a putrid smell from the beef and the work is done in shifts, including graveyard hours. The beef packing plant was outside the city limits and there was no public transportation. Refugees would attend English as a Second Language (ESL) classes during their off-time from work. This plant was one in which U.S. citizens were least likely to work. Lao refugees' willingness to work under these conditions strengthened their ability to succeed financially soon after their arrival. The refugees benefited, because the pay was, and still is, higher than that in other jobs, and insurance benefits begin after 90 days. As soon as employment was acquired, the refugees were terminated from the RCA program.

Another issue regarding the Lao culture was that women did not often obtain outside employment. Finding employment that would empower women to become more independent in the United States was a challenge. Their role in Laos had been to care for the children and the elderly relatives, to cook and clean, and to tend to the head of household. It was of utmost importance to devise a plan identifying individual strengths to encourage Lao females to enter employment. Seamstress was one job the women could do without a great deal of English, and employers were recruited to assist in teaching about job expectations. The women could not work in restaurants because of the language barrier. The beef packing plant began employing a number of Lao women, because very few jobs were available that did not require some level of English. The Lao females were strengthened in their skills, self-sufficiency, and acculturation through their employment. Women who were employed learned English more quickly.

The Lao culture provided much strength in the resettlement of the Lao refugees. Usually, the men and older sons of the family obtained employment first. Extended families would live together in one house until they earned enough income to afford a vehicle. Lao refugees who arrived earlier had already obtained a vehicle and carpooled new arrivals to the beef packing plant. All working members of the household pooled their income and paid cash for one car for the head of household or the oldest son. Then, they bought the next son a car, and so on, until all had transportation. The work was very hard at the plant, but with family members all working in one location, they were able to maintain employment even without public transportation. After initial needs were met, they saved enough money to purchase a home, with all working members of the extended family contributing. This eventually enabled the Lao to not live in overcrowded conditions and strengthened their ability to become homeowners relatively quickly.

In Amarillo, the Southeast Asians developed an enclave in a northeast neighborhood that was formerly military housing; when the airbase closed, the Asians bought the homes. The elementary school had a very high percentage of Asian students, and the high school, located in the north quadrant, was multicultural. Amarillo, by many standards, is still segregated, with the majority of Hispanics, blacks, and Asians living in the northern and eastern sections of town. The Caucasians tend to live in the central and southwest neighborhoods of the city. Integration within the neighborhoods is slow, but it is occurring more often now than in past years. The Lao resettlement in one area of the city strengthened their infrastructure by being available to provide new arrivals with assistance in close proximity.

The infrastructure developed by the Lao upon arrival in the United States was critical to their success in adapting. As refugees arrived in Amarillo, elders from the community would take newcomers under their wings and assist them in adapting to the United States. Many of the men affiliated with the government had been tortured and kept in "reeducation camps" in Laos. Most of the refugees had lived in refugee camps while waiting to be sent to receiving countries. Both type of camps were overcrowded, with disease and poor nutrition complicating the refugees' lives. Many of the Lao remained in these camps for years and on their arrival in the United States felt very isolated. Many had posttraumatic stress syndrome (PTSD). Our community has never been successful in intervening with mental health problems, because Lao culture does not recognize "counseling," even if Lao-speaking counselors had been available. Of course, there was not, and use of translators was not acceptable. The Lao resolve their problems within their family structure and would never speak of their trauma through a non–family member. The shared experiences of the elders and leaders in the Lao community were of great help in the resolution of problems that arose, and they were frequently called on by the resettlement agency to intervene. The Lao men empowered each other through "one-on-one" intervention. The men's abilities were respected, thereby strengthening their acculturation.

The resettlement of Lao refugee children presented a different set of problems. Children are taught to respect their elders, including parents and older siblings (Bempechet & Omori, 1990). This also pertains to teachers and anyone else in positions of authority. The younger children seemed to adapt more quickly than the older children, depending on the older children's experiences prior to arriving in the United States. There is definitely a hierarchy within the family that is recognized by all members. The cultural values of family unity and gain outweighs any personal desire. It was difficult to engage Lao parents in participating with the teachers and school system. Resettlement agency staff were often called in to mediate between the refugee families and school personnel. Increasing clashes with parents and culture occurred as children made new friends and learned Western ways. ESL classes were developed in the schools to smooth the children's transition. Teachers were challenged to learn about the Lao culture, and the resettlement staff had the major responsibility of teaching them.

Again, the already existing Lao infrastructure was critical to the successes of newly arriving refugees, providing information on cultural differences. In Lao adolescents who may have arrived as refugees during times of identity formation, feelings of isolation and the language barrier resulted in them making American friends slowly. In the United States, teens have many more freedoms than their Lao counterparts, resulting in loyalty issues between the Lao and American cultures. Lao parents became increasingly concerned about the changes children were experiencing as the youth started dressing in current fashions and wearing modern hairstyles. Not only did they begin to look differently but also they began to act differently. Some outward signs of stress include gang behavior and involvement with the juvenile justice system. Because the Lao tend to live in neighborhoods along with other Asian refugees, Asian gangs exist in those neighborhoods. Our city does have a number of gangs, usually defined by race, and each has its own "turf," normally in the neighborhoods in which gang members live.

People have a general view that all Asians are smart and very successful in school. As a culture, the Lao deem education important, and many attend college in the area. However, this cannot be said of all Asians. Experiences before coming to the United States, age, and rate of acculturation are all factors. The Lao are no different, and there are differences between American-born Lao and refugees born in Laos. American-born Lao youth cause much concern for their Laos-born parents. Some American Lao choose not to learn the Lao language, and their goals for the future are more independent. They may choose to move away from the extended family, which is considered the most important unit in the Lao culture. American-born Lao are the result of two merging cultures. Youth born in Laos maintain many of the cultural values of their parents. Although faced with two merging cultures, they seem to be strengthened by their abilities to choose from both cultures.

After having a child, a young woman may stay home for a year, then return to the workforce. A strength of the culture is that family members or friends often provide child care, rather than the use of a day care. Most Lao families have two parents working as a result of lower income jobs. Older Lao are concerned about the loosening of family ties and the loss of the Lao culture, which makes them feel fearful and more isolated. Due to age, they are less likely to be employable and therefore rely on economic support from their children. A strength of the Lao culture is respect for elders, and though some families do not remain close, the majority continues to support their elders.

The strength of niche building, as it relates to employment, means the Lao have been able to identify gaps in the community and have been successful in bridging those gaps. Many have opened restaurants that cater to both Caucasians and Asians. Grocery stores, hair salons, and nail salons are prevalent. Retail stores that serve the Asian population are successful and are located in the Asian neighborhoods. Their ability to work together as a family, with family members often working in the stores and restaurants, is one of the cultural strengths that empower the Lao to be successful. A strong infrastructure continues to exist here, and the Lao community is thriving.

Temples have been built in the United States because most Lao are Buddhist. However, some have converted to Christianity and attend Protestant churches.

CULTURAL VALUES AS STRENGTHS IN ASSESSMENT

The culture into which we are born helps us define the world around us and how to interpret what is happening in our lives. Although we may move beyond our culture, it continues to exert its influence throughout our lives. The Lao refugees come from a rich culture that empowers them to define who they are and where they fit in the universe. In working with the Lao, it is imperative that certain aspects of their culture be understood to assess more appropriately and empower them.

Family

The family is the central social unit in Laos. The "typical" family unit in the United States is a father, a mother, and their children. In Laos, the "typical" family unit consists of parents, their children, grandparents, married children, aunts and uncles, and frequently other relatives in the extended family. One strength of the Lao is they may live together, or at least in close proximity.

The patriarchal Lao family traditionally pays great respect to parents and the elderly. The father is charged with upholding family traditions and morals. The mother is most often viewed as maintaining the household, its budget, and family unity. If the parents are not present, the oldest child assumes the parental responsibilities. Grandparents, mothers, and older siblings care for children.

Religion

Religions among the Lao are as varied as those in the United States. There is no single Laotian religion, though generalizations can be made. Lowland Lao tend to be Buddhists, though other religious traditions such as Christianity, Islam, and Confucianism are in existence. Highland Lao tend to be animists, with smatterings of other religious traditions in existence.

One common theme among Eastern religions is a search for peace and harmony. This theme seems to permeate the Lao culture and can explain many of their actions and beliefs. It can be stated that the Lao seek peace and harmony from conflict, either in this life, or through reincarnation in the "next life." A great deal of respect is given to one's ancestors, and there is a good bit of importance given to visiting and caring for their tombs. For the Lao, pain of separation from their country is heightened by their inability to visit the graves of their ancestors. This practice of honoring ancestors is called "ancestor worship," but in this context, the word "worship" connotes more an act of commemoration rather than adoration. Buddhist monks have played the roles of teachers, counselors, healers, and community leaders throughout the history of Laos.

Death

Most Lao prefer to die at home rather than at a hospital. Burial is generally reserved for a person who has died of unnatural causes. Most Lao prefer cremation. A peaceful death with one's relatives nearby is seen as more comforting than death in a Western hospital.

Medicine

Traditional medical practices of most Lao are tied to religious beliefs. In Eastern medicine, evil spirits or "winds" create disharmony within the person who is ill. Thus, a shaman, holy man, or folk doctor is often asked to "prescribe" herbal medicines or prayers to help the sick person achieve harmony and, thereby, health. Invasive procedures including immunization and surgery are avoided.

Food

As with most ethnic groups, the Lao place great importance on hospitality and offering food to visitors. In many instances, the first thing a Lao might ask a visitor is not "How are you?" but rather "Have you eaten?" or "May I offer you something to eat or drink?" Favorite foods include sticky or sweet rice, *padek* (fish sauce), hot peppers, and lemon grass. In Laos, the family usually sits on the floor or around a low rattan dining table. Sticky rice is most often eaten by hand, but spoons, forks, and chopsticks may be used. The family does not begin eating until the head of the household is seated, and "grace" is said after the meal.

Education

Education, too, is quite different in Laos than what is encountered in the United States. The Lao place great value on education, but in many instances, adults and their children received little or no formal education in their country of origin. The school system that did exist in Laos was based on the French system that emphasized the lecture approach in classrooms. A good Lao student would not consider questioning the teacher or the methods in which information is taught.

Employment

The world of employment in the United States is very different from that in the mother country for most Lao people. The prospect of change and upward mobility at the heart of the American work ethic is an alien concept for most Lao. In their system, people most often worked in the same job their entire lives. In Laos, many jobs denoted ones station in life, so many Lao refugees who were members of the Royal Lao Army or otherwise allied with the Lao or U.S. government were reluctant to accept manual labor, which they believed was beneath them.

Social Greetings

The Western custom of shaking hands had become common between Lao men before the exodus of refugees in 1975. Lao generally do not shake hands with an elder unless the elder offers his hand first. Men do not shake hands with women, and women do not shake hands at all. The customary greeting among Lao is the *wai*, which consists of hands with palms together, raised from the chest or head, depending on the degree of respect one wishes to express:

Between equals: up to the chest
To a superior: up to the face

To a teacher or parent: up to the head
To God: over the head

Lao names are written just like most American names are written: first name, then family name. However, it is uncommon for a Lao to have a middle name. After marriage, a Lao woman takes her husband's family name. For the most part, titles such as Mr. are only used with the first name, and last names are used only in writing, not in speech.

It is considered offensive to touch a Lao's head, considered the most sacred part of the body. The feet have a lower status; thus, pointing or moving something with one's feet or putting feet on a table is considered very rude (Center for Applied Linguistics, 1981).

INDIGENOUS STRATEGIES AND WESTERN INTERVENTIONS

In this section, we compare Lao culture and health care, and the effects of Western medicine on the Lao culture. In Laos, people who lived in the cities had more familiarity with medical services, including doctors and hospitals. Those Lao who live in the country are very unfamiliar with modern medicine and often use folk cures for health problems that arise.

According to the World Health Organization, the life span of Laotians is 45.0 years for men and 47.1 years for women (Kemp, 2000). It can be posited that their lifespans will increase as the refugees are exposed to modern medicine. Barriers that arise for refugees who resettled in Texas include lack of transportation, language barriers, and the lack of knowledge of Western culture among the Lao, and lack of knowledge of Lao culture among medical service providers. Lao relationships build over time, and as a people, they are reluctant to answer personal questions. Because Lao refugees were immediately exposed to medical services upon arrival to the United States, it was necessary for translators to escort them to the clinic for their physicals. The translators explained the process and had few problems. They spent a great deal of time educating the clinic staff about the Lao culture.

One large difference between Lao and American culture is that the Lao do not want to know if they have a terminal illness or are dying. Conflicts arose with doctors who felt it was Lao patients' right to know what was going on; however, the patients did not want to know. The family was usually informed, but this information was kept secret from the patient. The doctors and nurses had a hard time understanding why the patient did not want to know and tried to talk the families into seeing how knowing would benefit the patient. The resettlement agency intervened and provided education to the doctors about the Lao culture and the fatalistic attitude of patients should they know their prognosis.

Mental illness in the form of PTSD was hardest to treat. In fact, in this smaller community, it was never treated by Western medicine. The Lao are very suspicious of "counseling," having never experienced it in their country of origin. Other barrier was the absence of Lao-speaking practitioners. Translators could not be used because of the intimacy of the questions. Most who needed services were older men who had been tortured in the camps; the translators were younger and could not, out of respect, translate this information for their elders.

Obtaining services through local doctors is the older Lao people's last choice. The younger Lao adjust more easily to taking their children and selves to the clinic, but the older Lao prefer to rely on folk medicines. Until they have reached an acute stage of illness, they do not present at the doctor's office. Therefore, prevention is difficult to impress on the older family members. Some suggestions to handle this include showing respect for the family members, particularly the males or head of households; explaining procedures but allowing Lao patients to take written information back to their community to have it explained to them; allowing the medical history to evolve; and respecting the modesty of women (Keovilay & Kemp, 2000).

Many Lao do not want to complain, and it is important to ask open-ended questions, because they are reluctant to say "no." Even the younger Lao retain some fears from their culture. For example, surgery is often avoided, because Lao doctors are not as well trained as United States doctors, so trust must be established, along with a great deal of information and education. Even having done so, the Lao are reluctant to let anyone do invasive procedures, probably a result of their earlier Buddhist and "spirits" beliefs.

In conclusion, there are many barriers to working with the Lao regarding the problems of health and treatment. The younger the Lao person, the more likely he or she will adapt Western medicine. The older the Lao person, the less likely he or she will accept. The elders continue to use folk medicine and only see a doctor as a last resort. However, educating the medical staff about Lao culture and learning specific techniques to establish a relationship with the Lao will make their jobs more effective. Hence, the Lao will benefit, too.

PRINCIPLES OF CULTURALLY APPROPRIATE PRACTICE

In working with any culture different from their own, social workers must be aware of their own cultural mores and traditions. Only by recognizing components of their own culture will they be able to work to their fullest potential with persons from other cultures. All social workers have prejudices, stereotypes, judgments, and assumptions about other cultures, based on where and how they were raised and personal experiences. It is not a failure to admit to having prejudices; it is only a failure if we refuse to believe we have any. Cultural competence comes from not being afraid to ask questions and educate oneself. Sometimes social workers may feel inhibited to do so because "they are supposed to know." It is here that the danger of stereotypes and generalizations persist.

It is not only important to know about the Lao culture but a social worker must also be able to distinguish what is cultural and what part is of an individual's personality. There are also many variations among Asian cultures, so one cannot assume because the Vietnamese do something one way that the Lao will do it the same way. If the culture is not well known, a social worker might develop a service plan that includes separating a daughter from the family. The Lao culture considers family unity and respect for elders to be the most important cultural factors, so a social worker will be working against the cultural mores of the client and family if he or she pursues a plan to separate a daughter from her family. This will only cause failure and blame of the client, when in actuality, the failure is the social worker's inability to devise a culturally appropriate plan. It is of utmost importance that a social worker speak with someone very familiar with the Lao culture, someone whom he or she can ask questions. Again, the resettlement agency and staff are a good resource, as are members of the Lao infrastructure.

A culturally competent assessment takes into consideration the degree of acculturation of the refugee. A newly arrived Lao refugee will be completely different than one who has been in the United States for years. It has been shown that refugees acclimated to both American and country-of-origin culture are the most successful (Hepworth & Larsen, 1993). Therefore, it is not the social worker's job to replace Lao culture with American culture, but to assist refugees in remaining comfortable with their own culture, and to help them adapt to American culture.

Language is the largest barrier in working with Lao refugees. The resettlement agency had to identify those Lao arriving in the community who could speak English. These individuals were hired as translators and case managers, because without overcoming the language barrier, very little progress could be made. Assistance from Lao who had resettled earlier was critical to the staff in empowering the new refugee arrivals and identifying strengths. Many elders in the Lao community volunteered their time to provide translation and drive clients to appointments and job interviews.

Problem solving varies among cultures, and the Lao tend to do all their problem solving within the extended family unit. They are not familiar with "counseling" and usually are reserved about asking for help. Trust develops over time, as does the social worker's knowledge about the family. For trust to build, it is important for the social worker to meet clients' immediate needs and identify strengths in the individuals. Upon arriving, the Lao refugees were immediately taken to their apartments, which were already filled with furniture, rice cookers, beds, and indigenous food. This strengthened the trust of the new arrivals by proving the social workers could anticipate and provide for their needs. It is also helpful during the initial assessment, always done with a translator or by a bilingual staff person, to communicate having shared thoughts and understanding about the refugee's plight. Paraprofessionals who resettled from Laos were highly effective in communicating this empathy to the refugees. Social workers must recognize the strengths in the tight-knit relationships that Lao staff establish with the refugees, and not view this as a threat to their authority.

During the assessment process of the Lao refugees, a social worker must keep in mind the strengths and the challenges of the culture. In general, maintaining family ties empowers the Lao to develop an infrastructure that supports their needs. Living in the same neighborhoods allowed the Lao to pool their resources upon arrival. Their ability to pool money to advance each member of the family is a result of their cultural norms. The inability to ask for help can be a weakness when there are resources available in the community to assist. Issues relative to PTSD are difficult to address, because problems in the Lao culture are resolved within the family and not via therapists or counseling.

To empower Lao refugees, resettlement staff mediated among employers, medical practitioners, landlords, teachers, and a host of other resources. The Lao had to be taught about American cultural values of assertiveness, confrontation, and persuasion that are very different from their own values of obedience, deference to authority, and cooperation (Hepworth & Larsen, 1993). Regarding employment, a system was developed in which the social workers made visits to refugees at work and contacted employers at 30-, 60-, and 90-day intervals. These contacts were important, because, at this time, problems viewed by the employer could be discussed. The social worker would then discuss with the refugee the problems that arose. Often, these problems resulted from cultural misinterpretation. Social workers could use these opportunities to educate the employers about the Lao culture.

The Lao worked their way up the ladder in the beef packing plant to supervisory professions, thus empowering later arrivals to work within the plant. The language barrier was lessened, and both parties had an understanding of the same culture. Prejudice still exists today at the plant, especially in circumstances in which the Lao work under a Hispanic supervisor, or the other way around. The majority of workers at the plant are Southeast Asians, including Vietnamese, a larger number of Hispanics, some Caucasians, and a few African American individuals. Some drawbacks to working at the plant include the economic and cultural security at this plant that can prevent refugees from seeking higher level jobs in the community. These workers are also less likely to become as proficient in English, because they can speak Lao at the plant.

The older Lao were more likely to remain at the beef packing plant to support their children. Sometimes they would work two jobs, because their children's future and education was so important to them. The younger Lao who began at the plant went to college at the same time. After getting their degrees, they were able to open their own businesses and/or move into higher level jobs outside the plant. This resulted in the older Lao finishing their working years at the plant, and the younger Lao leaving the plant to find success in the community.

CASE VIGNETTE

Somchin and Vilayphone were born in Laos, where they lived with their extended families. They were engaged in Laos. Vilayphone's father worked in the local medical school in the finance department, and her mother was a homemaker. In April 1979, Somchin and Vilayphone decided to escape to Thailand with her 6-year-old nephew. The trip took 2 days and involved their taking a taxi to an outlying town. There, they met other refugees and, together, they walked for 12 hours to a forest. In the forest, refugees from a variety of countries spent the night. The next morning, the escorts came and they all walked for 12 more hours, until they reached the border of Thailand; then, they were taken across the river by ferry.

After reaching Thailand, Somchin and Vilayphone were married in the refugee camp and ended up spending 18 months there. Somchin had been a dentist in Laos and was able to practice his profession at the clinic. Vilayphone worked as a pharmacist at the medical clinic in the camp. They had to buy their living quarters from a departing family, so it was fortunate that Somchin and Vilayphone had brought money with them from Laos in order to do this. The living quarters were described as a long building with one-room apartments and a long hall in the middle. Somchin, Vilayphone, and her nephew lived in these cramped apartments for the duration of their stay. They were treated somewhat better than many others, because they were educated and employable.

Vilayphone became pregnant in the camp, and her baby son was born dead. Within a week, a baby girl was placed with Vilayphone and Somchin. A woman living in their building had given birth and could not care for the baby. Adoption is never discussed within the Lao culture; it is kept a secret forever.

Finally, the United Nations processed out Vilayphone and Somchin. They went to Chicago to live with a Methodist church pastor who had sponsored them. Vilayphone remembers that they were offered hotdogs to eat. She took this literally to mean heated dog meat. Knowing no English, it was sometime before the pastor could explain that this was not the case. Their 6-month-old, adopted daughter remained in the refugee camp with

Vilayphone's parents, who had escaped after Somchin and Vilayphone. In Chicago, Vilayphone's first job was cooking at McDonald's. This job did not require any English, because she worked as a cook and had no interaction with the public. Somchin was able to work at a dental laboratory making dentures. He could not practice dentistry without going to school in the United States. While working, both Vilayphone and Somchin took ESL classes two times per week. Within 6 months, they could communicate some in English. They remained in Chicago for 1 year.

Vilayphone's parents, who resettled in Texas, brought their granddaughter. An Uncle sponsored them in Texas. Vilayphone and Somchin moved to Texas to be with her parent's and with their daughter. Vilayphone attended ESL classes at a junior college for another 2 months. Somchin found a job at a dental laboratory making dentures, and Vilayphone, at a hospital in housekeeping. She remained there for 4 months, then took a job at Levi Strauss, where she remained for 4 years. She continued to attend ESL classes at night at the junior college, as did Somchin. Vilayphone became pregnant with a second daughter in 1985, while she attended a technical institute to learn general office skills. She was then hired at a resettlement agency as a translator/secretary, where she remained until 1999. Their third daughter was born in 1987. Somchin continued working in the dental laboratory, until he decided to open his own dental laboratory in 1992, where he remains today. Finally, Vilayphone and Somchin had a baby boy in 1995, at which point they decided to have no more children. They opened their own Asian restaurant after Vilayphone left the resettlement agency. Vilayphone reports that both of their businesses are doing well.

Initially, Vilayphone and Somchin lived in the northeastern part of town, where they bought their first home. In the late 1990s, they bought a new house in the southwestern part of town and kept their original house as a rental property. They currently rent their old house out to newly arriving refugees.

Regarding Western medicine, Vilayphone reports that it is very different in the United States. In Laos, the French system is utilized, and doctors practice with an educational level equivalent to that of a high school graduate: 6 years of elementary school, 4 years of high school, and 4 years of "medical school." It takes much more training to be a doctor in the United States. Vilayphone states that surgical procedures are very "scary," that the Lao would rather leave the illness alone, and they hate having to see a doctor. Lao patients do not want to hear they have cancer or any other terminal illness. The family may choose to know, but the patient is absolutely not told. Vilayphone has been suffering from back pain for several years and refuses to have surgery. She reports that she exercises and takes an herbal medicine.

Vilayphone and Somchin were successful in acculturating to the United States. She states that she and Somchin were prepared for the many changes and invested themselves wholeheartedly in the process of becoming westernized. They persisted in learning English, which helped them get jobs sooner than most. Additionally, they came from a higher socioeconomic level than most, so they were better educated. Vilayphone talks of the people in the city seeing doctors, but people from the countryside in Laos may never have seen a doctor at all. Vilayphone and Somchin were young when they arrived as refugees, so they adapted to American customs quickly. Both had trades, she as a pharmacist and he as a dentist, prior to their arrival. The reunion of their extended family in Texas strengthened their supportive network.

A significant clash in cultural norms has caused estrangement between Vilayphone and Somchin, and their oldest daughter, who began asking many questions, because she knew she did not look like her parents. She is darker skinned and her facial features are very different. The more questions she asked, the more concerned Vilayphone became because she did not want to tell her daughter about the adoption. Eventually, they did tell her, when she was 16, because they were concerned that someone else would tell her. Their daughter began acting out and hanging around with a rough group of youth, possibly involved in a gang. She eventually left home, and they have never heard from her directly again. She is 21 years old, and her parents heard she is living with Vilayphone's sister in Dallas, Texas. The resettlement agency has an adoption division, and Vilayphone spoke often with the staff about what was happening. Vilayphone feels that her daughter feels rejected and lost. She has no information about her birth family and will most likely not ever have any. Vilayphone and Somchin did not know the birthparents directly. Intermediaries living in the camp brought the baby to them. Vilayphone and Somchin have always felt that she was their biological daughter, but once in the United States, American norms about adoption interfered with their cultural ways of secrecy.

Vilayphone and Somchin became Baptist after their arrival in the United States, and attend a Baptist church formed by refugees. They enjoy being in the Baptist church and participate fully in church activities. Vilayphone states her two older daughters speak a few words of Lao, but her younger daughter and son speak no Lao. They are not interested in learning, although Vilayphone reports they understand her perfectly when she speaks Lao to them. She states this is because the two youngest went immediately into public day care after their birth, and no Lao was spoken to them during the day. Now, they say that it sounds funny and giggle if Vilayphone asks them to respond in Lao.

Vilayphone states that they have gotten away from many of the Lao traditions, because her children do not like them. For example, a birthday party can go on for 4 or 5 days in the Lao tradition, but her children want to leave after 2 or 3 hours. They are used to American parties that may last only a few hours. They do not feel the need to interact with their Lao community and visit over so many days. Vilayphone is very proud of her children and wants them to be Americanized. She feels that they will be more successful if they live by American norms and culture.

Vilayphone and Somchin remain close to her parents and extended family residing in Texas. Their success in owning businesses and rental property is not the norm for many of the Lao refugees that arrive in the United States. They worked hard and succeeded in reaching the "American Dream," although they have done so at the risk of losing their Lao heritage.

CONCLUSIONS

This discussion of the history and adaptation of Lao refugees to the United States has included the issues, strengths, and challenges of their adaptation to a new culture. We have identified cultural values such as family unity, religion, respect and humility, employment, and medical adaptations. The merging of the two cultures results in acculturation and the retention of Lao culture, with the addition of westernized culture that empowers refugees to successfully adapt to living in the United States. The refugee's success in coping with racism and misunderstanding of their culture enabled them to become effective in niche building and developing skills and successful businesses. In conclusion, the Lao refugees have overcome extreme challenges, torn between two worlds, to adapt successfully to their new home in the United States.

REFERENCES

Bempechet, J., & Omori, M. C. (1990). Meeting the educational needs of Southeast Asian children. *ERIC Clearinghouse on Urban Education*, CUE Digest No. 68. ERIC Identifier: ED328644. Retrieved May 29, 2003 from *http://www.ericfacility. new/ericdigests/ed328644.ktml*

Center for Applied Linguistics. (1981). *The peoples and cultures of Cambodia, Laos, and Vietnam*. Washington, DC: Language and Orientation Resource Center.

Hepworth, D., & Larsen, J. (1993). *Direct social work practice*. Pacific Grove, CA: Brooks/Cole.

Keovilay, L., & Kemp, C. (2000). Health care beliefs and practices of Laotians. *Asian-American Health*. Retrieved May 1, 2001 from *http://www3.baylor.edu/~charles_ kemp/Laotian_health.html*.

UNHCR—Who is a refugee? Protecting refugees: Questions and answers. United Nations High Commissioner for Refugees, Public Information Section. Retrieved May 5, 2001 from *http://www.unhcr.ch/un&ref/who/whois.htm*.

U.S. Code: Title 8, Section 1101, No. 42. U.S. Code of Federal Regulations as of January 5, 1999. Retrieved May 29, 2003 from *http://www.bcis.gov/ipBin// pext.d11/inserts/51b_1/51b_21/51b_456=templates&fn=document-frame.htm# 51b_act101.*

U.S. Department of State. (2000). Bureau of East Asian and Pacific Affairs. September 2000, Background note: Laos, profile. Retrieved April 24, 2001 from *http:// www.state.gov/r/pa/bgn/index.cfm?docid=2770.*

CHAPTER 7

Hmong Children and Families

GWAT-YONG LIE
PAHOUA YANG
KALYANI RAI
PA Y. VANG

This chapter synthesizes the few available, recently published materials about the Hmong, including information accessible through Internet sources. The chapter leads off with a brief history of Hmong migration to the United States, followed by examples of ways that the group has adapted to life and circumstances in the United States. A subsequent section addresses problems and issues faced by Hmong people today. The resilience and fortitude of the Hmong community is highlighted in the section on cultural values and community strengths, which also addresses the salience of applying a culturally competent and strengths-based approach to assessment. The unique combination and application of indigenous and Western interventions are described in a later section, with a final section addressing the principles of practice indicated by the review of the literature on which this chapter is based.

Because of the circumstances under which Hmong people fled their homelands and resettled in other countries, including the United States, they are referred to as *refugees*. For the purpose of this chapter, the definition of *refugee* is as specified in the Immigration and Nationality Act (INA) 1952, Section 101(a)(42):

> A refugee is a person outside of his or her country of nationality who is unable or unwilling to return because of persecution or a well-founded fear of

persecution on account of race, religion, nationality, membership in a particular social group, or political opinion.

HISTORICAL BACKGROUND

Referencing the work of several scholars, Lo (2001) noted that over 5,000 years ago, the Hmong lived in an area known today as Iraq and Syria. Over time, they wandered away from the Middle East to other areas, including Turkestan, Russia, Siberia, Mongolia, Manchuria, Hunan, Tibet, India, Burma, Tonkin, and China. A French missionary, Father Jean Mottin (1980), suggested that the Hmong were in China even before the people known today as the Chinese. He noted that as the Chinese presence increased in numbers and political influence, the Hmong became more resistant to Chinese domination. Historical records document revolts and rebellions against the Chinese; in the fight to preserve their autonomy, Hmong people fled, moving southward beyond the valleys of the Yangtze and Yellow rivers, to higher and less hospitable terrain (Fadiman, 1997; Hones & Cha, 1999; Lo, 2001).

The Chinese called the Hmong the "Miao," the "Mien," or the "Meo"—derisive names variously translated as "barbarians," "people who sound like cats," or "wild uncultivated grasses." The Hmong themselves preferred to be called "Hmong," a name akin to other tribal names, such as "Inuit" and "Diné," all of which simply mean "the people" (Fadiman, 1997, p. 14).

By the beginning of the 19th century, persecutions, decreasing yields of lands worked, epidemics, and rising taxes prompted many Hmong to migrate to Indochina, although the majority remained in China (Fadiman, 1997). Altogether, about 500,000 Hmong relocated, mostly to the hills and mountains in the north of Laos, Vietnam, and, later, Thailand; still, the majority persisted and remained behind in China.

The next few decades were peaceful, with Hmong people practicing swidden agriculture, farming mountain rice and corn, and growing opium as long as the land was fertile and moving on to new sites when yields declined. Opium was an important cash crop for the Hmong. They kept less than 10% of the opium harvest for their own use. Few Hmong, aside from the chronically ill and elderly, were addicted. Opium was used to facilitate the ceremonial trances of *shamans* (Hmong folk healers) and "to dull the pain of headaches, toothaches, snakebites, and fever; to staunch diarrhea; and to ease the discomforts of old age" (Fadiman, 1997, p. 122); such uses still continue to this day.

The Geneva Agreements in 1954 partitioned Vietnam into North and South Vietnam. Anxious to stem the spread of communism in southeast Asia, the United States, as early as 1950, had engaged in covert military operations in Laos by providing military support to and helping in the training of Royal Lao Government Forces. A civil war erupted in Laos in 1958. Bound by the terms of the 1954 Geneva Accord, the United States (other signatories included the Soviet Union, North and South Vietnam, France, the Chinese People's Republic, Cambodia, Laos, and the United Kingdom) could not send in any of its own military personnel to intervene. Instead, the United States employed a secret guerilla army of Hmong soldiers recruited, trained, and armed by Central Intelligence Agency (CIA) personnel. These members of the Hmong Armée Clandestine were vital to U.S. military operations.

In the United States, the war in Laos was referred to as the "Quiet War" in contrast to the "Noisy War" being fought in Vietnam. Between 1963 and 1965, the Hmong Armée numbered about 35,000 soldiers. The estimates of Hmong casualty figures range from one-tenth to one-half; "some were soldiers who died in battle; most were civilians killed by cannon and mortar fire, bombs, land mines, grenades, postwar massacres, hunger and disease" (Fadiman, 1997, p. 133). Entire Hmong villages were decimated. By 1970, more than one-third of the Hmong in Laos became refugees in their own homeland.

In August 1964, the shelling of the American destroyer *Maddox* by North Vietnamese troops heralded the formal involvement of the United States in the Vietnam War. In February 1965, the United States began the first of several bombing raids, and in March, the first combat troops landed. By early 1973, both the United States and North Vietnam agreed to a cease fire, and the withdrawal of American troops was completed by March. Civil war between North and South Vietnam flared up again, and in 1975, Cambodia, Laos, and South Vietnam fell to the communists.

A mass exodus of Hmong refugees began, with many going to Thailand and others to the jungles of Laos. Huge camps were established in Thailand to accommodate the influx of refugees. More than 35,000 Hmong were housed at the camps in Thailand, but it is estimated that 15,000 others died *en route* (Hein, 1995). Resettlement efforts resulted in the first Hmong refugees relocating to the United States in 1976. It is estimated that by 1982, about 100,000 Hmong had been relocated abroad, and apart from the United States, host countries included France, Australia, Canada, Argentina, and China (Dao, 1982).

ADAPTATION TO THE UNITED STATES

Ranard (1988) noted that there were two waves of Hmong migration to the United States. The first large wave comprised about 50,000 and occurred around 1979–1980. The second wave took place about 10 years later, 1987–1989, during which some 28,000 Hmong refugees were estimated to enter the United States. By 1990, the U.S. Census records showed the Hmong population to be at about 90,000. In 2000, estimates were that the Hmong population would have more than doubled to about 250,000–300,000, with the majority residing in California (70,000–85,000), Minnesota (50,000–70,000), and Wisconsin (45,000–50,000) (Hmong National Development, 2000). About 58% of the Hmong population in the United States in 1995 was 17 years of age or younger (Hang, 1997).

Donnelly (1994, p. 184) described the experience for the older generation of Hmong who fled their home country to take refugee in the United States as follows:

> Hmong, like other refugees resettled to a new location, reconstruct as best they can their already understood social worlds, and overcome imperfections in the reconstruction by substitution and overlooking difference. In general, incoming Hmong refugees do not seek new lives, they seek the same lives in a new location, and where possible they use their new opportunities to bolster preexisting social conceptions.

In their attempts to recreate the tried, the true, and the familiar in new locations, the Hmongs encountered extraordinary challenges that often confounded their efforts. Accustomed to living in the mountains, and in plains with warm temperatures (around 90°F) and high humidity, the majority of Hmong refugees were resettled in areas with flat topography and freezing winters (e.g., Minnesota and Wisconsin). Furthermore, the Immigration and Naturalization Service (INS) had adopted a scatter placement plan to disperse refugees throughout the United States, "to encourage assimilation, and to avoid burdening any one community with more than its 'fair share' of refugees" (Fadiman, 1997, p. 185). In some cases, clans were split up, and nuclear families were placed in isolated rural areas. Even though local sponsors (e.g., Lutheran Social Services, Catholic Charities, and Church World Service) were available "to act as buffers between potentially hostile larger community and the Hmong" (Lucke, 1995, p. 93), conditions were sufficiently disagreeable to the Hmong involved that many left initial placement sites. They relocated to more temperate climes (e.g., California, North Carolina, and Texas), and to be closer to family, clan, and/or friends. These moves left government officials and local sponsors frustrated, feeling betrayed and concerned that such moves would only delay the Hmong attainment of self-sufficiency. In contrast, urban anthropologists framed such migrations as an adjustment strategy, as a retaking of control over one's life (Lucke, 1995).

Around the United States, most Hmong refugees were resettled in urban areas, because their sponsors were anxious for them to secure employment quickly and to receive the social service resources they needed to facilitate adjustment. Hmong families found themselves housed in inner-city neighborhoods with inexpensive rents, but high crime rates. For example, much of the Hmong population in Milwaukee, Wisconsin is concentrated in the inner-city area. According to Lo (2001), the Hmong population grew from 3,000, in 1988, to an estimated 15,000, in 2000, in Milwaukee. However, since 1990, there has been a steady movement out from these inner-city neighborhoods to a residential area in the northwestern sector of the city. About 95% of families living in the northwestern suburb are homeowners, whereas most of those living in the inner city are still renters (Lo, 2001).

Most Hmong refugees had few marketable skills on arrival in the United States. Many were soldiers and farmers, with an average of four to six children and elderly dependents to feed and support. In California, Minnesota, and Wisconsin, 65%, 70%, and 60% of Hmong families, respectively, were on welfare rolls (Fadiman, 1997). To augment family income, Hmong women were encouraged to market their needlework, *pa ndau*, beautiful appliqué and embroidery work traditionally intended for household use and ritual exchanges. In the process, "needlework intended for the market changed stylistically, alienated as it was from social and ritual use in Hmong households" (Donnelly, 1994, p. 185).

PROBLEMS FOR CHILDREN AND FAMILIES

Mental Health Issues

Posttraumatic Stress Disorder among Older Hmong

Many scholars (e.g., Chindarsi, 1976; Geddes, 1976; Lemoine, 1986) have admired the resilience of the Hmong people, that is, their capacity to transcend a history of upheavals and relocations, and still remain socially intact. O'Connor (1995) for example, was moved to note:

> Throughout their history of continual resettlement the Hmong have remained culturally separate and ethnically distinct from other southeast Asian peoples. . . . seldom socialize significantly with other groups in their countries of residence and very rarely marry non-Hmong. . . . The strength of the Hmong sense of ethnic identity and solidarity has been undiluted by hundreds of years of migration and a wide diaspora. (p. 81)

Still, the tremendous horrors of war are difficult to escape unscathed. Hmong refugees presented with a number of mental health issues, including a variety of anxiety disorders, combat stress reactions, and depressive symptoms. Not having the vocabulary to describe their mental health distress, they approached health care providers with frequent somatic or bodily complaints (Lin, 1983; Moore, Keopraseuth, Leung, & Chao, 1997). Similarly, Moore, Sager, Keopraseuth, Loo, & Riley (2001) noted a high prevalence of physical pain among Mien (Hmong) and Lao psychiatric patients, especially among those suffering from depression. Hmong refugees who were symptomatic often had complaints of headaches, backaches, not being able to eat or sleep, and a general feeling of "unwellness" or displacement. For the older Hmong, it was much easier to conceptualize a spiritual or physical hurt than a mental health disorder. As a result, the treatment of choice was likely to be an intervention recommended by the shaman, the indigenous healer, who often derived his healing prescriptions from the spirit world. The remedy often included a ceremonial offering to a particular spirit or spirits.

One of the most commonly diagnosed mental health disorders among Hmong refugees was posttraumatic stress disorder (PTSD) (Abe, Zane, & Chun, 1994; Kinzie et al., 1990; Mollica, Wyshak & Lavelle, 1987). Furthermore, it was not unusual to see a dual diagnosis of PTSD and a depression or anxiety disorder. Kroll et al. (1989) found an 80% prevalence rate of major depression among the Hmong presenting at a mental health clinic. It has also been found that patients with PTSD suffered twice as many traumas as did other psychiatric patients (Mollica et al., 1987). However, as Kinzie et al. (1990) noted, the prevalence of PTSD was underestimated even by well-trained and experienced doctors and counselors; over one-third of PTSD cases were not diagnosed as such in the initial interview.

The actual combat and encounter with war is only one aspect of the entire experience of Hmong refugees. Life in refugee camps prior to coming to the United States was traumatic. Aside from the horrific physical conditions, robbery, rape, and other kinds of maltreatment by the very people designated to help them were common occurrences. However, in order to survive and to overcome these life- and mind-threatening experiences, the process of grieving over multiple losses may be deferred, making grief work with refugee populations an important recovery and healing objective. The Hmong may also have unresolved grief around certain decisions made in times of crisis and feel devalued by dominant culture and their children's lack of appreciation of Hmong traditions and customs (Kemp, 2000).

Acculturation to life in the United States has also been difficult for many Hmong older adults. Many have had to adjust to a diminished status both within the family and in the majority society because of a lack of English-language proficiency, little of no formal education, and lack of employment opportunities (Boehnlein, Leung, & Kinzie, 1997). Even for those with basic English-language skills, there was a huge lack of context within which to understand difficulties that might arise. The process of acculturation may challenge long-standing traditions and values that enabled families to problem-solve effectively (Boehnlein et al., 1997). Different family members may find themselves at different points on the continuum of acculturation, and this may lead to "a sense of dysphoria and value conflict in family dynamics" (Moore et al., 1997, p. 142).

Children and Adolescents

According to the Commonwealth Fund (1997), Asian American adolescent girls were most at risk for the development of depression, with 30% of those surveyed indicating symptoms. For many traditional Southeast Asian cultures, disturbed behavior, particularly in children, is often seen as "willfulness" or a sign of physical illness (Carlin & Sokoloff, 1985). When depressed children do not exhibit physical signs, parents may perceive this as stubbornness or badness. Depressive symptoms may manifest as mood swings and irritability. The depressed child who spends most of the day sleeping may be seen as lazy or unmotivated, particularly if truancy becomes an issue, because the child cannot get up to go to school. Not being familiar with the many pressures of American adolescence, parents may also wonder why their children are stressed or depressed, particularly when compared with their own horrific war and relocation experiences.

Much like other refugee populations, Hmong children are certainly at risk for the development of some degree of secondary trauma caused by identifying or empathizing with the war victim. Children are also at far greater risk when the parents are so entrenched in their own maladjustment that they cannot give the appropriate support or parenting that children need to continue to thrive in this country. The anger and distrust of authority figures in adults as a result of their wartime experience can also influence how the children themselves view and respond to authority.

Physical Health Issues

The Minnesota Department of Health data on prenatal care between 1989 and 1993 reported that Hmong mothers were much less likely to receive early and frequent prenatal care than are other Southeast Asian mothers. As many as one-fourth of Hmong mothers began their prenatal care in the third trimester or received no care at all. According to the Department of Health index for measuring quantitative prenatal care, only 18% received "adequate care, while 37% received inadequate care or no care at all" (Minnesota Department of Health, 1994). The Department also noted that Asian births in Minnesota were 79% more likely than white births to be preterm, and 48% were more likely to be low-birth-weight deliveries. Additionally, it was noted that Asian/Pacific Islanders (undifferentiated by nationality or ethnicity) were overrepresented in teen births, accounting for 12% of births to females under age 15, 7% of births to females ages 15–17, and 6% to females ages 18–19. Given the still practiced tradition of marrying young, it is very probable that young Hmong females probably accounted for most of the teen births reported.

No epidemiological data on the extent or prevalence of HIV, sexually transmitted disease (STDs), or AIDS in the Hmong community. In 1995–

1996, Lao Family Community of Minnesota (2001a) staff conducted risk assessments on 146 youth and 123 adults; 15% of Hmong youth participants reported personally knowing a Hmong person with HIV or AIDS.

In the United States, a significant health risk for Hmong children and adults is hepatitis B. According to the Immunization Action Coalition (2001), Hmong immigrants were found to have chronic hepatitis infection at the rate of 18% compared to 11% for Chinese immigrant groups or 7.6% for Vietnamese immigrant groups. The concern about hepatitis B is that infected babies and young children are likely to develop chronic infection, which has a significant risk of leading to liver failure or liver cancer, usually in adulthood. Infection rates are high, and infected persons may be asymptomatic for many years. For this reason, all children 0–18 years of age should be immunized.

Another identified health risk for Hmong adults of both sexes is cancer. For women, the top five sites are lung, breast, colon/rectum, stomach, and liver. For men, the top five sites are lung, colon/rectum, liver, stomach, and prostate (National Cancer Institute, 1995). Beliefs about privacy and modesty hinder use of early screening methods, including breast examinations, mammography, or regular medical checkups. Lack of confidence in the efficacy of Western medical interventions, inability to pay for medical services, and alleged disrespectful and impersonal manners of medical service providers are often reasons offered to explain Hmong general reluctance to use mainstream medical facilities and services. With the younger generation, anecdotal evidence appears to indicate less resistance and more acceptance of Western medical interventions over indigenous healing practices.

Behavioral Health Concerns

In general, drug use among Asian and Pacific Islanders was found to be less frequent than that of non Asian populations (National Institute on Drug Abuse, 1995). Still less was known about use and abuse patterns among the Hmong. Sasao (1991), who reported findings summarized from community forums held in California, found that the most commonly used substances among Hmong people were alcohol, tobacco, marijuana, and amphetamines. He classified adolescents and adults to be at risk for substance abuse, and cited stress and peer pressure as risk factors. He also noted that substance use declined as Hmong youth and adults learned the consequences of substance abuse and voluntarily discontinued use. Overall, among Hmong people, risk factors for substance abuse include language and cultural barriers; unemployment or underemployment; educational, social, and health difficulties; racism/discrimination; increased acculturation into the mainstream and a concomitant loss of traditional cultural values and norms; intergenerational conflict; and diminished status and role reversal.

Economic Self-Sufficiency

The Hmong believe that a person's worth is not measured by how much money he or she has but by the size of the family and the amount of wisdom possessed. Coming to the United States, the older generation has had to adjust to a money economy in which employment is the norm to avoid poverty. However, because of a lack of proficiency in the English language, little or no formal education, and little or no employment experience (having been farmers most of their lives), the majority of Hmong ended up on public assistance. In contrast, younger adults have been successful, with many earning college degrees. From 1972 to 1998, some 118 Hmong persons received doctorates or other professional degrees; between 1984 and 1998, more than 2,000 Hmong earned baccalaureate degrees (Hmong National Development, 2000). Many Hmong have successful family businesses. In Wisconsin, there are more than 136 personally owned businesses, ranging from arts and crafts to video production establishments (Office of Refugee Services, 1999).

A community needs assessment survey carried out in Milwaukee, Wisconsin, in 2000, interviewed a total of 269 Hmong adults ranging in age from 18–72 years (Lie, 2000). The median gross total monthly income for families was $2,200, which would work out to about $26,400 per annum. The average size of families was two to four adults with one to four children. About 55% of respondents were members of families in which there were two income earners. About 18% of respondents lived in households of three to five income earners, and 13.4% lived in single–wage earner households. The poverty level in 1999 was $8,501 for a single individual, or $17,029 for a family of four (U.S. Bureau of the Census, 2001).

In 1997, Wisconsin was one of the first states to implement a work-based assistance program to replace welfare, affecting 31,336 families receiving cash assistance in Wisconsin. Of families impacted, an estimated 1,327 were Southeast Asian families, of whom 90%, or 1,194, were Hmong (Selkowe & Moore, 1999). The Office of Refugee services received reports of suicides in response to the introduction of welfare reform in 1996. Many people were desperate, believing that they had been stripped of their only source of income for their families. There was a strong belief among the Hmong community that the U.S. government had betrayed them by cutting off their only means of survival (University of Wisconsin—Milwaukee Community Action Scholars Project, 1997).

Selkowe and Moore (1999) also examined the impact of Wisconsin Works or W-2 (Wisconsin's welfare-to-work program) on Hmong families. Based on a convenience sample of 137 families, their findings indicated that close to the end of the allowable 2-year participation in W-2's employment positions, most Hmong aid recipients still lacked job skills, educational attainment, or language ability needed for employment. They were receiving little or no skills training through the W-2 program, and many reported being unable to communicate adequately with their W-2 caseworkers. Median income under W-2 was lower than under Aid to Families with Dependent Children (AFDC) for Hmong families. There were no adjustments for family size. Hmong families were not able to meet their basic subsistence needs. Four out of five Hmong interviewed felt that W-2 had made their family's life worse. About one out of three families ran out of food in the 6 months preceding the interview.

On the other hand, the response to welfare reform has not all been abysmal. Although official numbers are lacking, anecdotal evidence indicates that many Hmong with job training and preparation have been able to transition to fairly stable employment situations. A few others have relocated (Fadiman, 1997; Lo, 2001). According to Lo (2001), many Wisconsin families moved to North Carolina and Minnesota, hoping to buy cheap land and raise chickens for their eggs. However, business was not as promising as they had expected, and many returned to Wisconsin.

Family Life and Relationships

Youth Gangs

In 1994, *60 Minutes and Atlantic Monthly* portrayed Hmong and other Southeast Asian youth as gangsters, delinquents, and overall low achievers (Hang, 1997). Such media claims are reflective of a general public concern about increasing delinquency rates among Asian youth—a concern rooted in a generalized public image of Asians as the "model minority." Few question this image, and still fewer delve into understanding the sociostructural factors that have contributed to the delinquency of Hmong youth.

In 1998, the National Gang Crime Research Center reported that Southeast Asian gangs emerged as a form of support and companionship. Hmong children who became involved in gangs often pointed to the fact that their peer groups, be it gangs or not, were often other children very much like themselves—lost and caught between two worlds. In a study of Asian gang members ages 14–18 years, Wang (1996) found that despite criminal involvement, most of these children were not hardened criminals.

Hang (1997) implicated poverty and social upheaval as the two principal factors contributing to the malcontent expressed by Hmong youth in her sample. She noted that the bulk of Hmong refugees arrived in the United States when the country was in recession, and resettlement programs had been drastically cut. Available jobs were mostly located in the service sector, which generally paid minimum wage and required fair English-language skills. For many Hmong parents, even service-sector jobs were not available to them because of poor or no English-language skills. Those who did manage to secure minimum-wage jobs had to work more than one job to support a large family (average size five to seven members[1]). Parents were preoccupied with the business of surviving and had little time or patience for self-actualizing activities and time with others, even their own offsprings.

Intergenerational and Intercultural Conflicts

Intergenerational conflicts between immigrant parents and their children born or raised in the United States are not unique to the Hmong community. Several studies (e.g., Bishop, 1985; Boyer, 1991; Donnelly, 1994; Lucke, 1995; Lo, 2001; McInnis, Petracchi, & Morgenbesser, 1991) have documented the upheaval in family dynamics as a result of changed family structure and modifications in family relationships, values, and traditions after resettlement in the United States. Zhou and Bankston (2000) identified five issues over which parents and children often clash: parental authority, modes of teaching and punishment, views on American culture, role reversal, and gender-specific roles and expectations. Although these issues were identified in the course of work with Vietnamese refugee children in the United States, these were the same issues raised by parents in Lo's (2001) qualitative study of Hmong families.

Parental Authority

In many Asian cultures, filial obedience is an expectation. This obedience extends to adult children as well. Hmong children often see this expectation as excessive parental control. American society values critical thinking and query/inquiry, and Hmong children are socialized at school to be critical and inquiring. On the other hand, to question the decisions of elders in the Hmong community is highly disrespectful. Therefore, parents misunderstand this questioning as disrespect, while children become confused as to why parents are upset. Children might also see this response as a sign of rigidity and inflexibility. In an attempt to reign in "recalcitrant" offspring, parents may become increasingly restrictive and sometimes punitive.

Mental health issues and past war experiences may also play a big part in how some parents interact with their children. Parents who are struggling with their own mental health issues may not have the time or energy to parent the way their children feel they should. Consequently, children may see their parents as disengaged and uncaring.

---

[1] Selkowe and Moore (1999) reported that more than 50% of the 137 families interviewed for their study had five or more children under the age of 18, and nearly one in five respondents (18%) had eight or more children.

Modes of Teaching and Punishment

A personal attribute that is highly valued in Hmong society is modesty, and it is rare that a parent would pay a child a compliment. By the same token, Hmong adults are uncomfortable about receiving praise, whether directed at themselves or their children. When a compliment is paid, the "correct" thing to do is to deflect the praise. For instance, it would not be surprising to hear, "I don't think so!" in response to a compliment. The younger Hmong generation may construe such a response as insensitive and dismissive.

Furthermore, there is generalized concern that "praise" unnecessarily inflates the ego of those praised, leading to overconfidence and a "swollen head." As a countermeasure and character-building strategy, parents tend to "pick" on faults or mistakes. Unfortunately, children perceive such responses to be uncaring and hypercritical. Compounding the already-strained parent–child relationship is the "un-American" way in which Hmong parents express their love for their children. In meeting the material needs of their children, such as food, clothing, shelter, and safety, Hmong parents are exemplifying the ultimate expression of parental love and caring.

Many of the disciplinary methods (e.g., corporal punishment) used on Hmong parents themselves, who now use the same approach, are considered unacceptable and inappropriate in the United States. Physical punishment as a form of discipline in Asian American communities is apparently common. According to a 1997 Commonwealth Fund Survey, Asian American boys were most at risk for abuse, with 17% of those surveyed having experienced physical abuse. Parents are perplexed and confused by directives not to use the very approaches with which they were raised. Claiming that no other alternative is as effective as physical punishment, Hmong parents feel unjustly constrained. They cannot be good parents, because American society will not let them be good parents in ways they know how. Hmong parents do not look upon child abuse laws as protection of the child but rather as punishment of the parent. There is a saying among some parents in the Hmong community that American-born Hmong children are not really their children, but the government's.

Views on American Culture

Hmong parents and children clash over what is acceptable to adopt from the American culture and what is not. Subjects of disagreement include fashion, communication styles, and male–female relationships. It is not uncommon that points of contention may devolve into estranged parent–child relationships, disengagement, and alienation.

Hmong refugees often also find themselves having to choose between the values of two cultures: the American value that stresses individualism and independence, and the Hmong value that stresses group loyalty and family interdependence. This only exacerbates existing tensions and struggles between the older and younger generations. In addition, as more young Hmong Americans acculturate and "replace" Hmong values with American ones, they are perceived as rejecting Hmong "ways." This can often be the cause of marked distress for younger Hmong, who are accused of being selfish and a "sellout." Older Hmong may also worry about the continued integrity and viability of Hmong traditions and customs, and the future of the Hmong community as a whole.

Role Reversal

Traditionally, Hmong fathers were the head of the family, with mothers ranked next, with children at the lowest rung. Because of their command of the English language, many children serve as interpreters and cultural brokers for their parents. Daily-living issues such as taking care of bills, making appointments, and dealing with outsiders may also be entrusted to a child or two in the family. Parents who do not speak English or have a limited amount of knowledge about the school system may feel even more inept at dealing with school-related issues.

In some families, the mother may have replaced the father as head of household. The father who may not have been able to get a job that befitting his status in the old country remains unemployed. The mother, on the other hand, is less selective and may take on more than one job to support the family. The father's position as head of household may be threatened by the mother who is the principal, or in some cases, the only breadwinner. In some cases, the father may resort to violent means to assert his authority and affirm control.

Gender-Specific Role Expectations

As in most Southeast Asian cultures, women marry early and bear children. Males are pressured to perform well academically and groomed to assume leadership of the clan or family. Females are given mixed messages to do well at school or college and to be a "good Hmong girl." For example, some Hmong teenage girls complain about their parents' expressed interest in their academics and a concomitant expectation that they will marry young and bear many children.

Another hardship in this category is the changing roles among the adults themselves. Traditionally, Hmong mothers were more responsible for nurturing and caring for the children. Today, with more Hmong women working outside of the household, there is a tremendous need for men to assume more child-rearing and household responsibilities. Whereas the younger generation of men may be more responsive to this demand, the older generation is likely to be disdainful of those who do assume "women's" responsibilities.

CASE VIGNETTE

An adolescent continually told his parents that he was doing well in school and did not have homework because he completed it in study hall. Even though the school sent many letters home, the letters were always intercepted by the boy. The parents, who spoke some English, did not realize they could call the school to ask about their son's status. They were also unaware of the availability of parent–teacher conferences. School officials became increasingly incensed that the parents continually "ignored" them. It was not until a bilingual staff person called his mother that she became aware that her son had not attended school the entire semester. Both parents were extremely upset. They were particularly embarrassed that not only were they unaware that he had been truant but also that they had no idea where he was when he was not in school. They were also very concerned that they no longer had any control over their son's behavior, and that he did not respect them enough to do what they expected of him.

When the parents confronted the boy, they alleged that he had this "could not care less" attitude. He told them that he and his friends had been "hanging out" at an abandoned house, playing cards and listening to the radio. At about the time when school let out, they would head to the shopping mall, which they would avoid during the earlier part of the day to avoid getting reported to the school authorities. The parents were aghast; they were appalled to discover how devious their son had become. They interpreted his behavior as being ashamed of the fact that his parents did not speak English, then taking advantage of the fact. They blamed "American culture" for having "corrupted" their son; no Hmong adolescents would ever disobey their parents, skip school, and intercept/destroy messages from school authorities.

When they met with school representatives (teacher, principal, school social worker, and bilingual staff person) the parents were anxious, nervous, ashamed, and embarrassed. They were certain that the school authorities would expel their son, a decision that would cause them much grief and loss of face in the Hmong community.

CULTURAL VALUES AS STRENGTHS IN ASSESSMENT

Culture provides the interpretive system by which actions and reactions of others in relation to self (and, self to others) are understood. Therefore, to understand another's motivations and actions, and in turn, to decide how best to intervene, the service provider needs to "understand the meaning systems of those we help" (Saleeby, 1994, p. 352). Stories, narratives, and myths are the major vehicles for understanding "client's constructions of their individual and collective worlds" (Saleeby, 1994, p. 351).

Until the 1950s, the Hmong had no written language. Hmong history, values, beliefs, and practices were passed from generation to generation orally, through narratives and stories. Many elders today are still illiterate. Members of the generation now in their fifties are probably the first generation to learn the written version of the Hmong language. Because telling stories, narratives, and myths is second nature for many Hmong people, social workers need to learn how to listen to and use stories and narratives to strengthen Hmong individuals, families and communities.

A strengths-based approach examines meanings in terms of "what people know, and what they can do, however inchoate that may sometimes seem" (Saleeby, 1996, p. 297), and how these meanings figure in the lives of individuals, families, and communities. Specifically, the approach calls for looking at individuals, families, and communities in the light of "their capacities, talents, competencies, possibilities, visions, values, and hopes, however dashed and distorted these may become through circumstance, oppression and trauma" (p. 297). Applying a strengths perspective to early marriage involves framing the value of this practice in terms of the context in which this cultural institution emerged, and understanding both the meaning assigned to the practice and the resulting value that is attached.

Strengths that Hmong in the old country, as well as those who have taken refuge in the United States, include *resilience*, being able to transcend adversities of war and relocation; the existence of cultural values, such as being *family- and clan-centered*, because families and clans are important social supports and safety nets in times of crisis and need; a *rich cultural tradition*: in which the Hmong have passed beliefs, values, and practices from one generation to the next orally, using stories and narratives as a vehicle, and, more recently, through the written medium; the resolute *Hmong temperament*, as described by Fadiman (1997 p. 208) as "independent, insular, anti-authoritarian, suspicious, stubborn, proud, choleric, energetic, vehement, loquacious, humorous, hospitable, generous," which has helped the Hmong to respond to the hardships of life in the United States by becoming *more* Hmong rather than less so; and *spiritually centered*, because Hmong people practice ancestral worship and animism. This belief system and attendant practices have sustained them in times of chaos and ambiguity. The traditional Hmong way of life stresses balance and harmony with the earth and the surrounding world.

The family is the primary institution of Hmong society. Children are prized because they are the means by which the Hmong lineage is continued; they are the source of farm labor, and in the home country, where infant mortality rates were high, children were especially treasured. So it is not uncommon for Hmong households to have a large number of children present. However, the conception of adolescence as a significant development phase in the lifespan is novel to the Hmong. For the Hmong, one is either a child or an adult. The onset of puberty marks the shift from childhood to adulthood. Some begin adulthood as young as 12 years of age. However, the conception of adolescence as a significant development phase in the lifespan is novel to the Hmong.

The male-dominated family structure in the older generation is changing in the younger generation, in which more egalitarian relationships are increasingly the norm. In the old country, it was not uncommon for marriages to be arranged; however, arranged marriages are less often the case among the younger generation in the United States. Many Hmong men in the United States support more than one wife; they have one legal marriage and consider the others to be "Hmong marriage" (Lao Family Community of Minnesota, 2001b).

Early marriage is a cultural institution still valued by many Hmong parents. Soon after reaching puberty, a Hmong girl is considered eligible for marriage. Early matches in Laos were desirable for a variety of reasons, such as the high infant mortality rates, short lifespan, emphasis on large families, political and social connections that a bride could bring with her, and the extra helping hand she could provide to the family. Adolescent females and, less commonly, adolescent males were married at ages 14–16 years to ensure a longer reproductive cycle and, in turn, the perpetuation of the family. However, many state laws in the United States render such marriages illegal. Marriage of a "minor" female to a male age 18 years or older places the latter at risk of charges: contributing to the delinquency of a minor, and sexual assault.

A strengths-based approach to early marriage would call for the development and dissemination of new stories in the Hmong community. Although early marriage has helped to continue the Hmong lineage in the "old" country, the new context demands an *adjusted* response. It is simply postponing the marriage to a later time, when the female body is more developed, stronger, and more likely to result in live births and healthier, longer lived children. In addition, delaying marriage also protects the family from legal prosecution, preserving family integrity and privacy. After all, an intact healthy family is a premium Hmong cultural value

INDIGENOUS STRATEGIES AND WESTERN INTERVENTIONS

Linguistic and cultural barriers have made access to quality health care services difficult for Hmong refugees. Three linguistic barriers identified by Warner and Mochel (1998) were lack of proficiency in English, lack of trained medical interpreters, and lack of equivalent concepts in their native language. They also drew attention to cultural barriers, such as lack of knowledge about the Western health care delivery system, suspicions about Western medicine, and health care providers' lack of respect for Hmong culture and beliefs about health and illness.

A Western intervention that would be supportive of these cultural values about health care and healing would include collaborating with clan leaders to develop outreach services. These services would include providing professional Hmong–English–Hmong language interpretation; information about location of primary health care facilities in the neighborhood, and the programs and services available; and routine screening and physical examinations at Hmong-frequented sites (e.g., churches, community centers). Furthermore, instead of discouraging Hmong consultation of *shamans* and use of herbal remedies, social workers should consider working in tandem with *shamans* and the family to develop a plan for medication, healing, and recovery.

Giving consent for medical intervention, as O'Connor (1995, p. 87) noted, is not an individualized decision. Clan and community members constitute the decision-making body: "Individual Hmong are socialized not to attempt to resolve grave problems for themselves but rather to turn to the collective judgment of their extended families; consultation is the norm in all situations of any consequence and is virtually synonymous with decision making." O'Connor further noted that the Hmong self is "collectively developed and conceived, within the structure and mutual obligations of multigenerational family relations and clan affiliation." Therefore, in illness, it is traditionally Hmong families who "seek cures for sick family members, rather than the sick person seeking cures for himself or herself" (Bliatout, 1986, p. 361).

For the Hmong, rice is the primary nutrient and a staple. It also carries symbolic and ritual significance; the Hmong regard rice as their "staff of life" (O'Connor, 1995). To the Hmong, rice also has medicinal value. It may be served as a thin gruel, so that the sick person can drink it. A Hmong patient recovering and recuperating may ask to be served rice, a request that is likely to be denied; the Hmong find this practice "baffling, insulting, and dangerously foolish" (O'Connor, 1995, p. 88).

For the Hmong, disease has supernatural or spiritual origins. Organic causes are also recognized, but these do not necessarily rule out spiritual or supernatural factors. Core concepts of healing are concerned mainly with "invisible fluids and energies and with immaterial elements that need to be helped to reach proper balance"(O'Connor, 1995, p. 90). Loss or removal of body parts affects the souls that animate them and greatly interferes with passage of a Hmong person's spirit to the afterworld. Loss of a soul is a significant cause of illness. Geddes (1976, p. 98, as cited by O'Connor, 1995) observed that "in the majority of cases of sickness, soul separation is believed to be a factor." The soul may fail to return, or become lost or transmuted. Separation may be the result of any number of causes, including a curse, sudden fright, or having been ensnared by a malicious spirit.

The Hmong believe in the predestination of life. The length of each soul's lifetime in a given incarnation is predetermined by spiritual license. The length of time on the license determines how long the soul can live; when the license expires, the person dies (O'Connor, 1995). A Hmong *shaman* could bargain for an extension; however, if that extension is denied, nothing can be done for that person. As a consequence, many Hmong are resigned to their "fate," and are therefore wary that any intervention, including Western medical intervention, could make a difference.

A regimen of care typically consists of medicinal, physical, spiritual, and dietary measures. Recovering patients are commonly served traditional herbal medicines and health-promoting foods, and subjected to dietary restrictions. The *shaman* is likely to be consulted to restore the soul, and to conduct diagnostic and healing ceremonies. Among younger Hmong, adherence to and observance of traditional healing practices are on the decline as more and more turn to modern medicine and the accompanying technology.

Another example of an intervention that combines indigenous ideas with culturally responsive Western approaches is the Refugee Family-Strengthening Project (RFSP), started by the Wisconsin Office of Refugee Services, in 1995, in four different regions of Wisconsin (Vue, 1995). Each region covers at least three or more counties. These regions were chosen because of the large population of Hmong living in those counties. Project goals were to educate the Hmong community about the dynamics of domestic violence and how to prevent it; to provide intervention services, including counseling, case management, and education through workshops; and to provide in-service training for service providers.

The Project was strongly opposed by leaders in the Hmong community. At it inception, it was regarded as intrusive and labeled a "family wrecker." Indigenous leaders argued that domestic violence is a private family issue and should only be addressed within the clan system. They rejected any outside intervention and complained that the project was insensitive and disrespectful of Hmong traditions and customs. Project coordinators received hate mail with bullets enclosed (Vue, 1995).

The RFSP continues; it is currently in its sixth year of providing family-strengthening services to the Hmong community. Although there have been more than five tragic homicides after the Project started in 1995, it has accomplished much. Project staff learned many valuable lessons and continue to document many successful stories. The Project was able to reach out to clan leaders and hold several meetings with them. Because many couples and individuals turn to clan leaders for advice, leaders who are knowledgeable about the dynamics of violence, the pertinent laws and legal penalties, and helping resources could play a key role in spearheading the development of a community-based and culturally competent response to domestic violence. Additionally, by involving clan leaders in program development and implementation decisions, project staff were able to get community buy-in and participation.

By early 2000, the Project had served 777 clients, with 213 acute cases (Vue, 2000). According to site coordinators, increased caseloads meant that more victims were reporting the abuse. In addition, Hmong men who batter their wives are beginning to seek services to help them change. The Project is aiming for a Batterers Education Program in all the regions by 2002 (Vue, 2001).

PRINCIPLES OF CULTURALLY APPROPRIATE PRACTICE

Saleeby (1994, p. 358) noted that subjugated and vulnerable populations benefit from help "to restore and restory." Restoring and helping individuals, families, and communities restory is the process of developing the ability to gain power. This involves cultivating a sense of self-efficacy, providing validation of experiences, developing critical thinking, and fostering reflective action for personal and political change (Parsons, Gutierrez, & Cox, 1998). In other words, social work practice with Hmong people should be founded on empowerment methods and culturally competent strategies.

Cross, Bazron, Dennis, and Isaacs (1989) identified five essential elements of culturally competent practice: valuing diversity, self-assessment, the dynamics of difference, institutionalization of cultural knowledge, and adaptation to diversity.

Valuing Diversity and Challenging the Assumptions of "Cultural Deficit"

Effective outreach strategies build on proactive programmatic efforts that recognize and reflect cultural strengths of a community. The Hmong arrived in this country with strong extended-family ties and clan networks. They preserved cultural values, beliefs, and traditions in the face of adversity and change. This sense of communal efficacy should be acknowledged and affirmed.

The vast majority of adult Hmong, particularly those who are illiterate, still feel estranged from mainstream institutions, even mutual aid associations staffed by Hmong professionals. Going beyond the clan group for assistance is still difficult for both young and old. Social workers should consider taking information about the range, type, and availability of social services to the Hmong community, and presenting oral presentations, through an interpreter, on how to access services at sites where Hmong people gather (e.g., mutual aid associations and churches).

Cultural Self-Assessment

It is important for social workers to be careful not to impose their values, beliefs, and preferences on the family or child with whom they are working. A critical and honest self-evaluation should also probe for any biases or prejudices that the social worker may unknowingly harbor. At the agency level, conducting an audit for culturally biased or "color-blind" policies or practices is necessary to identify barriers that keep Hmong families and children away.

Dynamics of Difference

It is easy to misjudge another's intentions and actions based on learned expectations (Cross et al., 1989). For example, definitions of personal and social–professional boundaries differ. Hmong culture values affiliations. Hmong clients may expect social workers to reciprocate in sharing personal stories and to behave casually. Also, social workers may receive invitations to attend ceremonial events. The invitation, to the person issuing it, is an important expression of appreciation, trust, and respect. To attend a ceremony would reaffirm for the Hmong person the social worker's regard and respect for that client as a person.

Institutionalizing Cultural Knowledge

A practitioner is typically part of a larger whole—an agency or organization or system of care. An organization that values cultural competence would factor into its job evaluation and rewards system ways to support and reinforce those skills. Furthermore, organizational policies and operational manuals would emphasize the value placed on culturally competent service delivery.

Adaptations to Diversity

The purpose of adapting or adjusting the social worker's professional task and work styles to the expectations, preferences, and values of specific clients (Pinderhughes, 1989) is to ensure a more meaningful fit between the needs of Hmong families and children, and available services. This involves learning from and hearing clients but not utilizing them as our teacher. Thus, although it is important to conduct research to add to the existing knowledge about Hmong people, it is also critical to recognize that certain research conventions treat subjects as mere sources of data. Instead, the researcher should regard the research subject as collaborator and expert. The process and content of inquiry and the strategies for information gathering become a shared enterprise.

CONCLUSIONS

Effective outreach and intervention strategies for the Hmong community require sensitive and sensible attention to the values, beliefs, and practices of the community. An increased number of well-trained and competent indigenous professionals, particularly in the mental health and social services arena, does not absolve non-Hmong professionals of the responsibility for delivering culturally competent services. Non-Hmong service providers must continue to educate themselves about Hmong worldviews, mindful of the need to respond not only to diversity but also to the diversity that exists within that diversity.

REFERENCES

Abe, J., Zane, N., & Chun, K. (1994). Differential responses to trauma: Migration-related discriminants of post-traumatic stress disorder among Southeast Asian refugees. *Journal of Community Psychology, 22*(2), 121–135.

Bishop, K. A. (1985). *The Hmong of central California: An investigation and analysis of the changing family structure during liminality, acculturation and transition.* Doctoral dissertation, University of San Francisco, San Francisco, CA.

Bliatout, B. T. (1986). Guidelines for mental health professionals to help Hmong seek traditional healing treatment. In G. L. Hendricks, B. T. Downing, & A. Deinard (Eds.), *The Hmong in transition* (pp. 349– 364). New York: Center for Migration Studies of New York and Southeast Asian Refugee Studies Project, University of Minnesota.

Boehnlein, J. K., Leung, P. K., & Kinzie, J. D. (1997). Cambodian American families. In E. Lee (Ed.), *Working with Asian Americans: A guide for clinicians* (pp. 37–45). New York: Guilford Press.

Boyer, L. M. (1991). *The older generation of Southeast Asian refugees: An annotated bibliography.* Southeast Asian Refugee Studies Occasional Paper No. 11. Minneapolis: University of Minnesota, Center for Urban and Regional Affairs (CURA).

Carlin, J. E., & Sokoloff, B. Z. (1985). Mental health treatment issues for Southeast Asian refugee children. In T. C. Owan (Ed.), *Southeast Asian mental health: Treatment, prevention, services, training, and research* (pp. 91–112). Bethesda, MD: National Institute of Mental Health.

Chindarsi, N. (1976). *The religion of the Hmong Njua.* Bangkok: Siam Society.

Commonwealth Fund. (1997). Survey of the health of adolescent girls. Retrieved on February 11, 2002 from *http://www.cmwf.org/programs.*

Cross, T. L., Bazron, B. J., Dennis, K. W., & Isaacs, M. R. (1989). *Towards a culturally competent system of care: Vol. 1. A monograph on effective services for minority children who are severely emotionally disturbed.* Washington, DC: Child and Adolescent Service System Program (CASSP) Technical Assistance Center, Georgetown University Child Development Center.

Dao, Y. (1982). Why did the Hmong leave Laos? In B. T. Downing & D. P. Olnery (Eds.), *The Hmong in the West* (pp. 3–18). Papers of the 1981 Hmong Research Conference. Minneapolis: Southeast Asian Refugee Studies Project, Center for Urban and Regional Affairs, University of Minnesota.

Donnelly, N. D. (1994). *Changing lives of refugee Hmong women.* Seattle: University of Washington Press.

Fadiman, A. (1997). *The spirit catches you and you fall down: A Hmong child, her American doctors, and the collision of two cultures.* New York: Farrar, Straus & Giroux.

Geddes, W. R. (1976). *Migrants of the mountains: The cultural ecology of the Blue Miao (Hmong Njua) of Thailand.* Oxford, UK: Clarendon Press.

Hang, M. Y. (1997). Growing up Hmong American: Truancy policy and girls. *Hmong Studies Journal, 1*(2). Retrieved February 22, 2002 from *http://members.aol. com/hmong studiesjrn/HSJ-v1n2_hang.html.*

Hein, J. (1995). *From Vietnam, Laos and Cambodia: A refugee experience in the United States.* New York: Twayne.

Hmong National Development. (2000). *Population count.* Retrieved February 29, 2003 from *http://www.hndlink.org/popstats.html.*

Hones, D. F., & Cha, C. S. (1999). *Educating new Americans: Immigrant lives and learning.* Mahwah, NJ: Erlbaum.

Immunization Action Coalition. (2001). *Hepatitis B information for Asian and Pacific Islander Americans.* Retrieved February 22, 2002 from *http://www. immunize.org/catg.d/4190apia.htm.*

Kemp, C. E. (2000). *Mental health issues among refugees.* Retrieved February 22, 2002 from *http://www.baylor.edu/~charles_kemp/refugee_mental_health.htm.*

Kinzie, J. D., Boehnlein, J. K., Leung, P. K., Moore, L. J., Riley, C., & Smith, D. (1990). The high prevalence rate of PTSD and its clinical significance among Southeast Asian refugees. *American Journal of Psychiatry, 147,* 813–917.

Kroll, J., Habenicht, M., MacKenzie, T., Yang, M., Chan, S., Vang, T., et al. (1989). Depression and posttraumatic stress disorder in Southeast Asian refugees. *American Journal of Psychiatry, 146,* 1592–1597.

Lao Family Community of Minnesota. (2001a). HIV/STDs and the Hmong. Retrieved on May 27, 2003 from *http://www.laofamily.org/health/hmong_health.htm.*

Lao Family Community of Minnesota. (2001b). Hmong Families. Retrieved May 27, 2003 from *http://www.laofamily.org/culture/.*

Lemoine, J. (1986). Shamanism in the context of Hmong resettlement. In G. L. Hendricks, B. T. Downing, & A. Deinard (Eds.), *The Hmong in transition* (pp. 337–348). New York: Center for Migration Studies of New York and Southeast Asian Refugee Studies Project, University of Minnesota.

Lie, G.-Y. (2000). *A needs assessment survey of the Hmong community.* Report submitted to the Hmong American Friendship Association. Milwaukee: Center for Addiction and Behavioral Health Research, University of Wisconsin—Milwaukee.

Lin, T. (1983). Psychiatry and Chinese culture. *Western Journal of Medicine, 139*(6), 862–867.

Lo, F. (2001). *The promised land: Socioeconomic reality of the Hmong People in urban America (1976–2000)*. Bristol, IN: Wyndham Hall Press.

Lucke, J. J. (1995). *We all agree: A study of cultural consensus in a Hmong community*. Doctoral dissertation, University of Wisconsin—Milwaukee.

McInnis, K. M., Petracchi, H. E., & Morgenbesser, M. (1991). *The Hmong in America: Providing ethnic-sensitive health, education, and human services*. Dubuque,
IA: Kendall/Hunt.

Minnesota Department of Health. (1994). *Minnesota health profiles*. Minneapolis:
Minnesota Center for Health Statistics.

Mollica, R. F., Wyshak, G., & Lavelle, J. (1987). The psychosocial impact of war trauma and torture on Southeast Asian refugees. *American Journal of Psychiatry,
144*, 1507–1572.

Moore, L. J., Keopraseuth, K., Leung, P. K., & Chao, L. H. (1997). Laotian American
families. In E. Lee (Ed.), *Working with Asian Americans: A guide for clinicians*
(pp. 136–152). New York: Guilford Press.

Moore, L. J., Sager, D., Keopraseuth, K., Loo, H. C., & Riley, C. (2001). Rheumato-
logical disorders and somatization in U.S. men and Lao refugees with depression
and post-traumatic stress disorder: A cross-cultural comparison. *Transcultural
Psychiatry, 38*(4), 481–506.

Mottin, J. (1980). *History of the Hmong*. Bangkok: Odeon Store.

National Cancer Institute. (1995). *Surveillance, Epidemiology and End Results
(SEER) Program: Cancer statistics review*. Bethesda, MD: Author.

National Gang Crime Research Center. (1998). *Southeast Asian gangs*. Peotone, IL:
Author.

National Institute on Drug Abuse. (1995). *Drug use among racial/ethnic minorities*.
Bethesda, MD: National Institutes of Health.

O'Connor, B. B. (1995). *Healing traditions: Alternative medicine and the health professions*. Philadelphia: University of Pennsylvania Press.

Office of Refugee Services. (1999). *Wisconsin refugee resource directory*. Madison,
WI: Author.

Parsons, R. J., Gutierrez, L. M., & Cox, E. O. (1998). A model for empowerment
practice. In L. M. Gutierrez, R. J. Parsons, & E. O. Cox (Eds.), *Empowerment in
social work practice: A sourcebook* (pp. 3–23). Pacific Grove, CA: Brooks/Cole.

Pinderhughes, E. (1989). *Understanding race, ethnicity and power*. New York: Free
Press.

Ranard, D. A. (1988). Hmong self-sufficiency: Community differences. *America: Perspectives on refugee resettlement, 1*, 4–6.

Saleeby, D. (1994). Culture, theory, and narrative: The intersection of meanings in
practice. *Social Work, 39*(4), 351–359.

Saleeby, D. (1996). The strengths perspective in social work practice: Extensions and
cautions. *Social Work, 41*(3), 296–305.

Sasao, T. (1991). *Statewide Asian drug service needs assessment*. Sacramento: California Department of Alcohol and Drug Programs.

Selkowe, V., & Moore, T. (1999). *The impact of welfare reform on Wisconsin's
Hmong aid recipients*. Milwaukee: Institute for Wisconsin's Future.

U.S. Bureau of the Census. (2001). *Poverty in the United States, 1999*. Current Population Reports, Series P60-210. Washington, DC: U.S. Government Printing

Office. Retrieved May 22, 2003 from *http://www.census.gov/prod/2000pubs/
p60-210.pdf*.

UWM Community Action Scholars Project. (1997). *Welfare reform introductory interviews with the Hmong participants*. Milwaukee: University of Wisconsin—Milwaukee Press.

Vue, M. Z. (1995). *RFS program data report*. Madison, WI: Division of Economic Support, State of Wisconsin Department of Workforce Development.

Vue, M. Z. (2000). *RFS program data report*. Madison, WI: Division of Economic Support, State of Wisconsin Department of Workforce Development.

Vue, M. Z. (2001). *RFS program data report*. Madison, WI: Division of Economic Support, State of Wisconsin Department of Workforce Development.

Wang, Z. (1996). Is the pattern of Asian gang affiliation different?: A multiple regression analysis. *Journal of Crime and Justice, 19*(1), 113.

Warner, M. E., & Mochel, M. (1998). The Hmong and health care in Merced, California. *Hmong Studies Journal, 2*(2), 1–21.

Zhou, M., & Bankston, C. (2000). *Straddling different social worlds: The experience of Vietnamese refugee children in the United States*. New York: Educational Resources Information Center (ERIC) Clearinghouse on Urban Education, Institute for Urban and Minority Education, Teachers College, Columbia University.

CHAPTER 8

Asian Indian Children and Families

FARIYAL ROSS-SHERIFF
SHALINI CHAUDHURI

Viewed as family-oriented, affluent, intelligent, and hardworking, Asian Indians comprise one of the largest Asian population groups in the United States (U.S. Bureau of the Census, 2000). These immigrants of color represent religious, ethnic, linguistic, cultural, and socioeconomic diversity in the American mosaic. With the passage of the 1965 Immigration Act, the previous restriction on Asian Indian immigration was lifted, resulting in a dramatic increase of migration to the United States. Now numbering over 1.6 million, Asian Indians comprise one of the Asian groups with the largest population increase during the last decade of the 20th century. Despite the increasing numbers and relative professional and economic success of these first-generation immigrants, little is known about their history, culture, struggles, and distinctive strategies for adaptation to American society. In this chapter, we present historical background, demographic profile, and adaptation process of Asian Indians to American society. The discussion on adaptation focuses on religion, religious and ethnic organizations, and worldview of first-generation Asian Indians and their children, with examples of the Hindus, the religious group with the largest proportion of Asian Indians.

A case vignette is then presented to illustrate select issues that practitioners should consider for service provision to this population.

HISTORICAL BACKGROUND

The passage of the Immigration Act of 1965 marks the beginning of immigration of a large number of Asian Indians to the United States (Balgopal,

2000; Mogelonsky, 1995; Ramisetty-Mikler, 1993). Although there are early records of Asian Indians in the United States starting in 1790 (Balgopal, 2000) and of a sizable community between 1907 and 1914, Asian Indians in the United States today are primarily first-generation immigrants (Mogelonsky, 1995). The earlier group worked mostly in lumberyards or in laying railroads in the western United States (Takaki, 1989). The current first-generation Asian Indians came as students and professionals with temporary visas, obtaining legal permanent residency after the passage of the 1965 Immigration Act. After the 1970s, a number of Indian doctors immigrated to the United States to fill the shortage of doctors created by the Vietnam War. Additionally, those who have come since the mid-1960s sponsored their parents, siblings, and other relatives during the late 1970s and the 1980s. The momentum gained during the 1980s continued well into the 1990s and later years. Included among those who came are undocumented migrants. The most recent group of Asian Indians to arrive in the United States are highly skilled professionals, specializing in engineering, computer science, and information technology, who have been hired and brought to the United States to meet the great demands of the "tech market" in the 1990s. With the 1980 census, the separation of the Asian Indian population from the category "other Asians" has enabled demographers and researchers to study this group as a distinct population.

Like other groups of Asian immigrants, Asian Indians have a long history of struggles and hardships in the United States. Despite the resources they bring to America and their continuing contribution to American society, they have been harassed and ill-treated because of prejudices against them (History of Indians in the US, 2000; Takaki, 1989).

PROFILE OF ASIAN INDIANS IN THE UNITED STATES

Demographic Profile, Location, and Population Concentration

During the last decade of the 20th century, the population of Asian Indians in the United States doubled, from 815,447 in 1990, to 1,678,765 (U.S. Bureau of the Census, 2000), making it the third largest Asian population group following Chinese Americans (2,432,585) and Filipinos (1,850,314). Although Asian Indians are widely dispersed in the United States, their numbers have doubled in many places, including small states such as Delaware and Rhode Island. Georgia, Nevada, and Colorado posted an increase of over 200% (U.S. Bureau of the Census, 2000). There are populations in excess of 100,000 in the following five states: California, New York, New Jersey, Illinois, and Texas (see Table 8.1). A closer look shows significant Asian Indian populations residing in the following 10 metropolitan areas: (1) New York, (2) Chicago, (3) San Francisco/Oakland/San Jose, (4) Los

TABLE 8.1. States with an Asian Indian Population of over 100,000

State	Asian population	Percentage	Indian population	Percentage
California	3,697,517	10.9	314,818	0.9
New York	1,044,976	5.5	251,724	1.3
New Jersey	480,276	5.7	169,180	2.0
Texas	608,690	2.9	147,223	0.7
Illinois	423,603	3.4	124,723	1.0

Note. Source of data: *http://www.factfinder.census.gov/servlet/basicfactsservlet.*

Angeles, (5) Washington/Baltimore, (6) Philadelphia, (7) Houston, (8) Dallas/Ft. Worth, (9) Detroit, and (10) Boston (see Table 8.2).

Asian Indians are one of the most highly educated, wealthy groups in the United States (India Abroad Center for Political Awareness, 1999). According to the 1990 census, 87% of the Asian Indians had completed high school, with 62% having some college education. More than 58% held bachelor's or higher degrees—the highest percentage among all Asian American ethnic groups. Fourteen percent of Asian Americans in the United States were engaged in work related to science, medicine, engineering, and technology. A significant percentage (19.3%) held managerial, administrative, sales, and teaching positions. More than 5,000 Asian Indians held faculty positions at American universities (Project Impact, 2000).

Foreign-born Asian Indian women have the highest rates of education in the United States. The 1990 census, as cited in Kurien (1999), indicated that 49% had at least a bachelor's degree compared to 18% of the general American population, and 60% over the age of 16 were employed. Because many single women are in higher education as full-time undergraduate and postgraduate students, the percentage of married women in the labor force is likely to be higher. Along with Asian Indian men, these women also have high levels of education and labor force participation, resulting in high family incomes for the group.

The mean and median income of Asian Indians, according to the 1990 census, was $44,700 and $60,093, respectively, which is relatively higher than comparable figures for non-Hispanic white families. The discrepancy between mean and median household income can be explained partially by the fact that Asian Indian households have a high proportion of dual- and triple-income homes (India Abroad Center for Political Awareness, 1999). Asian Indians have carved out a strong financial, educational, and professional identity. Placing great value on education and economic security, Asian Indians go to great lengths to further their children's education. Saving money is a major part of the Asian Indian culture, and targeted

TABLE 8.2. Ten Metropolitan Centers with the Largest
Asian Indian Population in the United States

Metropolitan areas	Population
New York	400,194
Chicago	116,868
San Francisco/Oakland/San Jose	144,231
Los Angeles	104,482
Washington/Baltimore	88,211
Philadelphia	52,380
Houston	51,959
Dallas/Ft. Worth	49,669
Detroit	45,731
Boston	43,732

Note. Source of data: U.S. Bureau of the Census (2000).

saving—for education or retirement—is especially emphasized (Mogelonsky, 1995).

However, it is important to note that not all Asian Indians enjoy economic prominence and prosperity. The relatively high income of many first-generation, two-parent families masks growing poverty among the elderly and female-headed households. Seven percent of families and 10% of individual Asian Indians were below the poverty level (U.S. Department of Commerce, 1990).

Religious Affiliation and Ethnic Community Organizations

All the major religious traditions of India—Hinduism, Islam, Sikhism, Christianity, Jainism, and Buddhism—are represented among the Asian Indian immigrants. However, a vast majority of the Asian Indians in the United States are Hindus (Kurien, 1999; Williams 1988). A brief description of Hinduism is presented in the section on religion. The most visible marker of religious diversity is observed through the proliferation of places of worship—Hindu, Buddhist, and Jain temples, Sikh *gurudwaras*, and Islamic *masjids* (Eck, 1997). For example, according to Eck, over 30 Hindu temples were built over a period of two decades since the construction of the first ones in Pittsburgh and Flushing, Queens, in 1997. In addition to those built from the ground up, over 400 Hindu temples in the United States have been transformed from buildings such as warehouses, suburban homes, and former churches (Eck, 2000).

During the last three decades, the Asian Indians have created a number of national organizations and local voluntary associations to promote economic, social, and political causes of Asian Indians in America. Examples of these include the Association of Indians in America (AIA), the National Federation of Indian Associations (NFIA), the Global Organization of Indian Origin (GOIO), the Indian American Forum for Political Action (IAFPA), the Telegu Association of North America, the World Malyalam Council, the Kannada Kota, the New England Marathi Mandal, and the Gujerati Samaj. In keeping with the patriarchal and elitist nature of the local religiocultural associations, these organizations are dominated by upper-class, upper-caste males (Kurien, 1999). The local associations are based on religion, ethnic, and linguistic backgrounds in metropolitan areas with a concentration of Asian Indian immigrants (Eck, 1997; Kurien, 1999; Williams, 1988). In addition to data previously mentioned, two major reasons for such organizations, specifically, at the local levels, are "to preserve a sense of cultural identity and to facilitate the transmission of religious tradition to the next generation" (Fenton, 1988, p. 102). In an ethnographic study of the adaptation strategies of Asian Indians in the Silicon Valley, Gawlick (1997) found a social network of cultural support systems in Indian newspapers, magazines, stores, restaurants, and institutions for religious practice that promoted Indian culture and traditions.

Thus, the first- and second-generation Asian Indian populations in the United States represent immigrants with high levels of education; well-developed English-language skills; strong family ties focused around religion and community organizations; participation in a complex social life founded on home, work, and community ties; and an identification with religion and observation of rituals (Saran, 1985). Mogelonsky (1995) identified three segments, or subgroups, among them. In the first, the affluent group, the majority of persons migrated to the United States in the 1960s, led by a cohort of highly educated academics. These professionals, now in their 50s, are at the peak of their earning potential. The second group includes immigrants who came to the United States in the 1970s. Much like the first segment, the men are educated professionals. The major difference, however, is that these men are married to highly educated women who work outside the home. Furthermore, their children are most likely to attend college. The third group comprises relatives of earlier immigrants sponsored by established family members in the United States. Often "less well-educated" than members of the first two segments, members of this group are likely to run motels, small grocery stores, gas stations, or other businesses (Mogelonsky, 1995). An emerging fourth group includes undocumented immigrants and those living in poverty. Regardless of their economic status, all groups contain individuals and families who experience acculturation stress and related problems in the process of adaptation to life in America.

ADAPTATION TO THE UNITED STATES

Asian Indians have distinctly different cultural characteristics and world-views than those of the host American society. They experience stress and related adaptation problems in the process of adapting to American society (Ross-Sheriff, 1992). However, they have developed a complex web of social networks, and ethnic and religious community organizations in their adaptation process, with the specific goal of maintaining their culture, traditions, and distinctive Asian Indian identity in the United States. Adaptation[1] of first-generation Asian Indians can best be described as "adhesive adaptation," a pattern in which "certain aspects of the new American culture and relations with the host society are added onto the traditional culture and social network without replacing or modifying any part of the old" (Hurh & Kim, 1984, p. 35). The second and subsequent generations undergo further modifications as they become immersed in the American education system and lifestyles. Understanding the adaptation of Asian Indians requires an examination of their religious beliefs, worldview, and related cultural characteristics within the context of family and community.

Religion

India is a country with a Hindu majority. Thus, the representation of Hindu Indians in the United States is significantly greater than that for members of any other religious groups. Hinduism dates back to about 1500 B.C. and originated in the Indus Valley. The term "Hindu" is derived from the Sanskrit word *Sindhu*, which means the Indus River. Hinduism has given its followers or believers a body of social and doctrinal systems that extend to every aspect of human life, with a body of guiding principles of social living. Central to the understanding of Hinduism is the belief in actions reflecting good thoughts. A lifelong virtuosity frees the human soul from the painful cycle of birth and death. True salvation is eternal freedom and union with the cosmic power, the Absolute Whole. There is emphasis on the doctrines of "right behavior and right actions" leading to greater good for greater numbers of people. The Hindu population has been divided hierarchically into four castes or social groups ascribed by birth: *Brahmins*, *Kshatriyas*, *Vaishyas*, and *Shudras*. In addition to the primary gods, Shiva and Vishnu, thousands of gods and goddesses are worshiped.

---

[1] Adaptation is "the process in which immigrants modify their behaviors and attitudes in order to maintain and improve their life conditions compatible with the new environment" (Hurh & Kim, 1984, p. 35).

The rationale for these numerous gods and goddesses is the belief that every individual is at his or her own level of realization of the Supreme Being and needs a personal image of God that leads to the ultimate realization of *Brahma,* or Absolute Truth. Thus, Hinduism, to a believer, upholds the virtue of collective identity, while retaining the space for an intensely personal experience.

The ancient Hindu scriptures have divided the entire human life into four stages, or *Ashramas.* The first stage is *Bramhacharjya,* or chaste student, whose main goal is to acquire knowledge; then comes *Garhasthya,* or householder, who now needs to beget and have a family of his or her own to continue the family lineage and fulfill social responsibilities through professional contributions. Once having attained a certain age and accomplished all worldly duties, the individual becomes a forest dweller, or embarks upon *Vanaprasthya,* and renounces all his or her worldly possessions and become a *Sanyasi* (an ascetic). He or she now makes room for the next generation to follow the family tradition.

The Hindu scriptures set down in vivid detail the roles and responsibilities of every member of the family. The eldest male is considered the head and provides for the whole family. The eldest woman controls the activities within the household and is responsible for taking care of all the members of the family. The other members are assigned specific duties and responsibilities, and are controlled by the eldest male member of the family. The male child is considered to be the holder of the family name; the lineage is carried on through him. Thus, the relatively superior status of the male child has been sanctified historically by religion and remains valid today. The female child is expected to obey her elders and is groomed to take on the responsibilities of a wife, homemaker, and mother. In the process, female children and women learn to solve problems in their domestic and family roles. Hindu women are respected highly when they fulfill their responsibilities within their cultural context.

Because religion is a way of life for Hindus in India, and the total environment supports religious beliefs, many have taken it for granted. Not all consider themselves practicing Hindus when they arrived in the United States. However, many become more religious after coming to the United States. According to Saran (1985), Asian Indian immigrants with children turn to religion and religious practices "since they see this as a way of raising Indian consciousness in their children" (p. 42). Hindus generally set up a place of worship (*puja*) in their homes and worship as families or individuals in their homes and temples. Because Asian Indians are spatially dispersed in suburbs, they feel a greater need for congregational worship than they did in India. They use religion as a means of community development and a vehicle of transmission of culture (Williams, 1988). Women play critical roles not only in the socialization of children and management of their household but also in the social and religiocultural life of the household and the local community (Kurien, 1999). In the United States, religion continues to be a source of identity development and has profound impact on the worldview of individuals.

Worldview and Concept of Self among Asian Indians

Worldview is defined as the ways in which people "perceive relationships to nature, other people, institutions, and objects" (English, 1984). A person's worldview denotes his or her psychological orientation to life and influences how he or she thinks, behaves, makes decisions, analyzes events, and conducts social relationships. Asian Indians' worldview is also influenced by their religious and philosophical orientation to life. Unlike the Western mode of thinking, in which science and religion, natural and supernatural, and mind and body are viewed dichotomously, the Asian Indian worldview is typically characterized by unity and indivisibility.

The Asian Indian culture emphasizes significant values such as family/kin responsibilities, obligations, and filial piety; hierarchical order in carrying out responsibilities; sensitivity to the feelings of others; respect; and loyalty. Family needs have priority over individual needs. Group needs are emphasized, and value is placed on appropriate behaviors for all occasions. Disciplinary techniques invoking shame and guilt are used to pressure individuals to conform to the societal norms and to avoid embarrassing the family.

Asian Indians' worldview influences their self-concept. The concept of self is best explained in contrast with the Western concept of self, as presented by Roland (1984, 1988), who compared Asian Indians and the Japanese with Americans. The differences between the Asian Indian and the American concept of self can be conceptualized as differing gestalts of the integration of three subcomponents—individual, familial, and transcendental selves. Unlike the American self-gestalt, in which the individual self dominates, for Asian Indians, the familial self predominates. The transcendental self exists but is not overtly represented, and the individual self is emphasized least. The individual in social interactions represents the family or the ethnic, or religious group, and is not free to conduct relationships in a totally individuated way. Among family members, the familial self has "relatively open ego boundaries, and there is relatively little private psychological space around the self" (Roland, 1984, p. 176).

With migration to the United States, the Asian Indians' worldview and concept of self, specifically, that of children and adolescents, change with exposure to different expectations of family, school, and peers. Children and adolescents experience stress as a result of pressures from the conflicting expectations of the two worlds in which they live—first in the family, and second, among peers. Similarly, with participation in the labor force, in religious and ethnic community organizations, and with major responsibilities in socialization of children and management of the household, women's roles change in America. Women and their family members experience stress and have to make adjustments to traditional roles. Though their concept of self may change over time, many culturally distinct characteristics, which are the essence of the continuity of psychological, social, and self-understanding, endure over generations (DeVos, 1980). These characteristics serve as sources of strength as well as problems in America.

PROBLEMS FOR CHILDREN AND FAMILIES

Two major areas of difficulty for Asian Indian families that result in stress are intergenerational conflicts and gender roles within the cultural context. Some families learn to resolve their problems over time, whereas for others, stress from problems results in weakened family bonds and increased tension, resulting in deviant behaviors and spousal abuse. The Asian Indian cultural and religious ethos espouses subordination of children and adolescent to parental authority. In contrast, norms and expectations of the larger American society espouse individuality and independence from parents and family. This causes tensions and stress for both adolescents and their families. Parents are frightened by peer pressures regarding choice of friends, dating, drugs, and alcohol. They fear their children will lose their identity as Asian Indians, move away from the much-needed supportive and protective home environments, and bring harm to themselves. Adolescents, on the other hand, feel constrained by their concerned and "protective" parents and, in some cases, either withdraw or rebel against parental expectations. This results in deviant behaviors, problems in academic performance, alcohol and drug abuse, sexual promiscuity, and, in extreme cases, disassociation from family and community (Bhattacharya, 1998; Mohan, 1992; Saran, 1985). Mohan (1992) saw an association between intergenerational cultural conflicts, severe family problems, and resentment toward Asian Indian parents' unrealistic expectations of children and adolescents for school performance, and young adults' choices. Some of the issues arising from intergenerational conflicts are young adults withdrawal from family and friends by behaviors such as spending too much time watching television or on the computer, and just staying locked in their rooms. Other negative impacts are poor school performance, loss of appetite, depression, and general lack of interest in day-to-day activities. These issues are generally manifested through psychosomatic problems.

The Asian Indian worldview and culture ascribe roles and responsibilities that produce two central and widely recognized images of womanhood within Hinduism and Indian culture. The first is the conventional image of the obedient woman, whose influence is largely confined to the household. She is expected to be a "virtuous, self-sacrificing homemaker who enables the success of her husband and the academic achievement of her children through her unselfish actions on their behalf" (Kurien, 1999, p. 49). In their primary responsibility for the socialization of their children, parents take on major responsibilities in ethnic and religious community organizations. The second image is that of the well-educated professional woman, who participates actively in her community. Although both are respected, the former is the preferred and dominant model (Kurien, 1999). Execution of these roles places women in important positions and empowers them outside the home. Yet, at home, they are in a subordinate position, with multiple responsibilities and, often, little help from their spouses. The stress from these diametrically opposed, exacting, and unrealistic demands on women results in conflicts in the household and sometimes domestic violence. These women are unlikely to reveal their condition because of pressures to conform to their cultural roles and the fear that they would be viewed as "traitors to the community," affecting the model minority image (Dasgupta & Dasgupta, 1996, p. 385).

Another group of Asian Indian women who experience severe stress are recent immigrants. Many do not work outside the home, have no extended family support, and feel lonely and isolated. The literature on gender and migration of Asian Indian women is contradictory. Bhutani (1994), Rangaswamy (1996), and Rayaprol (1997) describe how immigration to the United States leads to greater empowerment and gender equity for women. Dasgupta and Dasgupta (1996) argue that in the process of developing institutions and establishing a positive ethnic and religious identity, Asian Indian women are more restricted and oppressed. Both sets of literature agree on the high levels of stress for women. In response to the need for culturally sensitive services for domestic violence victims, a number of shelters have been opened in major metropolitan centers with large Indian populations.

Asian Indians in need of social work support are most likely to come to the attention of professionals either through educational or health care systems. Service providers who are knowledgeable about Asian Indian religious and cultural beliefs are most effective with this population.

PRINCIPLES OF CULTURALLY APPROPRIATE PRACTICE

To work effectively with people from Asian Indian backgrounds, social workers not only need knowledge, understanding, and skills for culturally competent services but also an increased awareness of their own sociocultural backgrounds, assumptions, biases, values, and perspectives with regard to Asian Indian clients (Chandras, 1997). An understanding of the therapist's (in our case, school social worker's) feelings about his or her own social class, racial, ethnic, and religious characteristics, and points of convergence with or divergence from a patient (or client) is critical for therapeutic effectiveness (Windtrop & Harvey, 1981, p. 111). To increase the chances for successful interactions and a broadening of the use of services by Asian Indian clients, the culturally competent social worker needs to be sensitive and actively engaged in avoiding discrimination, prejudice, and stereotyping (Chandras, 1997).

Effective social work practice should include knowledge of the unique culture, history, values, and ethos that guide the Asian Indian community. An understanding and knowledge of the Asian Indian worldview enables the social worker to have a clearer understanding of the significance of certain life events over others and also engenders a psychological climate for barrier-free interaction with the client. Understanding the worldview serves as a reference guide for the social worker and enables him or her to attach appropriate meaning to the client's behavior. Specific elements of treatment intervention strategies (Tung, 1985) with Asian Indian clients include the following:

1. *Limiting the use of personal questions* during the intake interviews, because it may be threatening to Asian Indian clients. Asians Indians are not too verbal with strangers and maintain restraint with them. Thus, any disclosure on their part would require a level of comfort and trust that only comes with time.

2. *Orienting the client to the entire intervention program*, so that he or she accurately perceives the intervention process. Lambert and Lambert (1984) found that Asian immigrants who were better prepared saw their therapists as more interested and respectful, perceived more positive changes, and were satisfied with their adjustment.

3. *Focusing on the specific problem* of the client and helping him or her develop goals for the intervention.

4. *Acting as a mediator between the parents and the children*, such as when a teacher or concerned third party brings a child in for a presenting problem. After discussion with the youngster, parents are invited to discuss the youngster's presenting problem. The manner in which the social worker approaches the parents and presents the problem requires knowledge, understanding, and sensitivity to Asian Indian culture, specifically, in terms of roles, responsibilities, and decision making.

5. *Addressing the underlying problem* that may present as an academic or behavioral problem, there may be virtue in recognizing that, oftentimes, it may not be the school environment that is creating problems. The problem may originate in the family. The social worker needs to plot all the environmental concerns of the child to make an appropriate analysis of the problem and develop interventions.

The social worker needs to recognize that the child may experience an authoritarian environment at home. It is possible that the child may misguide or refrain from giving all information to the social worker for fear of punishment by the parent. Thus, the social worker has to earn the child's confidence and make him or her comfortable. Most often, adolescents create a protective cover around them and engage in a process of denial. They are particularly suspicious about any external help and may restrain themselves from accepting any help. The social worker has to apply special skills to help such a child, without disturbing the specific values and ethos of the Asian Indian family to which he or she belongs. There may be clients who have not discussed their problems with any other member of the family, or with anyone else from within the community. The client may perceive that any disclosure of his or her issues to other family members, or any other significant member of the community, may bring shame and dishonor to the family. Thus, involvement of the significant others may be undertaken only with the consent of the client. The following case vignette illustrates intervention by a social worker who effectively served a girl and her family.

CASE VIGNETTE

Lata, a 10th-grade, 16-year-old Asian Indian girl, does not like her name. Ever since she can remember, she has had to explain to her classmates what it means. She does not look or dress like her classmates. Her mother prefers to keep her hair long and plait it. According to her, school is for education and, as a student, it is preferable that Lata be as simple as possible. This is the way Lata's parents were brought up in India. Today, both her parents are very successful professionals. They believe that their success is based on "good Indian" upbringing and all the hard work they did when they were students. Lata, a very bright student, has done exceptionally well academically. She is part of the girls' basketball team and enjoys table tennis. However, Lata feels that her parents are too restrictive, and she reports having very few friends. Lata's teachers find her to be contented, well-adjusted, and generally obedient to both her parents and to authority figures.

For no apparent reason, Lata's grades started to deteriorate in the middle of 10th-grade. She shied away from any conversation, even with her parents, lost her appetite, and started to lose weight. Lata also stopped going to basketball practice and did not make the final team. The school social worker called Lata's parents and set up an appointment for all of them to visit the school to discuss Lata's social withdrawal and academic performance. Lata's parents felt ashamed that they had been called by the school social worker and told Lata a couple of times that they never thought that they would have to visit her school because of her grades. Nothing seemed to matter to Lata. She was interested only in sitting in her room and reading for hours on end.

The school social worker met the whole family on the assigned date.

The parents were very apologetic about Lata's failing grades. It appeared to the counselor that Lata's parents were only concerned about her academics and had little concern about issues that a teenager might face at school. They persistently directed the conversation toward how Lata needed to improve her grades and which career path she should choose. Lata was polite and maintained a pleasant disposition throughout the session but was reluctant to engage in the conversation. All efforts by the school social worker to involve Lata were unsuccessful. Lata's parents did most of the talking.

The next session involved only Lata. Though the school social worker informed Lata's parents about the session, they were not invited. She noted that although Lata's parents did not disapprove of the private session, they were somewhat uncomfortable. The school social worker explained to Lata's parents that she was concerned about Lata's emotional state, withdrawal from friends and family, as well as her deteriorating academic performance. Lata's parents reiterated that they loved their only child very much, had never neglected her, and would like her to do well in school.

The social worker was prepared with her notes before Lata came for the session. Lata seemed relatively relaxed but apprehensive. She resisted any personal conversation. The school social worker attempted to open up the conversation by asking, "Lata, I have heard that a lot of teenagers feel uncomfortable talking with their parents. Is that true for you?" The school social worker was careful to keep the conversation away from personal information. She was aware that in Asian Indian culture, adults act as guides, and Lata would not feel comfortable discussing intimate details. Lata relaxed considerably and slowly started talking about herself; she said that she could relate to some of the things that the social worker was talking about. It was hard for the social worker to understand how any 16-year-old could be so frightened of her parents. Lata's parents presented as being very open. They were successful professionals and had both earned graduate degrees in the United States. The social worker found Lata's fears of parental rejection unwarranted and decided to work with her in building up her confidence to face her parents and speak her mind. Lata's parents were informed of the session and were told that they possibly might need to return to the counselor's office for additional sessions. The counselor realized that Lata was reluctant to discuss such personal matters with her or her parents. It was also inappropriate to call Lata's parents and tell them what she had disclosed. There was a risk that Lata's parents might view the disclosure as a betrayal. The school social worker spent the next couple of sessions learning to understand Lata's family and cultural background. Because she was not aware of the child-rearing practices among Asian Indians, she tried to do some background reading. She was sensitive to the fact that though Lata presented as being more adjusted to the American way of life as a second-generation immigrant, her parents seemed to be deeply rooted in the Indian culture. The difficulty in communication between the parents and Lata was adding to the gap between the two generations in their acculturation process. The counselor was also trying to understand the larger community of Asian Indians that Lata's parents represented, along with the set standards of the community. Lata's parents were probably trying to fit into the shared mores and ethos of the Asian Indian culture. It was imperative that she become more knowledgeable about that culture.

During a later session, the school social worker approached the subject of support systems. She started by asking Lata questions about her relationships with friends, people at church, teachers, and relatives. Lata stated that she did not have any friends at school who would understand what she was going through. Additionally, her parents would be upset if she talked about her family with nonfamily members. She did not want to bring shame to her family. When asked if she had anyone with whom she felt comfortable talking, Lata mentioned her father's only sister, who lived very near. She said she had a warm relationship with her aunt and liked her very much. According to Lata, the aunt was close to the family and often socialized with her parents. The school social worker asked Lata if she had ever considered talking with her aunt about her problems. Lata said that she had thought about it but did not know how to approach her aunt. The school social worker advised Lata that they could work on how to approach her aunt and see whether they could reach a point where Lata felt more comfortable. After the next session, Lata felt ready to approach her aunt.

Lata's aunt came across as a warm and pleasant person. She openly communicated her concern for Lata's welfare and readily agreed to work with Lata and the school social worker. The session ended with Lata's aunt agreeing to intervene with her parents, without hurting their feelings or jeopardizing Lata's position at home. The combined session started out slowly. Lata was somewhat apprehensive, but after a few nervous moments, she started talking to her aunt. It had to do with a boy in her class from a different racial and religious background. She liked him and he reciprocated. How could she ever tell her parents? They would never approve of her liking a boy. She was also afraid that her parents would either send her back to India to live with her grandparents or become more restrictive if they found out that she was interested in an American boy. They wanted her to concentrate on her studies and go to a good college. Later on, when the time was right, they would find a suitable man for her to marry. But everyone she knew school had a boyfriend, and oftentimes she felt extremely left out and lonely. Lata had never had an open conversation with her parents, and her fear was that they would never understand this. Even when she started her menstrual cycle, all her mother told her was that she should stay away from boys. She felt that her parents were restrictive and would not allow her to grow up like her friends. Lata felt hopeless and lonely, and she found little meaning in her life. She confessed to her aunt that there were times when she felt like running away from home. Lata was rather uncomfortable after this self-disclosure and insisted that her parents should never know about her liking the boy.

The school social worker realized that she would have to learn more about the community, so that there would be a common ground where everyone could share concerns and exchange thoughts regarding Lata's welfare. She learned as much as she could about Lata's family structure, immediate and extended, both in the United States and India.

The school social worker assumed the role of facilitator during the sessions with Lata and her aunt. She was aware that any kind of cognitive restructuring would require a lengthy transitional phase to protect Lata's need to be in a nonthreatening environment. Thus, Lata, rather than hasten into any kind of confrontation with her parents, should allow her aunt to have some preliminary conversations with them. It was decided that Lata would approach her parents only after her aunt had set the stage. Lata's parents were informed about the sessions, but the content was kept confidential. There was tension within the family that had to be worked out. The parents were uncomfortable.

The school social worker set up a session with Lata, her aunt, and her parents. She prepared a detailed plan to assist Lata in openly speaking with her parents and decided to facilitate the session and provide input once Lata had completed her part. She started the session by exhibiting her awareness of Indian culture, along with those core issues associated with child-rearing practices among Asian Indians. Her familiarity with the Indian culture served to break down the barrier. Lata's parents responded in an open manner and slowly began to engage on a more personal level with Lata. The session ended on a positive note, with a commitment by Lata and her parents to continue to have open communication in which each would share their feelings and discuss personal issues.

Lata was asked to return after a few weeks to discuss her progress with her parents and her academic records. The social worker closed the case at the end of the semester, after reviewing Lata's improvement with her grades, and talking with her parents and teachers.

CONCLUSIONS

The rapidly increasing Asian Indian population in the United States has gradually created a sizable population that is experiencing stress and related mental health problems in the process of adaptation to American society. As the second and subsequent generations modify their culture and practices, cultural and intergenerational conflicts are likely to increase and intensify. By virtue of their minority racial and religious status, Asian Indians will continue to face sociopolitical oppression and related problems (Ramisetty-Mikler, 1993). These issues represent both an opportunity and a challenge in the delivery of social work services.

REFERENCES

Balgopal, P. R. (2000). *Social work practice with immigrants and refugees*. New York: Columbia University Press.

Bhattacharya, G. (1998). Drug use among Asian Indian adolescents: Identifying protective/risk factors. *Adolescence, 33*(129), 169–185.

Bhutani, S. (1994). *A study of Asian Indian women in the U.S.: The reconceptualization of self*. Unpublished doctoral dissertation, Department of Education, University of Pennsylvania, Philadelphia.

Chandras, K.V. (1997). Training multiculturally competent counselors to work effectively with Asian Indian Americans. *Counselor Education and Supervision, 37*(1), 50–60.

Dasgupta, S., & Dasgupta, S. D. (1996). Public face, private space: Asian Indian women and sexuality. In N. B. Maglin & D. Perry (Eds.), *Bad girls, good girls: Women, sex and power in the nineties* (pp. 226–243). New Brunswick, NJ: Rutgers University Press.

DeVos, G. (1980). Identity problems in migrant minorities: A psychocultural comparative approach applied to Korean and Japanese. In R. Bryce-Laporte (Ed.), *Sourcebook on the new immigration: Implications for the United States and the international community* (pp. 321–328). New Brunswick, NJ: Transaction.

Eck, D. (Ed.). (1997). *On common grounds: World religions in America* (CD-ROM). New York: Columbia University Press.

Eck, D. (2000). The Hindu experience in America. *Wilson Quarterly, 24*(3), 40–41.

English, R. (1984). *The challenge of mental health: Minorities and their worldviews*. Austin: Hogg Foundation of Mental Health, University of Texas.

Fenton, J. (1988). *Transplanting religious traditions: Asian Indians in America*. New York: Praeger.

Gawlick, M. (1997). Silicon Valley connections: Asian immigrants and sojourners: Adaptation strategies of second generation Asian Indians. *Journal of History and Computing Web Ring*. Retrieved October 2001 from *http://mcel.pacificu.edu/aspac/papers/scholars/Gawlick/gawlick.html*.

Kurien, P. (1999). Creating a Hindu Indian identity in the United States. *American Behavioral Scientist, 42*(4), 648–671.

History of Indians in the US. (2000). Retrieved October 2001 from *http://www.itihaas.com/independent/contrib3.html*.

Hurh, W., & Kim, K. (1984). *Korean immigrants in America: A structural analysis of ethnic confinement and adhesive adaptation*. Cranbury, NJ: Associated University Press.

India Abroad Center for Political Awareness. (1999). *The India Abroad Center for Political Awareness: Building a better America for future generations*. Retrieved October 2001 from *http://www.iacfpa.org*.

Indians in the USA—a success story. (2000). Retrieved October 2001 from *http:// www.cs.wisc.edu/~shubu/misc/indians-usa.html.*

Lambert, R., & Lambert, M. (1984). The effects of role preparation for psychothera- py on immigrant clients seeking mental health services in Hawaii. *Journal of Community Psychology, 12,* 263–275.

Mogelonsky, M. (1995). Asian Indian Americans. *American Demographics, 17*(8), 32–39.

Mohan, B. (1992). Trans-ethnic adolescence, confluence and conflict: An Asian In- dian paradox. In S. Furoto, R. Biswas, D. Chung, K. Murase, & F. Ross-Sheriff (Eds.), *Social work practice with Asian Americans* (pp. 189–201). Newbury Park, CA: Sage.

Project Impact. (2000). *Indian American community at a glance.* Available at Pro- ject Impact website: *http://www.project-impact.org/commResources/ pi_commResources_statistics.htm*

Ramisetty-Mikler, S. (1993). Asian Indian immigrants in America and sociocultural issues in counseling. *Journal of Multicultural Counseling and Development, 21*(1), 35–60.

Rangaswamy, P. (1996). *The imperative of choice and change: Post 1965 immigrants form India in metropolitan Chicago.* Unpublished doctoral dissertation, Depart- ment of History, University of Illinois, Chicago.

Rayaprol, A. (1997). *Negotiating identities: Women in the Indian diaspora.* Delhi, In- dia: Oxford University Press.

Roland, A. (1984). The self in India and America: Toward a psychoanalysis of social and cultural contexts. In V. Kavolis (Ed.), *Design of selfhood* (pp. 170–194). London: Associated University Press.

Roland, A. (1988). *In search of self in India and Japan: Toward a cross-cultural psy- chology.* Princeton, NJ: Princeton University Press.

Ross-Sheriff, F. (1992). Adaptation and integration into American society: Major is- sues affecting Asian Americans. In S. Furuto, R. Biswas, D. Chung, K. Murase, & F. Ross-Sheriff (Eds.), *Social work practice with Asian Americans* (pp. 27–44). Newbury Park, CA: Sage.

Saran, P. (1985). *The Asian Indian experience in the United States.* Cambridge, MA: Schenkman.

Sodowsky, G.R., & Carey, J. C. (1987). Asian Indian immigrants in America: Factors related to adjustment. *Journal of Multicultural Counseling and Development, 15*(3), 129–141.

Takaki, R. (1989). *Strangers from a different shore: A history of Asian Americans.* Boston: Little, Brown.

U.S. Department of Commerce, Economic and Statistics Administration. (1990). *Cen- sus of population: Asian and Pacific Islanders in the United States, CP 3-5.* Washington, DC: U.S. Government Printing Office.

U.S. Bureau of the Census. (2000). *The Asian and Pacific Islander population in the United States.* Washington, DC: U.S. Government Printing Office.

Williams, R. B. (1988). *Religions of immigrants from India and Pakistan.* New York: Cambridge University Press.

CHAPTER 9

South Asian Muslim Children and Families

FARIYAL ROSS-SHERIFF
ALTAF HUSAIN

Changes in immigration patterns during the last decade of the 20th century and the beginning of the 21st century have brought a new awareness of the religious diversity in America. Eck (1997) describes this diversity, as observed in the American landscape through Islamic *Masjids* (mosques), Hindu and Buddhist temples, *Sikh Gurudwaras* (temples), and related buildings in major cities all over the country. Though feared by some, this diversity is welcome as a source of strength by others. Americans are learning to affirm it and appreciate its potential (Unger, 1995). This chapter on the adaptation of South Asian Muslims to the United States (US) focuses on one of the major religious groups from Asia, namely, the Muslims.[1]

Muslim immigration to the United States has occurred over the last few centuries, but the largest numbers of Muslims immigrated to this country following the passage of the 1965 Immigration and Nationality Act (Nyang, 1998). Since then, Islam has become the fastest growing religion in the United States (Hadad, 1997; Mazrui, 1998). An estimated 6–10 million Muslims now call the United States their home (Nyang, 1998). Of these, 48% are a native-born population of African American Muslims. Two of the largest groups of Muslim immigrants are the South Asians, 24%, and the Arabs, 12% (Eck, 1997).

---

[1] "Muslim" refers to a person, whereas "Islam" is the religion.

The term "South Asian" is commonly used to refer to immigrants from countries such as Afghanistan, Bangladesh, Burma, India, Kashmir, Nepal, Pakistan, and Sri Lanka. Additionally, Pakistan, India, and Bangladesh are three of the five countries with the highest Muslim population in the world (see Table 9.1). Examination of Table 9.1 indicates that South Asia has the highest concentration of Muslims in the world. Among these countries, India and Pakistan have contributed the greatest numbers of immigrants to the United States.

Because South Asian Muslims trace most of their cultural norms and values to the advent of Islam in South Asia, they have a great deal in common. Thus, in this chapter, the term "South Asian Muslims" refers only to Muslim immigrants from India and Pakistan. Williams (1988) makes a similar case for the inclusion of only Indians and Pakistanis in a discussion on South Asians, noting that a majority of the South Asian population in the United States is from Pakistan and India. These two countries have a historical connection because they not only share a common border but also because Pakistanis lived as Indian Muslims under British rule until 1947.

HISTORICAL BACKGROUND

Tracing the flow of South Asian Muslim immigration to the United States is more complicated than that of their other Asian counterparts, such as Chinese, Filipinos, Japanese, and Koreans. For the most part, this complexity is rooted in confusion over how to classify South Asians generally, that is, the Indians and Pakistanis. The inherent diversity of South Asians stems from differences in their religions and in the color of their skin. At the turn of the 20th century, anthropologists in the United States recommended that Asian Indians be considered Euro Americans, owing to their Aryan ancestry. This classification might have been logical and acceptable for record keeping, but the reality of their dark skin did not "save Asian Indians from the rac-

TABLE 9.1. Top Five Countries with the Largest Muslim Population in the World

Country	Muslim population
[South Asia]	363,295,847
India	133,295,077
Pakistan	125,397,390
Bangladesh	104,603,380
Indonesia	196,281,020
China	133,100,545

Note. Source of data: *http://islamicweb/com* (1999).

ism of the anti-Asian movements of the first three decades of this (twentieth) century" (Fong, 1992, p. 11). In addition, there was considerable ignorance about the religious background of these early immigrants. Takaki (1989) notes that Americans referred to all Asian Indians as "Hindoos." This was an error, because the first arrivals were mostly Sikhs or Muslims from Punjab, a northwestern part of the Indian subcontinent. They eventually settled in California and worked on farms in the 1900s. Only a few considered themselves Hindu (Eck, 1997, Takaki, 1989).

Unlike their Chinese, Filipino, Japanese, and Korean cohorts of the same period, the South Asians applied for and were awarded citizenships based on their classification as Euro Americans (Fong, 1992). Between 1910 and 1920, a series of court decisions "ruled that, despite the Anthropologists' opinions, these were Asians and hence ineligible for citizenship"; furthermore, "some even had their citizenship revoked and were made stateless" (Fong, 1992, p. 12). A landmark ruling in 1923, *U.S. v. Bhagat Singh*, declared Asian Indians ineligible for naturalized citizenship. Finally, in 1924, the Immigration Act declared that "no one ineligible for citizenship may immigrate to the United States, thereby ending Asian immigration completely" (Nimmagadda and Balgopal, 2000, p. 32).

Although formal immigration was restricted, Muslim students from India and Pakistan entered the United States during the 1940s and 1950s, through cultural and scholarly exchange programs (Eck, 1997). Subsequent to the passage of the 1965 Immigration Act, even larger numbers of professionals and students entered the United States. Although many of the students returned home upon completion of their studies, a considerable number applied for a change of status from international students to permanent residents (Seth, 1995). Unlike the immigrants of the late 19th and first half of the 20th century, these immigrants generally came from urban settings in South Asian countries and were well educated (Das & Kemp, 1997). They took advantage of immigration legislation allowing them to sponsor their family members left behind in either India or Pakistan. Much of the immigration from India or Pakistan that occurred in the 1980s and 1990s was a result of family reunification, namely, naturalized citizens sponsoring their spouses and children, as well as their elderly parents and siblings, who in turn sponsored their own spouses and children (Balgopal, 2000). A profile of this later group indicates that not all were well educated and from urban areas.

DEMOGRAPHIC CHARACTERISTICS

Extrapolating from the Eck (1997) estimates, the total South Asian Muslim population in America ranges from 1.4 to 2.4 million, that is, 24% of the estimated 6–10 million Muslims (Ba-Yunus & Siddiqui, 1998). Although the census has a category available for Indians to identify themselves, there is no category for Pakistanis. They have the option of selecting the category "other," which groups them along with Bangladeshis, Burmese, and Sri Lankans (Nimmagadda and Balgopal, 2000, U.S. Bureau of the Census, 1992). There is no category for religious affiliation. This makes it difficult to estimate the exact number of South Asian Muslims in the United States. The largest group of South Asian Muslim immigrants who arrived during the second half of the 20th century did not follow an adaptation pattern similar to that of many of their Eastern European predecessors, who were uneducated and mostly farm workers. These South Asian Muslims are well educated and professional people. They have settled in suburbs around the United States. Today, high concentrations of South Asian Muslims can be found in six states, namely, California, Florida, Illinois, New Jersey, New York, and Texas.

As a group, South Asians who came after 1980, as a result of the family reunification laws and green card lottery, are different from their previous counterparts. There is a much greater chance that neither parent of these immigrant families speak English or have a college degree. Unlike their predecessors who arrived after 1965, these immigrants have not settled in suburbs but rather in neighborhoods with low-cost or public housing. There is a great likelihood that the children of these latest immigrants experience several challenges to their adaptation (discussed in a later section of this chapter).

Asian Indian and Pakistani Muslims demonstrate a linguistic diversity. Pakistan has four provincial languages, with Urdu as the national language. Indian languages are even more diverse, although the national language is Hindi, whose spoken form is understood with little difficulty by native Urdu speakers. Regardless of ethnic, cultural, or social diversity, or differences related to the time of immigration, one common factor among all Muslims is their religion and worldview prescribed by Islam. According to the normative teachings of Islam, the lives of Muslims are organized around their faith. "In Muslim communities religion is the structuring element of society which tends to integrate and harmonize all ethnic, cultural, racial, and linguistic particularities" (Azmi, 1997, p. 153). Muslims generally identify themselves by their religion, especially in communities where they are a minority group. For example, in a study of South Asian youth, Hutnik (1991) found that religion was the primary source of their identity, even before ethnicity, race, or national origin.

ISLAMIC WORLDVIEW

Muslims use the Arabic word *Allah* for God, which is the same term used by Christians in the Middle East. This term is used in the chapter. Although a comprehensive discussion of Islam and Islamic worldview is beyond the scope of this chapter, select critical concepts that would be helpful to social work practitioners are presented here.

The Islamic worldview enjoins mankind to live in peace, directs Muslims to do good, and forbids evil. *Allah*, the creator, has bestowed mankind with freedom to choose between leading a good or an evil life. An essential ingredient of a good life for a Muslim is to have *taqwa*, or a consciousness of *Allah* at all times, and a reminder to live within the guidelines provided by the *Quran* and the *sunna*, the teachings of the Prophet Mohamed. Because there is no universally accepted authority in Islam, the *Quran* and the *sunna* are subject to interpretation by a range of religious leaders and learned individuals. For example, Muslims who follow the *Sunni* interpretation of Islam rely on the interpretations of the scholars from the *Sunni* schools of thought. The *Shias* rely on the interpretation of their recognized religious authority. Various members of *Sufi* orders rely on their *Sheikhs*. Yet there is a unity in the diversity among the Muslim *tariqas* (sects).

Islam is a total way of life that includes economic, political, and social aspects. Islamic teaching does not accept the notions that dominate Western thinking about the separation of the secular from the religious. Muslim children and youth growing up in Western societies, such as America, experience stress because of the tensions that arise from conflicting values and mores of several cultures—the cultural values and expectations of significant adults in schools and social services (their teachers, counselors, etc.), the values of their culture of origin that they learn from their parents and extended family members, and the comprehensive normative teachings of Islam that they learn from their religious education teachers.

The cultures in which Muslims live are rich and diverse. According to Hamid (1996), this is "made possible by the fact that Islam's moral and legal code assures that everything is allowed unless it is prohibited, and not vice versa" (p. 124). It follows, then, that values of "local customs not in contradiction with any principle or law of Islam have been incorporated with ease in the cultures of the Muslim peoples" (p. 124). For South Asian Muslim immigrants to the United States, the resultant culture is a combination of the Islamic teaching, the culture of national origin, and the dominant American culture. Hence, South Asian Muslim children draw from at least four sets of values: (1) their family's culture; (2) the American society, as exhibited in the education system; (3) their peers and mass media; and (4) the teachings of Islam, which are considered the most important. There is likely to be more stress for families when the values that the children draw from the family culture are in conflict with the teachings of Islam.

Among the core values and concepts of Islam that have been articulated for South Asian Muslims are "*shariat* and *adab* (proper behavior in its plural form, rules or codes for behavior)" (Ewing, 1988, p. 5). Metcalf (1984), in her book *Moral Conduct and Authority: The Place of Adab in*

South Asian Islam, identifies *Adab* as the central key concept that encompasses a code of behavior for different individuals, which is described as "a concept of the well-constructed life, the harmonious life of a person who knows his relationship to God, to others, and to himself, and who, as a result plays a special role among his or her fellows" (p. vii). In South Asian Islam, "*Adab* means discipline and training. It denotes good breeding and refinement that results from training, so that a person who behaves badly is "without *adab* (*bey adab*)" (p. 5). *Adab* means etiquette, proper deportment that parents teach and expect their children to include in their daily life. The understanding of *Adab* also assumes that Muslims are capable of spiritual discipline, not only the correct outer behavior but also inner behavior. The *adab* for South Asian Muslims in America means seeking and learning to behave as Muslims, while at the same time internalizing the *sharia*, the concept of the right way in Islam, embodied in the divinely established body of law and code of conduct defined by the *Quran* and *sunna*. In the socialization process, parents train their children to be aware of their behaviors and expect deliberate and self-conscious efforts to live within the ethics of Islam.

Chung (1992) presents a number of character traits that are common to most people of Asian origin, including the South Asian Muslims. These traits are: self-control and restraint in emotional expression, respect for authority, well-defined social roles and expectations, awareness of social milieu, communal responsibility, high regard for the elderly, and the centrality of family relationships and responsibility. The expressions of grief, depression, and anger are not exhibited, even though they may be experienced.

Within the family context, the rights and responsibilities of each member are defined. For Muslims, the family bond is founded on mutual expectations of rights and obligations for every member of the family. Islam emphasizes a cooperative approach with regard to family cohesion. Each member is expected to contribute toward the overall family welfare, using his or her individual resources and incomes (Abd al Ati, 1977). Marriage is not only a formal contractual commitment between a husband and wife but also an informal commitment between the family members of each partner to help maintain and sustain the union. Islam charges the parents with the duty to "cherish and sustain their children, educate and train them" (Hamid, 1996, p. 73). Similarly, grown children are charged with the responsibility of looking after their parents. For Muslim immigrants, a strong family bond is essential to a successful adaptation experience.

Within the context of parent–child relationship, the dominant American culture encourages self-sufficiency, independence, and freely expressing oneself. The Islamic culture, on the other hand, calls on children to withhold outward expression of their feelings in deference to the wishes of the parents (Daneshpour, 1998, Haddad & Lummis, 1987, Hamid, 1996).

Muslim children, and even young adults, wishing to explore the dominant culture are caught between the old and the new, the traditional and the nontraditional, and the parents' wish to perpetuate Islamic norms. When children and youth are not able to navigate between conflicting expectations, mental health consequences may arise.

PROBLEMS FOR CHILDREN AND FAMILIES

South Asian Muslim families face challenges in the process of adapting to the American society at three levels—first as immigrants, second as immigrants from an Eastern society (i.e., Asia) and third as a religious minority in America. All immigrants experience the stresses and trauma associated with displacement and dislocation from their familiar social and cultural milieu. Immigrants from cultural, language, and social backgrounds that are different from those of the society of origin experience higher levels of stress than those who come to societies with similar background characteristics (Cox, 1983). Many Muslim immigrant families from Asia not only experience the stresses arising from migration but also differences arising from the norms of their culture of origin that are in some areas antithetical to the prevailing norms of the American society and institutions. Families from rural backgrounds with limited English-language skills, resources, and social supports have the most difficulty adjusting to life in America.

Certain groups of South Asian immigrants experience additional challenges and higher levels of stress based on (1) family characteristics, such as the parents' difficult work situation or extended family with grandparents; (2) low level of exposure to Western culture and the English language in their countries of origin; (3) limited skills and abilities to navigate the American culture and guide their children as they manage differences with significant people in their children's lives, such as teachers and peers; (4) insufficient family resources in the United States and a low level of comfort with the American way of life; and (5) lack of social support through Muslim and ethnic community organizations.

Children and parents experience stress in the process of becoming oriented to the larger American society. Whereas a majority of South Asian Muslim immigrants are well versed in English and well educated, a small percentage, especially women have little or limited English-language skills. When available, the parents might participate in formal orientation programs that range from English as a second language (ESL) classes at the local high school to parenting skills seminars at a community center in the neighborhood. On the other hand, through the school system, the children are enrolled in a formal socialization process. Here, the children are taught English and are directly exposed to the larger American culture through various programs and activities sponsored by the school. On the weekends, parents and their children may attend the local *masjid*, or Islamic center, where they are exposed to Islam, as well as their own culture of origin, through interactions with other Muslim immigrants from South Asia. Problems arise when the parents insist that the children should hold on to their culture of origin, be it Pakistani or Indian. The children, however, have more exposure to the larger American culture, as well as the ethics and practices of Islam, than to their culture of origin. They are caught in the middle, trying to learn the new American culture, retain what they know of their culture of origin, and practice what they can of the rites, rituals, and ethics of Islam (Mattson, 2000).

Specific problems arise around the celebration of holidays. The parents insist on celebrating holidays of cultural and religious significance, whereas the children cannot understand why they are not allowed to participate in the celebrations of American holidays such as Halloween, Thanksgiving, and Mother's and Father's Day. In addition, Muslim children often feel alienated in school because of the emphasis in class activities and projects on themes related to Christian holidays such as Easter, St. Patrick's Day, and Christmas. Muslim parents find it difficult to restrict their children's participation in holidays that have either Judeo-Christian or pagan origins and receive prominence in shopping mall displays, television programs, and the construction of arts and crafts in schools. Even when the parents try to make the Muslim holidays of *Eid ul Fitr* and *Eid ul Adha*[2] joyful and special occasions, the children realize that the dominant American society makes no mention of these holidays in the calendars: There are no special Ramadan sales and little or no mention of the celebrations in the media. To a certain degree, the high level of commercialism associated with various American holidays makes it difficult for parents not to get caught up in buying gifts for their children, thereby implicitly giving the holidays some significance. This debate around the celebration of holidays may have a negative impact on the parent–child relationship in some families, in which the parents are perceived as restricting their children from full participation in the larger American culture.

Family Structure

The immigrant family structure is another source of challenges. Within this discussion, two main issues deserve attention: mothers working or not working outside the home and the impact of grandparents living with the family. The economic situation may necessitate both parents working

---

[2] *Eid* (Arabic for day); *Eid ul Fitr* is celebrated at the culmination of *Ramadan*, the month of fasting; *Eid ul Adha* is celebrated on the 10th day of the *Dhul Hijja*, the month of the pilgrimage.

outside the home. Whereas some children who are accustomed to always having someone at home face difficulty coming home to an empty house, others may have a difficult time accepting that their mother is at home full-time and has no career outside the home. This latter arrangement may be difficult for young girls who may be starting to think about possible career choices, and could result in young women's lack of respect for their mothers' choice to stay home.

Then, there is the challenge of the grandparents living with the family. Immigrants who entered the United States in the late 1980s and 1990s availed themselves of the opportunity to sponsor their parents' migration to the United States under the family reunification portion of the immigration laws. Following both South Asian cultural tradition and Islamic injunctions to care for and respect one's parents, the sponsoring couples often arrange for their parents to live with them in their house. This arrangement poses several challenges. Living in crowded conditions may create stressful situations and have an adverse impact on intergenerational relationships. Although grandparents may be a source of support, their continuing presence may create intergenerational tensions within the family. The grandparents do serve two important functions, in that they help to transmit the culture and the language of origin to their grandchildren. Whereas parents might appreciate these functions, the children might shun insistence on the culture of origin, claiming it is old-fashioned or backward.

Peer Relations

The immigrant family faces challenges in the area of peer relations when trying to reconcile the perceptions and realities of practicing Islam in the US (Barazangi, 1996). Two areas of concern are the choice of friends and leisure-time activities. First, through their interactions with children their own age in the neighborhood, at school, and at the masjid, the immigrant children are making friends. From the parent's perspective, the difficulty arises when these friends are of a different gender, ethnicity, and culture. To preserve their culture of origin, South Asian Muslim parents often prefer that their children befriend other South Asian immigrant children and that the friends be from the same South Asian country.

Another common concern relates to religion. South Asian Muslim families show a preference for having their children befriend other Muslim children. Again, the degree of preference for same-religion over same-ethnic or -national background varies, but, in general, it seems that religion outweighs the consideration of friends from similar backgrounds.

Muslim immigrant families deal with stresses associated with finding appropriate entertainment and amusement for their children. Two issues emerge in the discussion of leisure time activities, namely, the nature of these activities vis-à-vis interaction among genders, and whether there should be adult or parental supervision. Reconciling or choosing what is acceptable in Islam and the culture of origin with the age-appropriate behaviors in the American tradition places a strain on family relationships.

Education and Career Choice

Children of immigrant families often experience stress when dealing with their parents in matters of education and career choices. Immigrant parents place a great deal of emphasis on education and high income for themselves and their children, and indicate access to quality education as a major reason for their decision to immigrate. The children are under pressure to choose a high-ranking college or university and to select careers in engineering, law, and medicine. For some families in which the home environment is not well equipped to prepare the child adequately for higher educational requirements, the child becomes distressed. On the other hand, pressure on the family to become financially secure may put a burden on the child and necessitate his or her working in the family business or at least some part-time employment while in high school or college.

Choosing a major can often be a source of strain between parents and children. Entering professions such as law or medicine normally requires that individuals declare their intention early and enroll in courses that will fulfill the law or medicine prerequisites. Failure to do so increases the risk of students having to spend more time at the university making up the coursework, thereby both increasing the financial burden on the family and delaying their ability to be wage earners.

Parents who were unable to pursue a certain career because of a lack of resources may exert pressure on their children to excel academically and accept the parents' choice of careers. Children may also be pressured to maintain a long-standing family tradition to pursue careers in certain fields. An immigrant child might be told repeatedly that all of his or her ancestors have been engineers, for example, and that this tradition must be upheld. Finally, parents also push their children into entering high-paying, high-profile careers as a means of securing a high income, with the assumption that more income equates to a higher quality of life. Children who want to pursue careers in social science or fine arts may face an uphill battle with their parents, because these careers are seen as low paying and are not given as much esteem.

MUSLIM AND ETHNIC COMMUNITY RESPONSE

South Asian Muslims have taken considerable advantage of the Constitutional guarantees of free speech and freedom of religion. It is worthwhile to note that in the last 4 decades, since the largest numbers of South Asian

Muslims entered the United States, a very strong religioethnic infrastructure has emerged. Earlier Muslim immigrants from Palestine, Lebanon, Syria, and Yemen established *masjids* (mosques) that served as "community centers, bringing people together for prayer, religious instruction, marriages, and funerals and for general activities such as dinners and bake sales" (Abu-Laban, 1991, p. 15). It was not uncommon to find that each *masjid*, while serving mainly as a house of worship, sponsored programs and activities geared toward a particular culture or ethnicity.

Since the passage of the 1965 Immigration Act, the Muslim population has increased substantially and become more diverse. Nyang (1999) has documented the evolution in the United States of formal and informal institution-building efforts at local and national levels, aimed at providing support services for both indigenous and immigrant Muslims. These include social and cultural groups at local *masjids*, youth summer camps organized at regional levels, and chapters of Muslim student associations at a large number of universities around the country. At local levels, support services for immigrant Muslims are intended to facilitate their successful adaptation to life in America, while maintaining their religious and cultural heritage. They focus on helping newcomers find employment, providing information on the quality of neighborhoods and schools, stressing the importance of religious education, and making referrals and recommendations for housing and medical services. At the regional and national levels, these organizations bring youth and young adults together to develop normative Islamic knowledge and practice, and provide support to foster Muslim identity.

PRINCIPLES OF CULTURALLY APPROPRIATE PRACTICE

Practitioners serving South Asian Muslim clients, in addition to helping clients, should attempt to understand their religious and cultural beliefs. The practitioner is reminded about the diversity among the Muslim populations and awareness of specific Muslim *tariqa* (sect) and the cultural practices related to the country of origin. Although social work practitioners are not expected to be totally knowledgeable about Islam, they may learn a great deal by listening to clients and trying to understand their worldview.

South Asian Muslims reflect interaction patterns of both the larger Asian population and those specific to an Islamic worldview. Cross-gender interaction is highly regulated out of respect and a concern for modesty. With regard to the interaction distance, an appropriate rule of thumb for Muslims is also what Chung (1992) has suggested for Asians, namely, that the social worker should "sit first and allow the Asian client to set the interaction distance" (p. 37).

In the South Asian Muslim culture, it is not uncommon for people to communicate without establishing direct eye contact. This phenomenon is even more obvious in relationships of power, for example, in the case of the practitioner and the client, or between a male and a female. Out of deference for the practitioner's expertise, the client may shy away from direct eye contact. Chung (1992) notes that "avoidance of eye contact between persons of higher social status is an Asian cultural norm and should not be misunderstood to indicate dishonesty or lack of confidence" (p. 36).

Along with active listening and prompting, social workers are trained to be deliberate in their communications with clients. In the case of the South Asian Muslim client, the practitioner must take extraordinary measures to keep the assessment phase as comprehensive as possible (Ross-Sheriff & Husain, 2000). In addition, "active listening and prompting require careful planning so that the worker does not interject personal biases or responses that reflect puzzlement or acceptance based on personal worldview" (Ross-Sheriff & Husain, 2000, p. 85). For example, in the literature, one of the stereotypes of Muslims is that they have a fatalistic worldview; that is, a client may not do her best to improve her condition because, according to the stereotype, the condition exists by the will of Allah; therefore, only Allah can improve that condition. Muslims do believe that everything happens by the will of Allah, but this does not preclude the individual Muslim from taking responsibility for his or her condition (Abd al Ati, 1977).

Muslims are exhorted to persist in improving their own condition through planned efforts and, ultimately, to leave the outcome of their efforts to Allah. Given an assignment by the practitioner, the clients might commonly utter expressions such as *insha'allah*, which in Arabic means "Allah-willing." The expression *insha'allah* connotes a sense of hope that the client's efforts will meet with success by the will of Allah. It is important for practitioners to take this into consideration in interpreting their client's responses and in adapting the service delivery methods to the social norms of their clients.

Involvement of family members may be helpful at certain stages during the service delivery, so that parents and siblings might serve to mitigate challenges faced by the client and facilitate the resolution. The following case vignette illustrates the challenges faced by South Asian youth and their families.

CASE VIGNETTE

Ali, a 16-year-old from Karachi, Pakistan, has been in the United States since 1995. His father, a high school graduate from Pakistan, migrated to the United States in 1993, worked hard to save money, and sponsored Ali, his mother, and his younger sister Jameela. Since his arrival in the United States, Ali has attended a public school, along with Jameela. His father owns a gas station and works 13–15 hours a day, 7 days a week. His mother stays at home; she did not finish high school and speaks very little English. Ali's mother hesitated to come to the United States, because she did not want to raise her children here. Now that she is here, she desires that both Ali and Jameela speak only Punjabi at home, and that they retain as much of their culture as possible. Ali's mother's knowledge of religious obligations is primarily based on what was transmitted orally by her family and other close relatives. His father, who believes that he is fulfilling his role as a provider by working extremely hard to save for his children's education, entrusts his children's upbringing and education to his wife. His work schedule leaves him little time for direct involvement with his children other than serving as the disciplinarian.

Ever since their arrival in the United States, Ali and Jameela have been struggling with the feeling that they will not really be accepted by other American youth. On the one hand, Ali wanted friends and eagerly tried to fit in, using bits and pieces of conversations of other youth that he had overheard. He found himself saying that he liked activities such as listening to music, going out to the movies, and even "partying" on Friday nights. Ali always felt uncomfortable speaking about things of which he had no knowledge, but in this case, he sensed that his non-Muslim friends were beginning to warm up to him because he was "just like them."

Onset of the Problem

Now, in the first half of his senior year in high school, Ali's academic performance has deteriorated. He seems withdrawn in the classroom. He has missed assignments in three out of five classes. The summer before his senior year, Ali became intensely concerned about his family's financial struggle in the United States. Ali and Jameela attended a camp for Muslim youth in July. They were both anxious, because their mother had told them not to get too close to those "American" youth. By "American," she was referring to American-born Muslim youth who did not speak Punjabi as a second language. Their mother often referred to the Muslim American children as being ill-mannered, having little respect for elders; in general, she cautioned her own children not to befriend such children.

To their surprise, at the camp, Ali and Jameela found Muslim youth who, despite being born and raised in America, had a very strong attachment to Islam. Even the Pakistani youth spoke fluent, accentless English and could understand only a little Punjabi. To Ali and Jameela, that scarcely seemed important at a camp, where the participants' first language was English and their native languages ranged from Farsi (Iran and Afghanistan) to Arabic (Middle East and North Africa) to Swahili (East Africa). Ali was especially pleased to hear the hopes and aspirations of some of the youth. He found them talking about their agenda for the future of Islam in America. Their goal was to use their respective future professions to contribute to the development of the Muslim community in America. Some shared their plans to become professionals in the fields of medicine, engineering, and law, whereas others spoke about becoming teachers and social workers. They spoke about practicing a balanced life, as prescribed by Islam.

Ali left the camp with a renewed sense of hope about what he would do in his own life. He realized that he had been wrong to think of the "American" Muslims as being farther away from Islam or being ill-mannered in their behavior. On the contrary, they seemed to link their identity directly with Islam. They treated each other with kindness and welcomed Ali and his sister Jameela without hesitation or ridicule, despite their accented English. Ali had approached his school social worker at the beginning of the fall term about his excitement in finding other Muslim friends at the summer camp and his desire to get a degree in social work. Eight weeks later, the counselor noted that Ali was quiet and did not respond to her attempts to reach him.

Assessment

Noticing Ali's decreased interest in studies and declining grades at the end of the fall semester, one of Ali's teachers referred him to the school social worker. She told Ali that it might help him to talk about his feelings. Ali was quite nervous about going to the social worker. He was embarrassed to talk to the woman with whom he had shared his excitement about finding other Muslim friends at the summer camp. Mrs. Y, the school social worker, welcomed Ali and set up an appointment for the following week after class.

Ali reported to Mrs. Y's office as scheduled but did not want to talk to her. Mrs. Y tried in vain to explore various areas of Ali's life. Ali responded to most of the questions with a simple nod of the head, sometimes mumbled "yes" or "no," but never really elaborated on any of the questions posed by Mrs. Y. Exercising restraint despite feeling frustrated with Ali's lack of communication, Mrs. Y scheduled another appointment for the following week. She wrote down questions that she had asked during the session and requested that Ali think about them and come back the following week. Mrs. Y told Ali that all of their conversations would be held in confidence. The promise of confidentiality did not lessen Ali's uneasiness to talk to a stranger about his problems.

Ali left school and came home much later than Jameela. He was ashamed to tell either Jameela or his mother that he had been referred to the social worker's office. His mother asked why Ali was late, and he said only that he was talking to a friend, without giving much more details. His mother reprimanded him, saying that she did not want him to stay behind after classes, and that he was to come straight home.

During the week, Ali thought about Mrs. Y's questions. What would he tell her about his father or mother, his culture and religion? Would Mrs. Y even understand what Ali was feeling? Even if she did, how could she help? At first, Ali had taken offense at some of Mrs. Y's questions. How could she think that Ali's problems stemmed from a relationship with a girl or involved exploring drugs or alcohol? Did she not know that those types of behavior were forbidden in Islam? If Mrs. Y did not know such basic aspects of Islam, how could Ali confide in her that part of his problems stemmed from his parents not being practicing Muslims?

Ali remembered back to the camp, when the other youth had talked about their interactions with teachers and counselors who knew little about Islam. He realized that he could help Mrs. Y become familiar with Islam, so that perhaps she could then help Ali with the school-related aspects of the problem.

Ali sat down and wrote out his answers. He had started not to care about college; though his family wanted him to get a professional degree, they did not understand or appreciate his interest in becoming a counselor. They had migrated in search of a better life for the whole family, and tradition held that as the oldest and, in his case; only the son, Ali would replace his aging father someday as the provider for the family. Ali's going to college to become a counselor would be a setback for his family. They could not afford the tuition expenses, four years of college would mean that Ali's family would have to make great sacrifices. Ali hated the idea of either spending the rest of his life dispensing gasoline and selling snacks at his father's gas station or having to get a degree in a profession just for money or prestige. Whenever he tried to talk to his father about his aspirations of becoming a counselor, Ali was told that his family had not migrated to America so that he could waste time studying trivial subjects. He was confused.

In addition, his family's emphasis on cultural Islam meant that Ali's life would be relegated to living as a Pakistani Muslim in America rather than living life like the confident Muslim American youth he had met at the camp. Ali was having difficulty trying to implement what he was teaching himself about Islam, because his own mother would not allow it. She thought he was being influenced by a more modern version of Islam and scolded him for adopting "American Islam." In reality, Ali was learning for the first time the teachings of Islam from teachers whom he considered scholarly. Unable either to practice his religion without cultural oversight or to pursue his desire to become a counselor, Ali found himself retreating from life more and more. Ali wrote about his difficulty with his family, his personal interests, and his feelings of helplessness.

Intervention

Ali felt much better having written out his answers and, in his excitement, even showed up 15 minutes early for his appointment with Mrs. Y. During the session, he found that the social worker not only appreciated his thoughtful responses to her questions but also offered to work with him on achieving his goals. She worked with him for the rest of the semester, guiding him with the challenges of pursuing his academic interests and his desire to continue learning more about his religion, while managing his differences with his parents.

CONCLUSIONS

Recent news reports indicate that Muslims in the United States are experiencing backlash and recrimination stemming from the September 11, 2001, attacks on the World Trade Center and the Pentagon. Although the 19 hijackers were allegedly Muslims of Middle Eastern origin, Muslims in the United States, both non-citizens and U.S. citizens of various national origins, races and ethnicity, have been targeted for profiling by government authorities. The number of hate crimes against Muslims has increased substantially (Council on American-Islamic Relations, 2002). South Asian non-citizens and U.S. citizens have become vulnerable to "verbal abuse, suspicious glances and in a small minority of cases, physical assault" and murder (Malik & Melwani, 2001). The South Asian victims of hate crimes have been of varied ethnicity and religious background. Various houses of worship, such as *masjids*, Hindu and Buddhist temples, and Sikh *Gurudwaras*, have received bomb threats and have had their property damaged by Molotov cocktails and graffiti (Malik & Melwani, 2001). Balbir Singh Sodhi, a South Asian adherent of the Sikh religion, was shot to death in Mesa, Arizona, because his assailant, who called himself a "patriot," mistakenly identified Sodhi's turban and beard with those of the followers of Osama Bin Laden. Rafiq Mohammed Butt, a Pakistani national who was detained in secret as a part of the indiscriminate round-up of Muslim men of "special interest" to the United States government, died of cardiac complications in the Hudson County Jail because he did not receive timely medical attention (Edwards, 2002). Bar Javad, a 30-year-old Pakistani national, was questioned and strip-searched by American Airlines employees on his way back to the United States from Pakistan via London (Robbins, 2001).

Notwithstanding the substantial rise in recent hate crimes misdirected at South Asian Muslims, there have been encouraging signs from some Americans affirming and appreciating the presence of Muslims in America. Despite their nearly four-decade-long existence in the United States, many South Asian Muslims do not feel fully accepted by the larger American society and feel they are treated as the "other." Today, more than ever, social work practitioners working with South Asian Muslim clients need to be aware of their demographic characteristics, history of migration, Islamic worldview, and various problems and challenges.

Practitioners need to acquire sufficient information to work effectively with Muslim clients. Given the overarching role that Islam plays in the life of a South Asian Muslim immigrant, the practitioner should strive to understand each client's worldview. One of the key elements of working with clients of this background is to explore their identity and their decision-making system. Which aspect of the multifaceted identity of a South Asian Muslim client is dominant? Is it the Islamic identity? Is it the culture of origin? Is it the family culture? Is it the culture of the South Asian family that has integrated into the American society? In terms of their decision-making system, which sphere of their worldview takes precedence or priority in helping them reach a decision? For example, does the client refer often to the Islamic view of the presenting problem? Does the client refer to "back home" or "our culture?" Or is the reference to "in our family?" Faced with a decision, which of these spheres takes priority and most likely influences the client's final choice of action?

Equally important is the practitioner's understanding of the client's religious, cultural, psychohistorical, and socioeconomic context. Depending on the level of rapport that is established between the practitioner and the client, eliciting helpful information about these various contexts should be a practice priority. A contextual understanding of the client also facilitates the acknowledgment and appreciation of the presenting problem as being multidimensional in nature.

In choosing appropriate models of social work practice with this population, practitioners should familiarize themselves with models that are culturally sensitive and consistent with essential Islamic beliefs concerning the afterlife, a trust in Allah as the ultimate source of healing, reliance on prayer as a part of the intervention, sanctity of life, family preservation, a collective versus individual identity, gender equity, and so on. The practitioner must realize that many Muslims do not separate religious life into the public and the private realms. Counseling approaches that are grounded in and do not depart from the Islamic law "would be infused with an ultimate concern with 'after life' consequences and might include forms of mediation, religious and spiritual invocation, pronouncement of guilt, and determination of acts of repentance and/or forms of punishment" (Azmi, 1999, p. 150).

Social work practice with South Asian Muslim immigrants is a challenge and an opportunity for growth of both the practitioner and the client. Members of this immigrant group have faced prejudice and racism because of their dark color and religious beliefs. The September 11, 2001, terrorist attacks make it more likely that, due to the backlash, these immigrants face an increased need for counseling and social work intervention to help them deal with their intense feelings of confusion, anxiety, grief, sadness, and depression. With their loyalty to America in question and having been falsely perceived as supporters of terrorism, it is likely that South Asian Muslim immigrants will need to seek help. The challenge, then, for managers and practitioners at social service agencies is to promote staff development in the area of cultural sensitivity and awareness of basic Islamic beliefs, as well as increase outreach among this population by hiring translators and South Asian Muslim community workers.

Overall, the helping relationship affords a tremendous opportunity for growth of both the practitioner and the South Asian Muslim client. By familiarizing themselves with South Asian Muslims' demographic characteristics, migration history, and Islamic worldview, practitioners will be better prepared to help their clients address the various problems and issues that South Asian Muslim immigrants face. In addition, in an atmosphere of mutual respect, cultural sensitivity, and, most importantly, an appreciation for Islamic beliefs, the client will also experience personal growth in seeking help from a non-Muslim, non–South Asian practitioner.

ACKNOWLEDGMENTS

Our special appreciation to Gail Desmond, MSW, of Howard University, and Ali Asani, PhD, of Harvard University for their critical comments in reviewing and editing this chapter.

REFERENCES

Abd al Ati, H. (1977). *The family structure in Islam.* Indianapolis, IN: American Trust Publications.

Abu-Laban, S. M. (1991). Family and religion among Muslim immigrants and their descendants. In E. H. Waugh, S. M. Abu-Laban, & R. B. Qureshi (Eds.), *Muslim families in North America* (pp. 6–31). Edmonton, Alberta: University of Alberta Press.

Azmi, S. H. (1997). Canadian social service provision and the Muslim community in metropolitan Toronto. *Journal of Muslim Minority Affairs, 17*(1), 153–166.

Azmi, S. H. (1999). A qualitative sociological approach to address issues of diversity for social work. *Journal of Multicultural Social Work, 7*(3/4), 147–164.

Barazangi, N. H. (1996). Parents and youth: Perceiving and practicing Islam in North America. In B. C. Aswad & B. Bilge (Eds.), *Family and gender among American Muslims: Issues facing Middle Eastern immigrants and their descendants* (pp. 129–142). Philadelphia: Temple University Press.

Ba-Yunus, I., & Siddiqui, M. M. (1998). *A report on Muslim population in the United*

States of America. New York: Center for American Muslim Research and Information.

Balgopal, P. A. (2000). Social work practice with immigrants and refugees: An overview. In P. A. Balgopal (Ed.), *Social work practice with immigrants and refugees* (pp. 1–29). New York: Columbia University Press.

Chung, D. K. (1992). Asian cultural commonalities: A comparison with mainstream American culture. In S. M. Furuto, R. Biswas, D. K. Chung, K. Murase, & F. Ross-Sheriff (Eds.), *Social work practice with Asian Americans* (pp. 27–44). Newbury Park, CA: Sage.

Council on American–Islamic Relations. (2002). *The status of Muslim civil rights in the United States 2002: Stereotypes and civil liberties*. Washington, DC: CAIR Research Center. Available at: *http://www.cair-net.org*

Cox, D. R. (1983). Religion and the welfare of immigrants. *Australian Social Work*, 36(1), 3–10.

Daneshpour, M. (1998). Muslim families and family therapy. *Journal of Marital and Family Therapy*, 24(3), 355–368.

Das, A. K., & Kemp, S. F. (1997). Between two worlds: Counseling South Asian Americans. *Journal of Multicultural Counseling and Development*, 25, 23–34.

Eck, D. L. (1997). *On common ground: World religions in America*. New York: Columbia University Press.

Edwards, J. (2002, August 26). Detainee's death blamed on lack of medical care: Jail rejects account. *New Jersey Law Journal*, 169, p. 800.

Ewing, K. (1988). *Shariat and ambiguity in South Asian Islam*. Berkeley: University of California Press.

Fong, R. (1992). A history of Asian American adaptation. In S. Furuto, R. Biswas, D. Chung, K. Murase, and F. Ross-Sheriff (Eds.), *Social work practice with Asian Americans* (pp. 3–26). Newbury Park, CA: Sage.

Haddad, Y. Y. (1997). A century of Islam in America. *Hamdard Islamicus*, 21(4), 1–12.

Haddad, Y. Y., & Lummis, A. T. (1987). *Islamic values in the United States*. New York: Oxford University Press.

Hamid, A. (1996). *Islam the natural way*. London: Muslim Educational and Literary Services.

Hutnik, N. (1991). *Ethnic minority identity: A social psychological perspective*. New York: Clarendon Press.

Malik, A., & Melwani, L. (2001, October 1). The backlash: Hope in the time of despair. *India Today*, p. 46.

Mattson, I. M. (2000, May 11–12). *To be resisted, embraced, or transformed: What America represents to Muslims*. Presentation at the Conference on Immigration and Religious Life in America, Georgetown University, Washington, DC.

Mazrui, A. A. (1998). Globalization, Islam and the West: Between homogenization and hegemonization. *American Journal of Islamic Social Sciences*, 15(3), 1–14.

Metcalf, B. (1984). *Moral conduct and authority: The place of Adab in South Asian Islam*. Berkeley: University of California Press.

Nimmagadda, J., & Balgopal, P. R. (2000). Social work practice with Asian immigrants. In P. R. Balgopal (Ed.), *Social work practice with immigrants and refugees* (pp. 30–64). New York: Columbia University Press.

Nyang, S. (1998). Islam in America: A historical perspective. *American Muslim Quarterly*, 2(1), 7–38.

Nyang, S. (1999). *Islam in United States of America*. Chicago: Kazi.

Robbins, M. A. (2001). Lawyers worry that authorities infringe on rights of Muslims, Arabs. *Texas Lawyer, 17*(30), p. 1.

Ross-Sheriff, F., & Husain, A. (2000). Values and ethics in social work practice with Asian Americans. In R. Fong & S. Furuto (Eds.), *Culturally competent practice: Skills, interventions and evaluations* (pp. 75–88). Boston: Allyn & Bacon.

Seth, M. (1995). Asian Indian Americans. In P. G. Min (Ed.), *Asian Americans: Contemporary trends and issues* (pp. 169–198). Thousand Oaks, CA: Sage.

Takaki, R. (1989). *Strangers from a different shore: A history of Asian Americans*. Boston: Little, Brown.

Unger, S. (1995). *Fresh blood: The new American immigrants*. Urbana and Chicago: University of Illinois Press.

U.S. Bureau of the Census. (1992). *1990 census of the population—General population characteristics*. Washington, DC: U.S. Government Printing Press.

Williams, R. B. (1988). *Religions of immigrants from India and Pakistan*. New York: Cambridge University Press.

CHAPTER 10

Latino Children and Families

MARIA ZUNIGA

The March 2001 U.S. Bureau of the Census initial report took demographers by surprise. Projections about the growth of the Latino population were dramatically smaller than the data count revealed. Latinos had reached approximately the same population size as the African American population. Latinos constitute about 12% of the U.S. population, or an estimated 35.5 million compared to 34.2 million African Americans. This has profound cultural and policy implications, (Cohn & Fears, 2001). It also raises a major challenge to social workers to be prepared to address the service needs of this group, with all its heterogeneity.

One of the major contributions to this growth is documented and undocumented immigration of Latinos, especially from Mexico. In the 1990, almost 1 million immigrants entered the United States through legal means, and at least 270,000 entered without documentation. Currently, 1 in every 10 Americans is foreign-born. However, in contrast to the major immigration epoch of the 1930s, when the majority of immigrants were from Europe, this present immigration is mainly from Latino countries. At least 20% of all legal immigrants and 67% of undocumented immigrants come from Mexico alone (Lindsay & Michaelidis, 2001).

Social workers must consider a variety of factors in sorting out Latino's heterogeneity: gender, phenotype, generation, acculturation, country of origin, as well as educational, occupational, and class differences (Comas-Diaz, 1997). To complicate these factors, they must discern whether a client is an immigrant, and if so, whether he or she gained entry through formal immigration channels. If the client entered the United States illegally, then adaptation themes take on another dimension for assessment purposes.

This chapter highlights the special stresses that Mexican immigrant children and families experience when they come to the United States. Within this group, the unique status of those who reside here without documentation is noted. The fear of being identified and sent back to the country of origin has a major impact on an immigrant's mental health. Social workers must not only be sensitive to these themes but also knowledgeable about the kinds of resources available to undocumented persons, and factors that will place them in jeopardy if they are to seek legal immigration in the future (Zuniga, 2001).

Aside from consideration of social assessment themes, workers must examine their own intervention roles, if they are to serve the Latino population in a competent manner. A case vignette elucidates the complexity of working with children and families who are Mexican immigrants, denoting the importance of stage of immigration and acculturation assessment, survival themes, and the special situation of those without documentation. Before identifying the themes for assessment, I present a brief overview of the history of immigration and demographics that characterize the Mexican immigrant population.

HISTORICAL BACKGROUND

Bean, Cushing, and Haynes (1997) report that, after World War II, immigration to the United States dropped tenfold, decreasing from over 700,000 per year during the first 20 years of the 20th century to less than 70,000 from 1925 to 1945. Then, for nearly 50 years, legal immigration increased, and during the 1980s and 1990s reached all-time highs set in the first 20 years of the 20th century. This latter surge was composed of legal, undocumented, and refugee immigrants. The 1986 Immigration Reform Act, which provided amnesty to those living here undocumented, the large majority of which were Latinos, contributed to this new immigration surge. The result was the largest increase of immigrants in U.S. history.

While antipathy and discrimination toward Latinos, especially Mexican Americans can be historically traced throughout the last two centuries (Acuna, 1972), this recent increase in Latino immigration has exacerbated negative feelings to Latinos in general and Latino immigrants in particular. Hayes-Bautista, Hurtado, Valdez, and Hernandez (1992), report that in California, Latino immigrants, mostly of Mexican origin, were being blamed for many of California's problems, even pollution, as scapegoating tendencies evolved, especially during the economic downturns in the 1980s.

Changes in Immigration Demographics

The change in national origins is also important. Prior to 1960, the majority of immigrants were from European countries or Canada. In the 1960s, this pattern changed when family reunification criteria rather than national origin quotas became the policy.

An important aspect of the changed immigration demographics is the differences in educational levels. Bean, Chapa, Berg, and Sowards (1994) point to the change in educational levels of recent Mexican immigrants compared to those who immigrated in the 1960s. Between 1960 and 1964, Mexican immigrants on average were 19 years old and had completed more than 8 years of school. Currently, Mexican male and female immigrants have completed less than 6 years of school, with an average age over 30. Consequently, these immigrants encounter a more difficult time becoming integrated into the United States than did earlier immigrants. They typically work in low-skill, low-paying jobs that restrict them to old urban areas with overcrowding and poor social conditions (Bean et al., 1994).

Although Mexican immigrants are dispersed widely, most can be found in a few states: California, Texas, Illinois, and even New York. As Engstrom (2000) notes, 70% of all immigrants now settle in six states: California, New York, Texas, Florida, Illinois, and New Jersey. It is fascinating that Mexican immigrants are now populating areas of the Eastern Seaboard such as North and South Carolina, where they find employment in various sectors, including poultry houses (L. Ewell, former City Manager of Raleigh, NC; personal communication, March 26, 2000).

For those immigrants who came legally, many became eligible for immigration under the family reunification provisions, the dominant route for Latinos. Engstrom (2000) describes the overwhelming number of Mexicans using this source to gain entry to the United States, with about 95% being sponsored by a family member.

My goal in this chapter is to elucidate what happens to immigrants, especially those who are undocumented, when they come to the United States. How do they adapt and cope with this new experience, situation, and culture? What stresses often characterize their experience? Importantly, what cultural resources or domains of strength soften this hard experience and enable them to succeed? To what should we be sensitive in determining how these experiences have affected children, adolescents, and entire family systems?

ADAPTATION TO THE UNITED STATES

The context in which the migration experience takes place is important for assessing what the immigrant brings with him or her in terms of preparedness and motivation for the this change. For some, it is a well-planned and thoughtful process that is viewed with optimism in the search for a better life. For others, it is being pushed out of their country, Mexico, because of the lack of economic opportunity.

Sluzki (1979) outlined five stages of migration, so that social workers would have a framework for identifying sources of family conflict. We can use this framework to assess where the immigrant family or individual is positioned along the immigration trajectory, and whether presenting problems are related to specific stage processes.

For example, in stage 1, the *preparatory stage*, the person or family makes the decision to leave. Is this decision made in an orderly and thoughtful manner, with everyone agreeing to this major change, or is it made at the last moment, without the opportunity to ritualize good-byes to family and friends? This latter kind of departure aggravates the grief and loss themes that naturally correspond to such a major life move. Members who have not agreed with the move may later blame the person who made this decision. Issues of loss and mourning are intricately woven into the immigration process and can heavily mire the family in dysfunctional dynamics if mourning is disallowed, incomplete, or extended.

It is not unusual for Mexican men to immigrate to the United States, leaving their families behind. They send money back to support the family, but children may see their fathers only once a year. The annual trek home for the Christmas holidays draws such heavy cross-border traffic that the new President of Mexico, Vicente Fox, established the Office of Peregrinos to oversee the safety and welfare of these sojourners, who are often robbed of the money and gifts they attempt to bring home. Moreover, the Mexican government's newly established office concerned with immigration issues has even developed survival kits and educational preparedness classes for those who will be crossing the border illegally, in the hope that this will mitigate the high death rates that occur annually in these border crossings.

The plight of mothers who come to work in this country to support their families, often leaving their children with grandparents, aunts, and uncles in Mexico, requires a tremendous amount of emotional stamina. Those who return home after long absences are saddened when they realize how much they missed in not seeing the growth and development of their children. If they leave when their children are young, they often find that their children may no longer relate to them as the parent.

The anguish that parents endure in this context needs to be acknowledged and considered an important assessment arena when the social worker discovers this splitting of family systems. If the parent, especially a mother, has not been able to return, how does she manage her worries about her children, and how does she manage this dreary separation?

In stage 2, the *act of migration*, a variety of circumstances may make the experience unique for each person or family. Some may arrive in the United States in a matter of hours, with a swift and peaceful plane trip. Others may undergo a treacherous journey to escape detection. For those who enter without documents, the horrors of exploitation, assault, and rape can be realities, replete with traumatic memories that impact their future ability to adapt and to cope. In San Diego County, tightened border surveillance has pushed immigrants crossing without documents to the eastern part of the county. In winter, dozens freeze to death as they cross mountainous terrain; in the summer, this same trek takes them through desert-like conditions in which many die of dehydration and exposure annually. For those who are able to complete the journey, memories of relatives or friends who died in the process result in tremendous grief and guilt issues. An assessment must consider what this crossing experience was like, and whether trauma was part of this process. These kinds of trauma lurk in the immigrants' psyches, contributing to depression and anxiety that is not easily eradicated from their new lives without intervention.

In stage 3, the *period of overcompensation*, Sluzki (1979) points out that there often is a honeymoon period after entry into the new country that negates the losses that have actually occurred. It is a time when the person or family is in a heightened task-oriented stage, unable to recognize the incongruity of the cultural situation. However, they eventually experience the lack of fit with accustomed values, roles, and expectations, and those of the new society as they confront many fatiguing conflicts and pressures. Many families react by rigidly hanging on to old cultural patterns and rituals. However, the problems soon begin to raise their ugly heads.

In the fourth stage, *period of crisis or decompensation*, symptoms begin to be noticeable; conflicts become more overt and heightened. Often, the family is drawn into interaction with societal institutions because of child abuse, family violence, or some other issue or need that highlights their crisis. Resources they could call on in the old country to address such issues are typically not available. It is not unusual that conflicts between children and parents come to a head as the younger generation integrates new values and roles that threaten the family's cultural framework. The family system is dramatically challenged to undergo a new configuration of values and styles that allow them to keep some of the old but integrate new ways of thinking and behaving that will enable them to cope more effectively in this new society. This is a major challenge for families to address. Often, if one spouse has more readily entered into societal roles due to employment, the other spouse, who is not acculturating at the same rate, will be left behind, creating a spousal cultural chasm that exacerbates couple and family problems. If the woman rather than the man has employment opportunities, then role and gender conflicts will challenge these traditional families.

In the fifth stage, *transgenerational impact*, the family's ability to work through an integration process of new and old values, behaviors, and coping mechanisms enables the younger generation to function in society in a viable manner. If a value and behavior revision has not occurred, the younger generation may experience culture clashes within their family or the larger social culture, sometimes resulting in delinquent behaviors.

The issue of gang phenomena is not new for immigrants. Gangs evolved on the Eastern Seaboard and in the Midwest during the immigration epochs of the early 20th century (Morales, 1995). In those days, gang phenomena were related to poverty, family dysfunction, and unemployment, to name a few variables. For Mexican immigrants, the reality of gangs is also related to poverty, family breakdown, poor housing, alcoholism, drug addiction, major chronic illness, and more family members' involvement with law enforcement and correctional agencies (Morales, 1995).

For Mexican families this is a major risk issue for the youth. It is a theme that the social worker must examine in families with adolescents or even upper-age-latency children who may be "wanna-be" gang members.

Sluzki's framework (1979) helps the interventionist to consider what these immigrants experience and the price they pay for their journey, whether freely chosen or imposed on them by economic necessity. This enables the human services worker to evaluate the themes outlined previously, to discern how to offer services that provide problem-solving processes for addressing the needs, conflicts, or grief reactions that are causing maladaptation. This framework enables therapists to trace back those painful experiences the immigrant may resist processing because of major guilt, remorse, or even trauma suffered in the dangerous journey of undocumented entry (Cervantes, de Snyder, & Padilla, 1989).

Although isolation is an issue of concern with any client, it imposes a heavier impact for an immigrant who has already suffered familial, cultural, resource, and network losses. The competencies demanded in their new country, such as language skills, how to obtain employment, and, for undocumented persons, how not to be detected by the Border Patrol, begin to pile up and overwhelm the individual or family system.

Hostile Reactions

As noted earlier, mass immigration provokes many different reactions from governments and their citizenry. The dynamic increase of Latino immigrants, especially those without papers, has often resulted in very hostile and discriminatory attitudes. In San Diego, during the 1990s, these negative attitudes fostered such a high degree of xenophobia that two young men decided to "hunt down" Mexicans. They were later brought to trial for shooting and killing someone they assumed to be an undocumented Latino. This person was a legal resident of Mexican origin. In another case, five teens in a San Diego suburb were charged as adults in the brutal attacks on migrant workers, 60 years of age, at an encampment. The migrants were stomped on, shot with BB guns, and pelted by rocks, requiring hospitalization (Moran, 2002). The point here is to underscore the hostile and even lethal reaction that Latino immigrants often encounter when they cross to the United States. A social worker must consider to what extent a Mexican immigrant experiences this hostility and how he or she copes with these emotional and, at the extreme, physical assaults.

An ecological perspective (Germain & Gitterman, 1980) is used to assess the interplay between immigrants and this new environment into which they have been thrust. How do cultural, economic, health, and educational systems impact these new immigrants? The ecological theme of adaptation is the centerpiece for examining their experiences. This includes a focus on identifying the strengths those individuals present that can be easily overlooked. Importantly, assessment for cultural strengths is particularly pertinent. How did these immigrants cope before, and how can they learn to cope anew in this stressful situation? This perspective provides a focus for comprehending how individuals view themselves or their identities in light of this new cultural context. How do they evaluate their skills or competencies; what networks or supports are called upon as resources to curb their isolation? How do they carve out a mode of functioning independently, despite all the barriers that impede this goal? Importantly, In utilizing the four domains of an ecological view, a person's identity, autonomy, relatedness, and competence are themes that guide this examination (Germain & Gitterman, 1980).

PROBLEMS FOR CHILDREN AND FAMILIES

Educational Demographics

As a group, Latinos do not fare well in educational systems in the United States. In 1996, about 40% of Latinos ages 25 to 29 had not graduated from high school or obtained a high school equivalency degree, compared to only 7.4% of whites and 14% of black young adults. Within-group differences indicate that both immigrant and native-born adults of Mexican descent have much lower levels of educational attainment compared to adults from Central and South American, and Cuban origins. In 1993, 47% of Mexican-origin young adults ages 25 to 34 had not graduated from high school compared to 16% of Puerto Ricans living in the United States. Other Latino subgroups also tend to have higher rates of college completion than those of Mexican origin.

At the other end of the educational continuum, when we examine preschool attendance, we see that Latino children are the least likely to be enrolled in early childhood programs. In particular, those children whose mothers' first language was Spanish were least likely to be enrolled. These are children of immigrants. Hispanic 3-year-olds were only about half as likely to participate in early childhood programs as non-Latino, white, or black 3-year-olds (Roderick, 2000). As Roderick notes, preschool is valuable, because it promotes early school success, improves health and behavioral outputs, and facilitates literacy environments in the home. The fact that Latino children have a lower preschool participation rate indicates that they will enter kindergarden without the behavioral experience of having been in a formal school. This then mitigates their ability to have a platform of skills that readies them for early school success (Roderick, 2000).

This theme is exacerbated by the fact that Latino children also are less likely to come from families in which mothers actively teach them reading and numerical skills to prepare them for school. For example, 61% of Latina mothers of preschoolers reported that their children could identity the primary colors, compared to 73% of black and 91% of non-Latinos. Moreover, Latina mothers were only half as likely compared to whites to report that their preschoolers could recognize letters, 31% versus 61%, and count to 20, 39% versus 66%, respectively (Roderick, 2000). This evidence highlights the "catch-up" mode that characterizes members of this group even before they enter kindergarden. In light of the national trend of increased expectations for student performance at all levels of education, this scenario is a pessimistic one (Roderick, 2000). It suggests that those who work with Latino families, especially immigrant families, take a proactive role in supporting and facilitating aggressive educational pursuits by parents for their children.

Health Care Needs

An important area for Mexican children and families is their health and access to health care resources. Latinos in the United States encounter substantial barriers to health care. For example, they are most likely to be uninsured even though they have the highest labor force participation in states such as California (Hayes-Bautista et al., 1992; Suarez, 2000). The present issues around the increased use of managed care and national increased costs for health care magnify the problem for this group. As noted before, the low educational levels that characterize the group of Mexican origin are also correlated with increased health risks. For instance, less-educated people are less likely to use preventive health care. As Suarez notes (2000), those with less education tend to be less likely to have employment that offers adequate wages and health insurance.

Health and Poverty Correlations

Low educational levels are also correlated with poverty. Approximately 27% of Latinos were living in poverty in 1998 compared to 8.6% of whites. This complicates health issues, because low-income groups tend to have higher fertility rates, which necessitate more prenatal health care. This coupled with the fact that either their employment typically does not provide health insurance or their immigration status may indicate they are ineligible for health care, means that they have less access to health care, although their needs are in fact greater. The enactment of the Immigrant Responsibility Act of 1996 means that immigrants not living in the United States prior to August 1996, now have restricted access to health care. For undocumented immigrants, all public health resources are off limits (Suarez, 2000). Although elaboration on this important theme is beyond the scope of this chapter, suffice it to say that not speaking English, and culturally related health beliefs and practices contribute to this complicated health care reality for Latinos in general and Mexican immigrants in particular.

CULTURAL VALUES AS STRENGTHS IN ASSESSMENT

Immigrant Networks

One of the cultural values characteristic of Latino groups can be utilized in the attempt to adapt to the United States. The value of the collective and the importance of the group enable immigrants to seek out support from this collective system. As DeAnda (1984) has remarked, they have been able to utilize familial or friendship networks in this new country and be guided by those who already know how to manuver with facility within these new systems. It is not uncommon for immigrants to settle in a town in which friends or family have already settled. Having cultural brokers who teach one "the ropes" about where to rent, how to find employment, or jobs that will not demand legal documentation are some of the networks DeAnda has noted that facilitate immigrants' adaptation. These resources break the isolation and may provide contacts that also result in social and recreational connections, especially for families that have children. They also provide immigrants with a comfortable option that utilizes their relations to others as a resource.

Special Assessment Themes for Undocumented Families

Often, immigrants have to contend with the hostility of the receiving country. Yet the hardships they face to get to the United States speak to the power of their value of family and the importance of sacrificing for family and community. Acknowledging this aspect of their motivation enables them to realize that despite their dire circumstances, they are viewed by social workers as honorable for the sacrifices they make. The theme of sacrifice is particularly pertinent for those mothers who leave children behind as they struggle in this country to assure their financial support, and give up the experience of seeing them grow. Acknowledging the nobility of this sacrifice enables immigrants to view their struggles in a more positive light and supports a value that is part of their cultural heritage.

Some reference has been made to the plight and special stressors of immigrants who come to the United States without legal documents. The social worker must examine this area with sensitivity and concern. Because deportation is such a major risk for families, and especially the fear that parents will be separated from their children if they are picked up from their job or off the street, this constant fear challenges their sense of trust. It is critical that social workers underscore the fact that, in their role, they have no obligation or motivation to deport anyone without documents, or to call authorities such as the Immigration and Naturalization officials or the Border Patrol, also known as *La Migra*. The social worker may have to repeat this and to display by behavior that he or she is someone to trust.

INDIGENOUS STRATEGIES AND WESTERN INTERVENTIONS

If this trusting relationship has evolved, the social worker can gingerly explain the need to know more about the immigration trek to discern the kinds of anguish, fear, or even trauma the immigrants have undergone. Talking about these experiences is often a helpful way to unburden the individual; it also is a way to discover the strengths. The practice principle is that the social worker is asking for information that will help immigrants adapt; that he or she is not asking these intrusive questions out of curiosity; this may need to be explained in a concrete manner.

If trauma has been part of the experience, the social worker may need to refer individuals for mental health intervention from a facility that is not public, because immigrants would be ineligible for these kinds of services. Agencies such as Catholic Social Services or private, nonprofit organizations that provide bilingual counseling services are appropriate referrals.

If the social worker can offer therapeutic support him- or herself, assignments such as asking clients to write journals in their native language or write pieces about their immigration experience so that they can be discussed in counseling, are helpful devices that allow the immigrant to think about and describe an experience in a private way, before sharing this with the social worker. Falicov (1998) identifies a useful kind of intervention, narrative therapy, as enabling immigrants to examine what their experiences have been like, so they can share the stresses/pains of this process for healing purposes.

Given the yearly 400–600 deaths that occur, for example when immigrants traverse the border between Mexico and the United States (Sanchez, 2002), the clients have a variety of traumatic experiences that they have endured and often kept to themselves. Cervantes et al. (1989) identified posttraumatic stress disorder (PTSD) as a not uncommon difficulty that characterizes the mental health issues of these sojourners. Because children are sometimes included in this border crossing, therapists need to assess for PTSD in undocumented families. Did one of the immigrant group they crossed with die due to exposure or dehydration? Were they held up by bandits? Who was beaten, and how fearful were they when this occurred? Was anyone in their group raped? Even if the individual him- or herself was not hurt, witnessing this kind of trauma and not having any power to control it leaves lasting psychological injury that can intrude on the ability to adapt.

The role of spirituality in the life of most Latinos should be called on especially when it relates to death and trauma themes. Assessing whether clients have a special ritual or saint they call upon during times of emotional upheaval might offer one support mechanism the therapists can use to therapeutically address trauma. For example, use of *mandas*, or a promise or commitment to undertake a series of prayerful rituals, is viewed as a special spiritual intervention with particular power (Smith-DeMateo, 1987; Zuniga, 1998).

If social workers encounter enough clients who are immigrants, the idea of a *platica* group, or a group to discuss how they contend with their new experiences, is another format that enables immigrants, especially those without documentation, to discuss the anxieties, embarrassments, and fears they encounter in their new society. The value placed on the family group and the sense of the collective in Mexican culture can be utilized to motivate individuals to participate in a group. For those who have few contacts, a group experience with other Spanish-speaking immigrants may encourage the kind of networking and socializing that will help break down the isolation.

In Portland, Oregon, the Latino community utilizes paraprofessionals, or *promotoras*, immigrants who assess and help Latino families, and especially women, who are fearful of seeking help from mainstream agencies. The use of women who have experienced domestic violence and now are paraprofessionals has been particularly successful in reaching distrusting immigrants in need of support and problem solving (Connelly, 2000). In Mexico, health promotion and prevention formats typically offered by women who are *promotoras* is a common strategy. This demands that agencies organize their resources, so that this kind of service becomes available to this group. The collaboration in Portland among churches, nonprofit organizations, political entities, and community leaders has resulted in a safe-house for Latina and immigrant women, some without "papers," suffering domestic violence. This kind of partnership or collaboration demands that social workers take the lead first in advocating to have needs of those who are undocumented addressed. Then, social workers must provide leadership in the development of resources that will be needed to support this new kind of service provision (Connelly, 2000).

Parents' Advocacy for Their Children

The use of problem-solving groups for Mexican immigrant parents is another intervention format that enables parents who feel powerless to use their mutual needs and concerns about their children as the avenue to seek more viable resources. Children are a critical aspect of family life. For Latino families, the importance of children is evident by the larger families that characterize Latino populations. For example, social workers in grammar schools have found that reframing parents groups into cultural parent–teacher associations (PTAs) ensures that Mexican parents participate in school meetings that are crucial for their children (R. Martinez, school social worker, who facilitates a Spanish-speaking parent group in her middle school; personal communication, May 3, 2000). The reliance on sociability and the value of interpersonal relations that emanate from their culture contribute to the viability of group use. Use of the needs of children as the frame that necessitates group participation draws on immigrants' cultural values on the importance of children. Social workers design the group so that there is time for eating and socializing as part of the group format.

In San Diego, California, the need to teach immigrant parents of various ethnicities the value of knowing how to work with school systems in the education of their children contributed to the development of a Parents Institute, a nonprofit agency that collaborates with schools in training parents about school culture, the rights of their children, and school law and policy. The training teaches parents how to have a dialogue with a teacher or school principal. The goal is to help these immigrant parents develop communication and advocacy skills that ensure their children the quality education that is their right (Teacher–Parent Institute, n.d.).

The goal of empowering immigrant parents is a critical one. In San Diego, Mexican, mainly immigrant, parents sought the support of a private, nonprofit Chicano advocacy group to help them negotiate with a school principal the parents felt was unresponsive and difficult. As a group, these parents quickly learned how to take their needs to higher bureaucratic authorities. The outcome was that they successfully had this principal removed from their school. This process taught these parents about school policy and procedure, and importantly, that with some community support, they could be heard and effect positive changes. Thus, the roles of social workers in addressing the needs of these immigrant families are diverse, flexible, and necessarily creative.

PRINCIPLES OF CULTURALLY APPROPRIATE PRACTICE

Because survival issues are so paramount in the lives of so many Latino clients, social workers must ready themselves to recognize that family or individual concerns may prioritize survival themes before other pertinent items of need. Moreover, trust issues particularly related to the undocumented status of some clients or family members demand that social workers learn how to discuss these themes in an honest and supportive fashion. They should clarify immediately their role and the fact their agency does not mandate reporting to immigration authorities. Acknowledging that these are areas of fear especially for families who are fearful of being split up if detected, enables clients to know that an agency is safe.

Similarly, if clients need services, for example, from government sources that could jeopardize their future request for immigration processes, social workers must attempt to find alternative modes of service delivery, such as seeking resources from private agencies. If the situation demands use of the government resource, the social worker is obligated to inform the family that this could jeopardize any hopes of legal immigration. The point is that social workers need to become informed about immigration law and access to resources such as the National Council of La Raza (NCLR; *http://nclr.policy.net*), which provides legislative updates for its agency affiliates and interested parties. In this manner, clients will be able to make decisions, with full knowledge of all the implications.

So many Latino families and individuals follow a traditional format of values, especially related to gender and parental roles. Social workers must learn to respect and support these roles. Choosing to speak to the father first in deference to his patriarchal role in the family may be difficult for a feminist worker, but it is the culturally appropriate mode of communicating.

When professionals can work with the entire family, this allows for a format that easily follows the value of family to which many Latinos subscribe. It also ensures that the resources different members can offer will be available to help the social worker problem-solve. Falicov (1998) has highlighted how structural family work is culturally sensitive and effective with many Latino clients.

Interventions with the family also provide the forum wherein social workers can teach members new modes for adapting in this new culture. For instance, parents may be taught how to communicate with their children in a more informative manner. When there are acculturation conflicts between children and their parents, teaching parents how to share their developmental experiences with their children helps both generations to clarify expectations and areas in which problem solving must take place.

Social workers must assess whether a family or Latino client uses religious or spiritual resources. Identifying a church community, or a religious or spiritual belief system that can be harnessed for extra support, enables the social worker to use a format with which clients feel comfortable while they are learning new Western modes of intervention.

In this same vein, combining the use of cultural formats to which

Latino clients are accustomed with intervention formats, such as group work, which are Western aspects of social work, contributes to an effective intervention strategy to which Latino clients will respond more effectively. Although school systems or agencies may not always be prepared to pay for coffee and Mexican sweet bread, as an example of promoting the Mexican value of sociability, asking parents to bring these kinds of items displays the social workers awareness of the importance of this eating ritual.

The following vignette illustrates some of these needs and interventions. Although the scenario depicts the role of a social worker in a medical setting, it also highlights the various roles she took on in addition to her normal medical social work role.

CASE VIGNETTE

The Garcia Family: Role Flexibility

The Garcia family came to the attention of the Spanish-speaking, European American social worker when the father, Hector Garcia, age 28, was brought to the hospital after a severe car accident. His spinal cord had been so damaged that he was paralyzed from the waist down. He had been married to his 26-year-old wife for the past 8 years; he had a daughter, age 7, and a son, age 4. He lived with his nuclear family, as well as his mother. All members of the family except for the children were in the United States without legal papers. The two children had been born here.

Hector was in the landscaping business with his younger brother, and their business enabled this extended family to fare well; the business had two pickup trucks; one driven by each brother. They were able to support their mother, and the younger brother had just married and moved to the adjoining house, near his brother Hector.

The social worker had to provide some crisis intervention services both for the patient and the family, because this severe accident was such a shock to everyone. Part of the focus was on helping Mr. Garcia to address the loss of his ability to walk, function independently and work to support his family. Because there were no male social workers to which she could refer the case, and since she was the only Spanish-speaking social worker, she worked with Mr. Garcia on some very sensitive issues. She learned to discuss themes with him very carefully, so that he would be able to develop a trusting relationship with her. Given that part of his loss was his ability to have normal sexual relations with his young wife, and that he and his wife had been trying to have another child, his paralysis took on an even more significant theme of loss. However, before she could do any therapeutic work with Mr. Garcia, both he and the family felt that the first order of business was how to continue to run their landscaping business.

Respectful of Mr. Garcia's priorities, the social worker facilitated a family conference to sort out how to continue to run the business without Mr. Garcia's presence. One format chosen was for the younger brother to come in every other day to consult with his brother on how to address the needs of their clients now that Mr. Garcia could not work.

Another outcome was that Mr. Garcia's wife would take on some of the administrative and phone work with clients that he used to undertake, so that they could inform their clientele of the time adjustments they would need to catch up given the accident. Although Mrs. Garcia spoke broken English, she was motivated to help in any way she could. In addition, during her visits, she was to consult with her husband on a daily basis as to how this part of the business was functioning.

An important aspect of the social worker's role was to enable Mr. Garcia to maintain his role as head of the family. Given all the major losses he was enduring, the importance of maintaining and strengthening this role was seen by the social worker as a critical way to address Mr. Garcia's cultural proscriptions regarding his family responsibilities.

However, a reality that was producing major anxiety for the entire family was to what extent they would be at risk of being identified by immigration authorities, because they did not have medical insurance and could not pay the expensive hospital bills. The social worker assured them that the hospital personnel had no intention of reporting them to the Immigration or Naturalization Service. The credit department worked with them on a format for monthly payments, knowing that the costliness of the hospital stay would be beyond their means.

A particular crisis-ridden event occurred during a visit with Mr. Garcia's mother, when she became distraught about the entire family being sent back to Mexico, or her fear that her two grandchildren, who were citizens, would be kept in the United States by the social service authorities, while the rest of them were forced to leave. As the social worker spoke with her, it came to her attention that since the accident, now 3 weeks hence, the grandmother had not allowed the children to go to school or preschool, because she feared the authorities would take them.

The social worker contacted the school and set up a meeting with the brother, the grandmother, the mother of the children and the school counselor. The school clarified their policy and verified that there was no intention on their part to make any reports, because this was outside of their jurisdiction. A plan was established so that the grandmother would ensure that the children went to school each day, and she would also pick them up from school to enable their mother to take on more of the business responsibilities.

The social worker also set up several meetings with Mr. Garcia and is wife, because he felt that he was now failing his wife by not being employed and by being unable to function independently. The social worker facilitated several couple sessions that enabled them to clear the air about their pain, sorrow, and commitment to each other. In between one of these sessions, she obtained the services of a physical therapist and a male translator, so that Mr. Garcia could be educated and ask questions about his physical losses and, particularly, about his sexual abilities. The social worker felt that her relationship with Mr. Garcia could become jeopardized if she attempted to be the translator for this sensitive session. She felt, that utilizing the resources of male staff would allow this very traditional man to maintain his dignity. He would also have the ability to seek out the information he needed to know about his sexuality and sexual-relations issues given his disability.

When Mr. Garcia was getting ready for discharge, the social worker held several family sessions, educating the family on how to take care of his needs, and identifying the areas that would be stressful for all of them. She also taught Mr. and Mrs. Garcia how to respond to their children's questions, so that they could give them correct information in a manner that would not alarm them. She also took on some normal discharge planning processes, including future visits with the physical therapist. She set up an important referral, a visitation plan by their parish priest, who had visited the family at the hospital. The family agreed that they would continue to work with the priest as counselor, to address future areas of anxiety.

After Mr. Garcia was discharged, he called the hospital to indicate his appreciation to the social worker for all her help. He indicated that on his arrival home, he was surprised to find that a ramp had been built to allow wheelchair access. School personnel had organized staff and parents, purchased lumber, and had volunteered time to build this access for Mr. Garcia and his family.

Debriefing

Although these roles appear to be commonsense types of activities to undertake, they highlight several themes. One, the social worker knew how to follow cultural themes in being sensitive to Mr. Garcia's role as a male, father, and husband. In her work, she attempted to support this traditional role, because it held such great meaning for this man at this time of crisis in his life. She also found alternative routes to address familial issues, recognizing the importance of working with the entire family in their problem-solving forays and that their survival needs had to take priority. She understood the importance of sexual issues in this kind of case and found alternative ways to provide the needed service and provide information, but in a manner in which Mr. Garcia could save face and not feel humiliated by her presence. Also, she was not afraid to extend her work to another important system for this family: collaboration with the school in helping to alleviate the family's fears and anxieties about deportation issues. Moreover, she noted the role of the family priest and utilized this important person to establish future counseling support that the family would undoubtedly need. This is particularly important when immigrants cannot access public counseling services.

For the family, this tragic accident was coupled with legitimate fears about being deported and having the family split apart. This latter fear was less realistic, but there have been some cases of family disruption when parents are deported to Mexico and their children, who are citizens, are placed in foster care under the public social services agency. Helping the family to know which fears are real and which ones may not be well grounded is one of the services social workers can offer these families. The medical debt may become a theme in the future, if this family attempts to seek legal documentation from the Immigration and Naturalization Service.

In this situation, medical care was not an option but was required to save the life of this father. Social workers are cautioned that in less drastic situations, if a family can forgo a public resource and obtain private kinds of services, this is the option the social worker needs to ferret out.

Social workers need to become knowledgeable about the various policy issues that immigration law presents. Utilizing resources such as the National Council of La Raza's website links offers almost daily updates on policy changes that affect Latinos, especially those who are immigrants. There is a growing literature on immigration policy and issues evolving in social work journals and books (Hulewat, 1999; Munz & Weiner, 1997). Social workers need to enter this arena, if it is new to them, to become educated about both policies related to immigration and psychosocial crises that immigrants have to address when they come to live in the United States. To be culturally competent in serving immigrants, one has to make the commitment to become knowledgeable about their unique needs, while also examining personal attitudes and feelings about immigrants, especially those who are in this country without documents. Our job as social workers is to provide resources to people in need, regardless of their immigrant status. We cannot allow our personal bias or prejudices about this sensitive issue to impede our work; if we do, we are actually functioning in an unethical manner, (Zuniga, 2001).

CONCLUSIONS

This chapter has elucidated the multiple and complex needs that immigrants encounter when they are new to this country. Sluzki's assessment scheme offers an adaptation model that helps the social worker to discern at what level of adjustment their clients' problems emanate. The particular barriers Latino immigrants encounter were noted, with special attention to the antipathy that is often present toward them, especially if they are here without legal documentation. Cultural resources that can be called up to enable clients to adapt more successfully include identifying networks of family or friends that can teach them the ropes of adaption to their new city. Identifying natural supports such as religious services that provide culturally driven rituals is a critical asset to utilize. Interventions such as family, group work, or the use of *promotoras* again offer contexts that are culturally comfortable for clients, whereas teaching them Western modes of intervention, such as talk therapy, may be more difficult. Educating oneself about the traditional roles to which these immigrants adhere enables the social worker to utilize these role scripts to ensure an atmosphere of respect and comfort. Knowing immigration laws regarding utilization of public resources is critical to ensure that social workers do not unwittingly endanger future immigration prospects. Moreover, knowing how to refer alternative resources imposes on workers the need to be knowledgeable about community resources, especially those that are private. Social workers must be sure that they do not allow negative personal feelings about undocumented immigrants to counter their ethical obligation to ensure access to resources for those in need.

REFERENCES

Acuna, R. (1972). *Occupied America: The Chicano's struggle toward liberation*. San Francisco: Canfield Press.

Bean, F., Cushing, R., & Haynes, C. (1997). The changing demography of U.S. immigration flows: Patterns, projections, and contexts. In K. Bade & M. Weiner (Eds.), *Migration past, migration future: Germany and the United States* (pp. 121–152). Providence, RI: Berghahn Books.

Bean, F., Chapa, J., Berg, R., & Sowards, K. (1994). Educational and sociodemographic incorporation among Hispanic immigrants to the United States. In B. Edmonston & J. S. Passel (Eds.), *Immigration and ethnicity: The integration of America's newest arrivals* (pp. 114–129). Washington, DC: Urban Institute Press.

Cervantes, R. C., Salgado de Snyder, V. N., & Padilla, A. M. (1989). Posttraumatic stress in immigrants from Central America and Mexico. *Hospital and Community Psychiatry, 40*, 615–619.

Cohn, D. V., & Fears, D. (2001, March 7). Hispanics draw even with blacks in new census. *Washington Post*, p. A1.

Comas-Diaz, L. (1997). Mental health needs of Latinos with professional status. In J. Garcia & M. Zea (Eds.), *Psychological interventions and research with Latino populations* (pp. 142–165). Boston: Allyn & Bacon.

Connelly, L. (2000). *Sociodrama: "Promotoras."* Workshop, Families Working Together Against Violence, 2nd Annual Power in Partnership Conference, University of Portland, Oregon.

DeAnda, D. (1984). Bicultural socialization: Factors affecting the minority experience. *Social Work, 29*(2), 101–107.

Engstrom, D. (2000). Hispanic immigration at the new millennium. In Pastora S. J.

Cafferty & D. Engstrom (Eds.), *Hispanics in the United States: An agenda for the twenty-first century* (pp. 310–369). New Brunswick, NJ: Transaction.

Falicov, C. J. (1998). *Latino families in therapy: A guide to multicultural practice.* New York: Guilford Press.

Germain, C., & Gitterman, A. (1980). *The life model of social work practice.* New York: Columbia University Press.

Hayes-Bautista, D., Hurtado, A., Valdez, R. B., & Hernandez, A. C. (1992). *No longer a minority: Latinos and social policy in California.* Los Angeles: UCLA Chicano Studies Research Center.

Hulewat, P. (1999). Resettlement: A cultural and psychological crisis. In P. Ewalt, E. Freeman, A. Fortune, D. Poole, & S. Witkin (Eds.), *Multicultural issues in social work: Practice and research* (pp. 669–678). Washington, DC: National Association of Social Workers.

Lindsay, J. M., & Michaelidis, G. (2001, January 5). A timid silence on America's immigration challenge. *San Diego Union-Tribune*, p. B7.

Morales, A. (1995). Urban gang violence: A psychosocial crisis. In A. Morales & B. Sheafor (Eds.), *Social work: A profession of many faces* (pp. 433–463). Boston: Allyn & Bacon.

Moran, G. (2002, June 27). Migrant attackers to be sentenced. *San Diego Union-Tribune*, pp. B1, B9.

Munz, R., & Weiner, M. (1997). *Migrants, refugees, and foreign policy.* Providence, RI: Berghahn Books.

Roderick, M. (2000). Hispanics and education. In Pastora S. J. Cafferty & D. Engstrom (Eds.), *Hispanics in the United States* (pp. 123–174). New Brunswick, NJ: Transaction.

Sanchez, L. (2002, June 24). Memorializing border crossers. *San Diego Union-Tribune*, pp. B1, B4.

Sluzki, C. (1979). Migration and family conflict. *Family Process, 18,* 379–390.

Smith-DeMateo, R. (1987, February). *Multicultural considerations: Working with families of developmentally disabled and high risk children: The Hispanic perspective.* Paper presented at the Conference of the National Center for Clinical Infants Program, Los Angeles, CA.

Suarez, Z. (2000). Hispanics and health care. In Pastora S. J. Cafferty & D. Engstrom (Eds.), *Hispanics in the United States* (pp. 195–236). New Brunswick, NJ: Transaction.

Teacher–Parent Institute [pamphlet]. (n.d.). San Diego, CA: Author.

Zuniga, M. (2001). Working with Latino families: Ethical considerations. In R. Fong & S. Furuto (Eds.), *Culturally competent practice* (pp. 47–60). Boston: Allyn & Bacon.

Zuniga, M. (1998). Families with Latino roots. In E. Lynch & M. Hanson (Eds.), *Developing cross-cultural competence* (pp. 209–245). Baltimore: Paul Brookes.

CHAPTER 11

Cuban Children and Families

EDGAR COLON
GISELA SARDINAS

There are over 17 million Latinos in the United States, more if the number of residents without official documentation could be counted. At current rates of growth, Latinos will be the largest minority group in the country by 2050 (U.S. Bureau of the Census, 2001). The second largest group is people from Central and South American countries. Their growth has greatly increased cultural diversity within the Latino population generally. The presence of Puerto Ricans, the third largest group, is facilitated by the Commonwealth status of their island and freedom of movement to the mainland. Many Puerto Ricans virtually commute, at least on a seasonal basis, between San Juan and the major cities of the East Coast and the Midwest. Cubans comprise a small and specialized population that is quite distinct demographically and politically.

The Cuban population is the third largest group of Latinos in the United States. According to the most recent U.S. Bureau of the Census report (2001), approximately 170,000 native-born Cubans reside in the United States. Cubans trace their ancestry to Spanish and African cultures (Bustamante & Santa Cruz, 1975; Ortiz, 1995). The largest immigration of Cubans to this country began in 1959.

At present, the Cuban population has concentrations in New York and New Jersey and, most heavily, in south Florida. The south Florida community has established a strong political and business base, creating its own banking institutions, professional services, newspapers, and educational institutions (Perez-Firmat, 1994). However, Cubans have paid a very high price for their "success." Their loss of motherland, separation from family and loved ones represent some of the emotional baggage Cubans carry with them.

The Cuban American population in the United States is a unique population whose cultural and ethnic reality is complex. Due to the political turmoil that occurred with the takeover of Cuba by Fidel Castro in 1959, there have been several waves of Cuban immigration to the United States. The reasons for the departure of Cubans and the experiences of these individuals in this country have contributed to the complexity of the lives of immigrant Cuban American families and children. Moreover, the sustained and substantive reliance by Cuban immigrants on Spanish language, and Cuban values and beliefs, thereby promoting adherence to traditional Cuban culture, is also an important confounding factor (Zuniga, 1992).

Our purpose in this chapter is to provide social workers and other helping professionals with an understanding of the sociopolitical and immigration experience of Cuban children and families. We contend that the attainment of an understanding of this experience will enable social workers to engage in the development of culturally competent assessment and intervention planning work. The ecological, strengths-based practice framework presented provides a conceptual model for the provision of culturally sensitive individual, group, and community services within Cuban American communities.

The chapter begins with a brief historical overview of the immigration waves of Cubans to the United States from the post-Castro period of 1953 to the present. We contend that understanding the unique aspects of this history provides the reader with an important context for understanding the adaptation issues confronted by Cuban immigrant families and children. A second section discusses problems and issues facing Cuban children and families in the United States. A discussion of adaptation issues faced by Cuban immigrant children and families follows this section. A subsequent section describes relevant Cuban values and beliefs, providing a cultural lens for viewing these issues. Finally, a discussion of Western versus indigenous intervention strategies provides a context for an illustrative case vignette and a list of practice principles.

The relative success of Cubans in the United States must be understood in terms of the sociohistorical and political context of the Cuban immigration after the rise to power of Castro. Moreover, the significance of the Cold War period (1945–1990) and United States foreign policy must considered. The following section briefly describes each of the important immigration waves that characterize the history of Cuban immigration to the United States.

HISTORICAL BACKGROUND

Post-Castro Regime Immigration Wave (1953–1959)

Upon the rise of Fidel Castro to power, the established political, social, and economic structure of the island of Cuba changed significantly

(Torres, 1994). In contrast to earlier Cuban dictatorships, the communist government of Fidel Castro promoted a social shift in Cuban societal norms, values, and social expectations, more in line with Marxist socialist ideals.

During this wave, Cubans began to arrive in this country in significant numbers. Approximately 144,000 Cubans immigrated to this country during this period (Rogg, 1974). Lack of trust, suspicion, and uncertainty about the future were issues faced by most Cubans at the time. Fear of harassment and political persecution were primary reasons for Cubans leaving the Island.

Freedom Flight Cuban Immigration Wave (1965–1973)

By the end of 1965, Fidel Castro announced that the Camarioca capitol port located at the northern coast of Matanza Province would open to Cubans wishing to live the island. Cuban exiles residing in the United States arranged for the transport of relatives, family, and friends who wished to leave the island. This transportation led to many death and tragedies, because boats were loaded beyond safe capacity. Approximately 5,000 individuals left Cuba before the negotiations between Castro and the United States that resulted in freedom flights or airlifts from Havana to Miami.

On a more personal level, I experienced the impact of this particular immigration wave because it was during this time that my family and I immigrated to the United States. I was a child when my family sought to leave Cuba, and I recall the pain my family and I felt when we left Cuba. The family, although disillusioned with the Castro regime, still held strong feelings of loyalty to Cuba and to friends and extended family.

While still in Cuba, soon after our family filed a petition for permission to leave Cuba, my father lost his job. Subsequently, he went to work in a government agricultural field for no pay. This was a usual outcome for individuals and families filing petitions. In addition, prospective Cuban immigrants faced many negative consequences as a result of wanting to leave Cuba, including personal persecution by Castro loyalists and physical punishment by Cuban troops.

Marielitos Wave of Immigration (1980–1990)

After the storming of the Peruvian Embassy by 10,000 Cubans seeking political asylum, Bernal (1982) reported that the U.S. government began diplomatic negotiations with the Cuban government within a matter of days. The outcome of these negotiations opened the way for 135,000 Cubans to immigrate to the United States over a 5-month period. The immigration agreement between the United States and Cuba led to the orderly migration of Cubans to this country, until Castro broke off the agreement in 1990.

These Cuban immigrants left Cuba from the Port of Mariel, which is why this particular group of immigrants is called the *Marielitos*. Many first- and second-generation Cuban Americans used this term to disparage this group of Cuban immigrant families comprised primarily of working-class and unemployed individuals. A large percentage of these immigrant families were also of African Cuban heritage.

Extraordinary Economic Hardship Period of Cuban Immigration (1990–Present)

The most recent phase of Cuban immigration began to coalesce in 1990. At this time, the Cuban economy began its period of added economic difficulties after the disintegration of the Soviet Union. Given the economic blockades maintained by the United States, the years from 1990 to the present have led to extraordinary economic hardship for the Cuban people. Consequently, many Cubans have increasingly taken risks and lot their lives or limbs in attempts to leave Cuba. During this immigration wave in the summer of 1994, thousands of Cubans attempted to cross the Straits of Florida on makeshift rafts, trying to escape capture by the Cuban coastal police.

ADAPTATION TO THE UNITED STATES

Thomas (1971) notes that many Cuban Americans argue that the Cuban American success story required a high price for many immigrant Cuban children and families. Despite the fact that many Cubans are successful professionals and entrepreneurs in business, Novas (1994) agrees with this assertion. The Cuban American success story is illusory for many Cuban immigrant children and families.

For the many Cuban immigrant families, the loss of the motherland, and separation from family and loved ones is a high price to pay for freedom. Moreover, the "emotional baggage" of deep resentment and hate toward Castro and his supporters is also a high-price item for personal freedom. McGoldrick (1996) cites Coco Fusco's (1995) *English Is Broken Here* to illustrate the many difficulties faced by Cuban exiles through the years.

> Americans often ask why Cubans exiled or at home, are so passionate about Cuba, why are discussions are so polarized, and why are emotions so raw after thirty-three years. My answer is that we are always fighting with the people we love the most. Our intensity is the result of the tremendous repression and forced separation that affects all people, who are ethnically

Cuban, wherever they reside. Official policies on both sides collude to make a change practically impossible. (p. 3)

In summary, the life experiences of the different groups of Cuban individuals that participated in each immigration wave provide a clear picture of the adaptation issues faced by Cuban immigrant families and children. The experience of each Cuban immigrant family is linked to the wave during which it left Cuba, the sociopolitical conditions in the United States, and the nature of U.S. diplomatic relations with Cuba during the time of migration. The adaptation issues affecting the lives of the Cuban immigrant are discussed in terms of the differences in reception and adaptation experiences of early and recently arrived families.

Early-Arrival Immigrant Families

The fact that the post-Castro (1953–1959) wave of Cuban immigrants comprised primarily white, upper-middle-class professionals with business skills and experience made it easier for them to find success in this country. However, the social adaptation experience of this particular group does not tell the whole story.

Bernal and Flores-Ortiz (1982) contend that when these immigrants came, the United States feared threats of communism close to its shores and loss of economic control of the island. Therefore, this country opened its doors to Cubans fleeing the Castro regime. During the course of this period ending in 1970, the U.S. government provided some resettlement assistance, job training, and small-business loans. These early Cuban immigrants were able to embrace these opportunities and succeed.

Recent-Arrival Immigrant Families

On the other hand, during the later Cuban immigration waves, from 1980 to the present, this country was, and continues to be, less willing to provide social and other support to groups of Cuban immigrants such as *Marielitos* and *Balseros*. The adaptation issues faced by these waves of Cuban immigrants provide an example of the difficulties in adaptation faced by more recent Cuban immigrant children and families.

Because the United States has imposed economic sanctions against Cuba, these two countries continue their polarized, ideological battles. More importantly, the old, well-established Cuban American communities have been resistant to providing economic or emotional support for their comrades in Cuba. However, most recently, an increasing number of Cuban Americans are softening political barriers and seeking greater contact between Cubans in America and those in Cuba. Given their shared social and political history, these two communities are engaged in an intense and embattled kinship (Bernal, 1982).

The life experiences of the *Marielitos* and *Balseros* immigration waves are very different from those of earlier Cuban immigrants, who arrived in this country at a time when they were welcomed and supported. The majority of these immigrants came from a racially mixed, lower socioeconomic background. Upon their arrival in the United States, many of these immigrants confronted the negative effects of discrimination and racism.

PROBLEMS FOR CHILDREN AND FAMILIES

The nature of the ever-evolving sociopolitical relationship between the United States and Cuba provides a context for understanding the social problems of immigrant Cuban children and families. The relationship has shifted from active support to detention and police control of Cuban immigrants. The success of Cuban immigrant children and families in this country is of necessity associated with the nature of the migration experience of the Cuban people and the historical context of United States–Cuban diplomatic relations (Bernal & Flores-Ortiz, 1980).

American racism and discrimination have impacted the lives of these later immigrant families. The *Marielitos* and *Balseros* immigrant families have not received a warm welcome. In the case of these immigrant groups, Cuban American leaders feared that their image and presence would tarnish the Cuban American image as model individuals (Bernal & Flores-Ortiz, 1980; Perez-Stable, 1981). Furthermore, with the maintenance of a strong sense of anti-Castro sentiment that continually ripples through the fabric of Cuban American families and communities, and is often directed at these individuals, these Cuban immigrant families and children have been given a difficult task.

Because of the many losses experienced by Cuban immigrant families, Cuban Americans have become tenacious in preserving their language, heritage and culture. Researchers further note that for the second and succeeding generations of Cubans born and raised in this country, the tenaciousness of Cuban elders has been a source of familial conflict.

CULTURAL VALUES AS STRENGTHS IN ASSESSMENT

The diversity of literature speaks of the importance of the family within Latino culture (Canino & Canino, 1982; Torres, 1994). The Cuban family is a primary source of social and economic support. It is also the medium through which individuals engage in the unique Cuban cultural processes of gender-role socialization and ethnic identity formation.

The Cuban family tends toward an extended family structure (Garcia & Marrotta, 1997; Garcia-Preto, 1994). The structure of the Cuban family tends to be patriarchal, giving great power and responsibility to the male head of household. The Cuban family is viewed as the focal point of mutual aid in the Latino community, based on the cultural norm of *personalismo* and the fact that nonfamilial organizations are not generally trusted (Garcia & Marrotta, 1997).

In Cuban culture, *la familia* (the family) and interdependence among its members is highly valued. Cuban families have strong ties to each other and have maintained many of the qualities of the extended family system. Cubans depend more on the family than on professionals for services, emotional support, and advice. Within Cuban society, an important support network maintains the family system. Along with material, moral, and spiritual responsibilities of the godparents toward the godchild, functioning as a form of indigenous social security, Cubans family members within the nuclear and extended family form a pattern of mutual respect and help. In the Cuban family system, a network of mutual kinship, as serious and important as that of natural kinship, provides a strong source of individual and group support (Molina, 1983).

Because of the centrality of the family in Cuban community life and the adhesion of generations under the concept of *pater familias* (male domination), decisions about the behavior of an individual in the family are usually the result of a group process overseen by the men (Colon, 2001). The Cuban family differs from the Anglo norm of autonomy by emphasizing interdependency, and mutual help and support in time of need (Solomon, 1982).

Respect and the maintenance of personal dignity in everyday social interactions are other important values in Cuban culture. The value of respect oftentimes characterizes the nature of social interaction between Cubans and professional non-Cubans. As is true of many Latino groups, Cubans respond better to social interactions, particularly in the workplace, after a brief social conversation has occurred, before the formal, more businesslike discussion. The interaction may consist of a simple inquiry about how the individual is feeling today. The type of initial interaction sets the emotional climate for a more relaxed, warm future interactions.

The value of *personalismo* (personalism), which means valuing personal relationships that are trusting and supportive, is also an important factor in the ability of Cuban families to cope with social distress and economic uncertainty. Cubans, as is true of many Latinos within other subgroups, tend to favor and respond better to a congenial, personal manner than to an impersonal interest in their problems. Cubans relate more effectively to people than to institutions; they object and do not respond well to formal, impersonal structures and environments.

Within this context, the practitioner can begin to understand the importance of Cuban norms and values. In particular, the cultural values of *dignidad* (dignity), *respeto* (respect), *personalismo* (personalism), and *familismo* (familism) can be best understood in the context of the unique group and interpersonal dynamics that occur in Cuban immigrant families. An understanding of these and other important Cuban values provide intervention opportunities for practitioners. The social worker can then work with the Cuban immigrant child and family through the acknowledgment of the importance of their values and worldview.

In summary, the values that guide Cuban culture have influenced Cuban immigrants' social interactions with others in American society and within established Cuban American communities. The social experience of many of the less-educated and less-skilled Cuban immigrant individuals and families requires that they draw personal strength from traditional Cuban values. In particular, the value of loyalty to family and dedication to the good of Cuban communities provides a source of strength for these vulnerable Cuban immigrant children and families.

CULTURE AND DIVERSITY:
A STRENGTHS-BASED AND ECOLOGICAL PERSPECTIVE

The ecological perspective is uniquely suited for practice with vulnerable Cuban immigrant children and families. Within a biopsychosocial, cultural, and spiritual context, this perspective provides a framework for understanding how Cubans interact throughout the life cycle. The practitioner is able to identify strategies indigenous to the immigrant Cuban child and family.

The ecological perspective reflects the integration of theories of human development and behavior across the life cycle. Moreover, the reciprocal interaction that occurs between individuals and their environment, and the influence that culture and ethnicity have on Latinos across the macro-, meso-, and micro-levels, is emphasized.

The experience of the newly arrived Cuban immigrant is complex and disruptive of the usual adaptive balance or goodness of fit required for human adaptation. An effective, non-Western-based approach to practice emphasizes the adaptive interaction with all elements of their environment. The use of an approach that views the experiences of the Cuban immigrant as static and linear fails to take into account the reality of this individual's level of human interaction with the environment.

In summary, a strengths-based and ecological social work practice approach that considers the interconnectedness and interrelatedness of the Cuban families and American society provides the practitioner with a means for understanding the nature of the problems and issues of these families, in the context of Cuban values, family roles, adaptive responses, and coping strategies (Pinderhughes, 1989).

INDIGENOUS STRATEGIES AND WESTERN INTERVENTIONS

Contemporary social work views human needs and problems as generated by the transactions between people and their environments. The goal of social work practice is to enhance and restore the psychosocial functioning of persons, or to change the oppressive or destructive social conditions that negatively affect the interaction between persons and their environments. Failure to recognize the client's strengths is partially due to the Western norm of cultural blindness, or the melting-pot ethos (Solomon, 1982). Effective practitioners must act on the social work commitment to respect human diversity, placing all clients in their own cultural context, and to draw upon a strength perspective.

Pinderhughes (1989) argues that the Western concept of culture often views the culture of others as a static phenomenon. This view of culture suggests that the unique characteristics of a diverse group are unchanging. Moreover, a static view of culture leads to labels and other symbols of cultural belonging as fixed and not altered by the changing reality of group development. The identification of indigenous strategies is based on the recognition that the cultural reality of the Cuban immigrant child and family is not static but dynamic. This view clearly supports the use of indigenous strategies for working with Cuban immigrants.

The Western view does not account for the sociopolitical and historical experiences of the immigrant Cuban child and family. McGoldrick (1996) notes that to understand the meaning of ethnicity for a particular group, one must go beyond simply identifying the individual's place of origin. An indigenous intervention approach assesses the socioeconomic status, racial background, religious affiliation, political status, and immigration experience of the Cuban immigrant family and child in the United States.

Cuban cultural interactions serve as protective factors for the family. Shared traditions and values have kept Latinos together as an ongoing, distinctive community despite devastating poverty, high unemployment, decrepit housing, and poor health status. Cuban culture provides the means for a family to view the world.

It is important that the process of developing indigenous interventions in relation to the Cuban family include an assessment of the level of acculturative stress being experienced by the individual and the family. The social worker must assess internal and external factors that either increase or decrease the subjective experience of stress and, as a result, mediate the risk of stress-related diseases. External factors that can be assessed include current individual and family social and economic conditions. External factors might include individual temperament, problem-solving skills, sense of internal control, and self-esteem. Many of these external factors must be related to the experience of Cuban families in acculturation.

Issues of Family Acculturation

The most common and problematic consequence of acculturation for the Latino immigrant is the breakdown of traditional cultural and family norms. For Cuban and other Latino immigrants, acculturation may take the form of challenges to traditional beliefs about male authority and supremacy, role expectations for men, and standards of conduct for women. Given these challenges, the Cuban immigrant family's ability to accept, conform, or adhere to new standards of conduct is affected. Moreover, it is during periods of individual cultural adaptation that acculturative stress is most pronounced. The Cuban child and family's inability to handle this stress can result in individual and family withdrawal and isolation.

Family Structure and Social-Role Functioning

Indigenous strategies consider the individual and group meanings that family members associate with roles in the family, the local community, and the greater society. In this regard, it is important to note Cuban immigrant families' strong sense of family and loyalty to homeland that supports individual and group decision making in the context of the family and the larger community. Therefore, the associated historical experiences of prejudice and discrimination must also be viewed through this lens. Finally, the social worker must expand the boundaries of intervention beyond Western models, which may not take into account the particular cultural factors of a group (Colon, 2001).

Indigenous strategies that can best address the social realities of the Cuban immigrant family must also consider the social–relational and interactive nature of the Cuban family system. In particular, given the strong value of *familismo*, family centeredness, and the highly interdependent structure of the family, a family-systems- based strategy must affirm both individual and family accomplishments, while building on the strength and resilience engendered by strong traditional values based on goal mutuality and group membership. Because many recently arrived Cuban families left Cuba after achieving a strong sense of personhood based on professional and personal success, the affirmation of these roots of origin is critical to the development of treatment strategies that account for the indigenous reality of these individuals. Consequently, the task ahead for the social worker is to understand better the life transitions, environmental pressures and interpersonal processes that are unique to the Latino community. Although this general model of intervention moves us in the right direction, it becomes more complicated when we look at the specifics.

PRINCIPLES OF CULTURALLY APPROPRIATE PRACTICE

The practice of social work with culturally diverse and oppressed Cuban immigrant populations requires the use of affirming intervention approaches, which must take into account the daily social realities confronted by the members of these populations. The following practice principles provide guidelines for practitioners involved in the development of implications essential to practice with the Cuban immigrant child and family:

1. Social workers must seek to develop alternative paradigms of knowing these realities to enhance their ability to assist Cuban immigrant families and children in telling their powerful stories.
2. When working with Cuban immigrant children and families, social workers must participate in self-exploration designed to overcome personal biases and to develop integrative ethnic identity.
3. Social workers must engage in communication patterns that achieve appropriate self-disclosure, when therapeutically necessary.
4. In the context of a dynamic, constantly changing environment, social workers must therefore assess the Cuban immigrant's interaction.
5. Social workers must assess issues in family functioning of the recently arrived Cuban child and adolescent.
6. When using models of social work and psychotherapeutic intervention, social workers must exercise caution to ensure that they affirm the adaptive strength and resilience provided by Cuban values and beliefs.
7. Social workers must maintain a view that assumes the Cuban immigrant client possesses untapped reserves of mental, physical, and emotional resources. They must work with the client to call on these personal resources to develop, grow, and overcome their problems.
8. Social workers are reminded that the client's perception of his or her life problem, as well as their own understanding of the perception is complex and variable. All people do not necessarily experience particular events or processes in the same way as either negative or positive.
9. Social workers must affirm the adaptive strength and resilience provided by Cuban values and beliefs.

In summary, traditional models of helping often ignore the interdependent, mutually supportive aspects of Cuban immigrant group norms and individual values. Cuban immigrants have experienced unique diversity within their self-identified group—racial, ethnic, sexual orientation, gender, or special status (mentally or physically challenged). The social worker must call upon his or her understanding of the cultural dictates, roles, values, and complex relationships that comprise the lives of these multidiverse people.

CASE VIGNETTE

A Cuban immigrant family arrived in this country as part of the *Marielito* immigration wave in 1990. The trip on a makeshift raft from Cuba was very turbulent and dangerous. Several of the individuals on the raft died of dehydration, and some drowned. Upon the arrival of the family in the United States, there were no friends or relatives to welcome the family. When the Immigration and Naturalization Service contacted these individuals about assistance with housing the family, the response was negative. Within 6 months, the family was able to locate a temporary shelter in a low-income Cuban community. They moved into the shelter with few belongings. After a few weeks of residence in the shelter, they found that no one in the community would speak to them. The family members felt both hostility and resentment.

Moreover, the family experienced many problems with finding employment for the father and assisting the two young children, ages 6 and 10 with their adjustment difficulties in school. While in school, the children experienced harassment about their inability to speak the English language. Second- and third-generation Cuban American children could not identify with them. While in Cuba, the father had had a drinking problem. Because of the difficulties that confronted the family, the father again began to drink heavily. His increased drinking created significant conflict among all the family members.

In working with this family, the social worker must take into account the important role of the family in Cuban culture. Based on a strengths-centered and ecological approach, the family must be helped to draw on its strengths as a family system. The role of religion would also be an important avenue to explore when assessing the impact of problems in social functioning of the family. It is important to assist the family to identify supports the will help family members deal with the sense of loss and social isolation each is experiencing. The social worker must assist in solving the adjustment problems of the children within the school system. He or she will need to educate teachers, counselors, and others about the values and social reality of the family. Therefore, the intervention strategies that best address the social needs of this family must take into account the multisystemic issues affecting the family in its interactions with various health and social service agencies. An effective strategy to assist this family is the use of genograms, culturagrams, and eco-maps in helping them find a vision and solutions for themselves. Affirmation, *familismo*, and a welcoming environment are also intervention tools that give the provider an opportunity to assess and best help Cuban families.

The social worker must develop indigenous strategies that consider the roles of extended family members and individuals in friendship groups. These individuals might be called upon to help the family address its problems. The identification and engagement of natural support systems is also of value when working with Cuban families. Moreover, the ability to work is important to the Cuban immigrant family. It is important, therefore, for the social worker to discuss the issue of work and the reality of feelings surrounding the loss of employment possibilities.

Finally, for Cuban families, it is important to consider the reality of their status as recent arrivals to the United States. While developing indigenous strategies, it is critical that the practitioner understand the social reality of these families. It is therefore essential that indigenous strategies include discussion of feelings associated with social situations in a sensitive manner.

CONCLUSIONS

We have described the issues and problems that immigrant Cuban children and families confront within the social context of the sociopolitical and immigration experience of the population. An ecological, strengthbased, affirmative practice framework is presented as a means of enhancing the helping professional's understanding of effective, indigenous, and culturally sensitive assessment and intervention strategies in working with Cuban children and families.

Given the multidimensional and dynamic aspects of Cuban culture, social workers must be open to expanding their clinical interpretations of Cuban conceptions of gender, race, and class. They must be able to move beyond an exclusively intrapsychic or sociocultural view to a strengths-based one. This shift in paradigm thinking requires the flexibility to reach for a collective or systemic perception of assessment and intervention as opposed to an individualistic one. This approach allows the practitioner to integrate individual treatment with family, group, and community dynamics that are consistent with Cuban culture.

When working with the Cuban immigrant child and family, the use of a strengths-based and ecological approach must consider the human experiences of family members. Therefore, gender, color, sexual orientation, religion, age, disabling conditions, culture, income, social class, and social status issues require consideration. The experiences of the Cuban family translate into values and perspectives that shape a worldview quite different from that of the dominant Western societal paradigms. The search for an alternative indigenous, culturally sensitive paradigm is at the core of the search for the source of strength, creativity, wonder, and power inherent in the everyday lives of these diverse children and families.

REFERENCES

Bernal, G. (1982). Cuban families. In M. McGoldrick, J. K. Pierce, & J. Giordano (Eds.), *Ethnicity and family therapy* (1st ed., pp. 187–207). New York: Guilford Press.

Bernal, G., & Flores-Ortiz, Y. (1980) . *Latino families in therapy: Socio-historical and cultural differences.* Unpublished manuscript, University of California, San Francisco.

Bustamante, J. A., & Santa Cruz, A. (1975). *Psiquiatria transcultural.* Havana: Editorial Cientifico Tecnica.

Canino, I., & Canino, G. (1982). Culturally syntonic family therapy for migrant Puerto Ricans. *Hospital and Community Psychiatry, 33,* 299–303.

Colon, E. (2001). Multidiversity and Latino communities. In G. Appleby, J. Hamilton, & E. Colon (Eds.), *Diversity, oppression and social functioning* (pp. 120–128). Boston: Allyn & Bacon.

Fusco, C. (1995). *English is broken here.* New York: New Press.

Garcia, J., & Marotta, S. (1997). Characterization of the Latino population. In J. Garcia & M.C. Zea (Eds.), *Psychological interventions and research with Latino populations* (pp. 1–14). Boston: Allyn & Bacon.

Garcia-Preto, N. (1994). On the bridge. *Family Therapy Networker, 18*(4), 35–37.

McGoldrick, M., Giordano, J., & Pearce, J. K. (Eds.). (1996). *Ethnicity and family therapy.* New York: The Guilford Press.

Molina, C. (1983). Family health promotion: Conceptual framework for "La Salud and El Bienestar" in Latino communities. In S. Andrade (Ed.), *Latino families in the United States* (pp. 35–44). New York: Planned Parenthood Federation of America.

Novas, H. (1994). *Everything you need to know about Latino history.* New York: Plume/Penguin.

Ortiz, V. (1995). The diversity of Latino families. In R. Zambrana (Ed.), *Understanding Latino families: Scholarship, policy and practice* (pp. 18–30). Thousand Oaks, CA: Sage.

Pinderhughes, E. (1989). *Understanding race, ethnicity, and power: The key to efficacy in clinical practice.* New York: Free Press.

Perez-Firmat, G. (1994). *Life on the hyphen.* Austin: University of Texas Press.

Rogg, E. M. (1974). *The assimilation of Cuban exiles: The role of community and Class.* New York: Aberdeen.

Solomon, B. B. (1982). The delivery of mental health services to Afro-American individuals and families: Translating theory into practice. In B. A. Bass, G. E. Wyatt, & G. J. Powell (Eds.), *The Afro-American family: Assessment, treatment and research* (pp. 62–73). New York: Grune & Stratton.

Thomas, H. (1971). *The pursuit of freedom*. New York: Harper & Row.

Torres, M. (1994). Beyond the rapture: Reconciling with our enemies, reconciling with ourselves. In R. Behar & J. Leon (Eds.), Bridges to Cuba [Puentes a Cuba]. *Michigan Quarterly Review, 33*, 419–436.

U.S. Bureau of the Census. (2001). *The Hispanic population in the United States: March*. Washington, DC: U.S. Government Printing Office.

Zuniga, M. E. (1992). Using metaphors in therapy: Dichos and Latino clients. *Social Work, 55*, 55–60.

CHAPTER 12

Dominican Children and Families

EDGAR COLON

Currently, approximately 31 million Latinos live in the United States (U.S. Bureau of the Census, 2001). Demographically, Latinos in the United States are relatively young, because of immigration by younger people seeking work and their high fertility rate. The Latino population is on average 8 years younger than African Americans, and fully one-third of all North American Latinos are under the age of 15. The image of Spanish speakers as a predominantly rural, farm-oriented people is prevalent in many western states, but on the East Coast, urban residence for Spanish speakers is the norm. In fact, nearly 85% of all Spanish speakers in the United States live in urban areas (U.S. Bureau of the Census, 2001).

Based on the present rate of growth, during the new millennium, the Latino population group will become the largest multidiverse minority group in this country (Hayes-Bautista, Hurtado, Valdez, & Hernandez, 1992). This amazing statistical trend projected by the U.S. Bureau of the Census (2001) predicts that by 2050, the Latino population will reach approximately 81 million, approximately one-fourth of the U.S. total population. This population growth trend does not take into account the illegal immigrants residing in many U.S. cities. In addition, it does not reflect a numeration of Latinos who marry Anglo Americans. In an attempt to assimilate into American society, many of these individuals tend to choose the label Caucasian as opposed to the categories based on nationality and race when responding to census reports. Other groups not accounted for in this trend are Mexican and South American persons that identify themselves as indigenous Indians and choose the category American Indian.

This chapter describes issues and problems related to the immigration experience of Dominican children and families in the United States. Given the particular social, economic, and political vulnerabilities confronted by Dominican children and families, the focus of the chapter is on strategies for the development of assessment and intervention strategies within the context of an empowerment and ecological–theoretical framework.

A discussion of select Dominican cultural values for effectively assessing immigration-related issues and problems affecting the lives of Dominican children and families is presented. For social workers and other helping professionals wishing to work with Dominican families and children, a discussion of strategies for the development of indigenous and Western interventions is followed by a discussion of culturally sensitive principles for such interventions. The chapter concludes with an illustrative case vignette.

HISTORICAL BACKGROUND

The Dominican population is now one of the largest Latino minority groups in the United States. Since the 1960's, the migration of Dominicans to the United tates has been primarily to the northeastern region of the nation, with the largest concentration in New York. The most recent estimates place the number of Dominicans living in New York and surrounding northeastern states at approximately 153,078 (U.S. Bureau of the Census, 2001). An important historical period during the Dominican exodus into the United States is the 30-year span of time during which Rafael Trujillo was President of the Dominican Republic (Grasmuck & Pessar, 1996). The dictatorship of Trujillo ended with his assassination in 1961.

Some individuals migrate to the United States seeking economic opportunities. Others flee oppressive regimes, and religious and political persecution, and a small percentage of individuals leave their native land to better their education and professional experiences and then return home. The available research contends that for many Latino families, living in the United States represents obtaining a place in the sun and a place to be free of political and economic oppression. This individual perception of life in the United States seems to be particularly true for Central and South American individuals and families. Many of these individuals left their homeland because of significant levels of fear and emotional anxiety experienced because of continued political oppression and/or acts of terrorism by their government.

The opportunity to migrate to the United States offers potential and promise. However, one of the costs is the need for families to adapt to their receiving community contexts. Once in the United States, poverty is a way of life for the majority of Latinos who live in this society, and their inability to access resources keeps them locked in a cycle that is oppressive and demoralizing.

A driving force behind the rapid increase of Dominicans in this country is the worsening political and economic situation in the Dominican Republic. In general, Dominicans who have immigrated to the United States have been of lower socioeconomic status. Dominican immigrant families, upon arrival, confront a scarcity of jobs even when they are willing to accept extremely low wages. Consequently, these families also find themselves relegated to substandard housing. For many families, the inability to understand and speak English keeps them on the periphery of mainstream society.

This is especially true of dark-skinned Latinos who, according to the available research, are more highly segregated from non-Latino whites than are light-skinned Latinos (Massey & Bitterman, 1985; Massey & Denton, 1992). The darker their skin, the more difficulty Latinos experience in finding housing (Scott, 1996; Yinger, 1991) and the more likely they are to earn low wages (Colon, 2001).

The arrival of Dominican children and families in the United States has occurred in three distinct waves. Three somewhat different groups comprised these waves of immigration (see Table 12.1). The shared experiences of these Dominican immigrant groups and other immigrant groups are the difficulties and hardship of adapting to life in the United States.

In regard to the characteristic help-seeking behaviors of each distinct Dominican immigrant group, the Trujillo era immigrants have been less willing to accept the assistance of formal health and mental health systems. However, the post-Trujillo era group are more willing to accept such help. Finally, the *Flotilla* do actively seek assistance and support from such systems (Paulino, 1994). Given the difficult historical social reality faced by all recently arrived immigrants into this country, particularly for Dominicans, several adaptation issues confronted by the Dominican family are discussed.

ADAPTATION TO THE UNITED STATES

As reported in the *National Association of Social Workers News* (November 1998, p. 15), the number of Latino children in the United States has surpassed the number of African American children. Given this trend, the

TABLE 12.1. Three Waves of Dominican Immigration

Immigration group	Time period	Characteristics
Trujillo era	1930–1961	Established professionals in Dominican society with strong ties to social, economic and political power
Post-Trujillo era	1960–1980	Middle- and working-class Dominicans
Flotilla era	1982–1986	Very poor members of Dominican society

United States Bureau of the Census has reported that by the early part of the 21st century the general population will include more individuals of Latino than of African American heritage.

Many Latino children and adolescents experience "culture shock" hastened by anxiety that results from losing all familiar signs and symbols of social intercourse. "Culture shock" is the result of a series of disorienting encounters that occur when an individual's values, beliefs, and patterns of behavior are influenced by the differences in these elements in the dominant society (Furnham & Bochner, 1986).

The vast diversification and multiethnicity within racial groups of Latino subgroups that have migrated to the United States make it difficult to generalize about the experiences of Dominican immigrant families. However, it is clear that the cultural experience of the Dominican immigrant family is influenced by a unique history and the nature of the political relationships between the immigrant's nation and the United States. These factors characterize the social reality of the Dominican immigrant family (Congress, 1994). These issues are important when considering the social issues affecting this population. Ultimately, the management of these historical and political issues significantly influences the recently arrived Dominican families' ability to gain acceptance into mainstream culture.

Lack of English-Language Proficiency

Recently arrived Dominican families experience economic and social powerlessness. Because of lack of English-language fluency, many Dominican families are unable to locate employment and therefore provide for basic needs such as food and shelter. For a culturally proud ethnic group, this social situation has caused much social, economic, and psychological distress. Shortly after their arrival in this country, many Dominican families realize that their hopes and dreams are unattainable. The available research suggests that language barriers and unfamiliarity with American customs, rules, and norms contribute to the Dominican immigrants' sense of powerlessness (Torres & Bonilla, 1993). In addition, the impact on the lives of Dominican immigrant families of discrimination and prejudice against foreigners and people of color in American society is a factor that also contributes to a sense of powerlessness and social isolation. Hayes-Bautista et al. (1992) add that the antipathy by the general public and policy makers toward the plight of Dominican immigrants further exacerbates threats to their psychological well-being.

Acculturation Stress

Dominican immigrants experience high levels of psychological stress and fear because their undocumented status while in this country increases the family's sense of powerlessness. Ortiz (1995) reports that others stresses experienced by the Dominican family include separation from family, relatives, and country of origin; the relocation issues related to language and cultural incongruity; and the practical aspects of housing and employment (Padilla, 1999). The impact of these stresses on the lives of Dominican immigrant families and children is particularly significant (Melville & Lykes, 1992).

Many of these immigrant families struggle to survive on low incomes and live doubled up with grandparents or other relatives for several years, until they are settled. When the children finally arrive, they must make an enormous adjustment, learn a new language, reacquaint themselves with their parents, and make the transition to the new environment and its school system. Often, those who come from rural areas have a greater adjustment to make. Many of these immigrant families retain their belief systems, often leading to antithetical attitudes toward the use of American helping systems (Giordano & Giordano, 1977).

Social Isolation and Loss of Social Support

It is clear that given the available research literature and census data on the Dominican population in this country, this population is living with a high level of economic and social risk, resulting in social isolation and the loss of significant social supports (Burnette, 1997; Torres-Salliant & Hernadez, 1996; Tran & Dhooper, 1996; U.S. Bureau of the Census, 1993;). With regard to the social functioning of the undocumented Dominican family, the experience of social isolation and loss of social supports contribute in significant ways to feelings of personal despair (Drachman & Ryan, 1991). Additional negative consequences for the undocumented Dominican family result from the avoidance of interactions with local institutions such as schools, hospitals, and police to avoid deportation. These Dominican families also use institutional health resources only episodically, and only when a health emergency arises. Moreover, others criminally victimize these families on a continual basis, because they will not turn to police or the criminal justice system for help.

This social reality is further compounded by the Dominican immigrant children and families' struggle to gain access to educational opportunities to develop competence in the English language. Grasmuck and Pessar (1996) contend that these critical factors contribute in significant ways to high underemployment rates within this population.

Intrafamilial Conflict between Dominican and American Values

As many newly arrived Dominican families seek to retain traditional Dominican values, Dominican parents may react by limiting the mainstream experience of Dominican youth with peers, therefore creating intrafamily conflict (Aponte, 1993). Consequently, the Dominican child confronts the difficult task of adapting to social values in two conflicting social and cultural situations while attempting to navigate the resulting confusion and conflict with the parent. (Lefley, 1984; Thomas, 1967).

Given the demands of acculturation for the rapid acquisition of English by Dominican youth versus the parents, additional conflict in interpersonal communication may emerge. In summary, traditional Dominican families tend to resist the need to transition to American family values and patterns. While these families undergo the demands of a new, often hostile culture, intrafamily communication conflict hinders the process of acculturation by the family system.

The Immigration Experience of Dominican Youth

Given the significant increase in the number of immigrant Latino youth in the United States, the attempt by Dominican youth to adjust to the migration experience deserves special attention of social workers and other helping professionals. Dominican immigrant youth are at great social risk. Given each family's need to accomplish the essential tasks of educational achievement, social development, and family socialization, these families confront significant psychological and emotional upheaval. The scant available literature on the migration experience of Dominican children suggests that they experience behavioral problems and have difficulty integrating into the social fabric of American society.

Given the view held by many Dominican youth that they are victims of discrimination, many of them also experience significant psychological and emotional distress. These youth often view the American way of life as hostile to their tradition of family unity, personal warmth, and respect for elders. In particular, given the history of racism in American society based on skin color, dark-skinned Dominican youth often feel disrespected and devalued by others outside of their family. For these youth, Paulino (1994) notes, life can contain a significant degree of high emotional distress. As a way of adapting and coping with this difficult social reality, these youth attempt to protect their self-respect. Many Dominican youth are unwilling to call themselves American or to let their language, traditions, and way of life disappear.

Legal Status

Clearly, the social stigma that is oftentimes associated with the legal status of the Dominican immigrant family can significantly affect important social relationships that support the social and emotional development of Dominican youth. Upon his or her arrival, the Dominican youth soon experiences the negative racist attitudes of non-Latinos. The impact of these attitudes toward racial, linguistic, and cultural differences causes psychological and emotional distress among Dominican youth and families. In response, the Dominican immigrant family can either develop the capacity to deal with these issues or become dysfunctional. A dysfunctional response may result in social interactions between children and parents, children and grandparents, husbands and wives, relatives, and siblings that are fraught with communication problems and crises in parenting (Lum, 1999).

The undocumented Dominican family is at particular risk for psychological and emotional distress, because oftentimes these families live in constant fear of deportation. The impact of such fear is detrimental to the functioning of the family (Congress, 1994). Because of its undocumented legal status, the employment market exploits the family. Family members must often take menial, low-paying jobs, including housekeeping, gardening, factory work, or hotel domestic service positions. The exploitation of the undocumented worker often leads to very low wages, no health care insurance, and long working hours. The Dominican family system itself is further negatively affected by the employment experience of the adult working members.

Among these families, Pinderhughes (1989) notes that Dominican immigrant women assume multiple roles within the family system. This family adaptation response leads to role confusion for these women as they attempt to act independently and carry the same the same burdens as their male counterparts. More importantly, these women are often are unable to adhere to traditional Dominican values that are in conflict with those of the larger society. These women experience strong ambivalence between maintaining the desire and motivation to stay in the United States or return to their homeland. Pessar (1987) contends that the ambivalence is centered on a sense of loss of social, economic, and political rights, and the privileges accessible in the United States as opposed to those available in the Dominican Republic. A closer examination of immigration data reveals that Dominican women have consistently been able to immigrate at a higher rate than Dominican men. There are several reasons for this social phenomenon. Dominican women have emigrated at a higher rate than men entering the labor market throughout the world. This immigration pattern is consistent with the general sociopolitical flow of women entering labor markets (Rosario, Goris, & Angeles, 1990).

AN ECOLOGICAL AND EMPOWERMENT PERSPECTIVE FOR ASSESSMENT AND INTERVENTION PLANNING

Colon (2001) suggests that the empowerment approach to social work practice is an effective approach to understanding the diversity issues that influence the lives of the Dominican child and family. The use of this perspective enhances the social work practitioner's understanding of the institutional, systemic, and interpersonal stresses that dominate the lives of many Dominican immigrant families. This practice approach also supports the practitioner's development of an indigenous, culturally congruent basis for clinical assessment and intervention planning.

The ecological perspective provides a basis for assessing the problems and issues affecting the functioning of Dominican family systems. While considering the vast diversity of experience among all Dominican immigrant families, the practitioner can engage in the development of empowering strategies consonant with the uniqueness inherent in Dominican culture, history, and structure.

Dominican immigrant families live in various parts of the country. The Dominican population also exhibits different births and mortality rates, and achieves different levels of income and educational status. In addition, the influence of traditional Dominican culture in interaction with multiple social factors exerts a significant influence on the social functioning of the family system and the individual members.

It is important that the social work practitioner recognize that the Dominican immigrant family is influenced, promoted, and shaped by its cultural heritage. Dominican culture, language, and ethnicity are overt expressions of family identity (Colon, 2001). However, these factors are not the sole determinants of the values, beliefs, and behaviors of the Dominican family. Dominican culture is not a static entity. The experience of social adaptation among Dominican families has strongly influenced the social reality of Dominican children and families. While engaged in working with Dominican families to address social service needs, the practitioner must view Dominican culture as an ongoing process in which Dominican individuals steadily rework new ideas and behaviors within a cultural framework (Anderson & Goolishian, 1992).

Within the context of the successes and failures associated with this ongoing process of cultural adaptation, the practitioner is able to engage with Dominican immigrant families in developing effective adaptation strategies. In essence, it is important for helping professionals to maintain the view that Dominican culture is not a material phenomenon. Dominican culture involves the constant interaction of beliefs, behaviors, and emotions within a changing environment.

Dominican families also experience a social reality of cultural transition. Traditional families consist of all family members born in the family of origin. A traditional family consists of parents and grandparents with strongly held traditional beliefs living with westernized, younger family members. Americanized families are those families in which all members are fully acculturated, loosely adhering to traditional beliefs.

Traditional Dominican immigrant families identify along four specific cultural orientations. Lee (1996) posits a model of family development that involves four cultural orientations, including traditional families, transitional families, bicultural families, and "Americanized families." He argues that these cultural orientations are useful for understanding the Dominican immigrant family's position in the cultural transition–acculturation process. Based on these four cultural orientations, Lee contends that the Dominican immigrant family is a traditional family in transition. While considering the length of residence of family members in the United States, the Dominican community is a transitional family attempting to acculturate to a dominant society and the resulting intrafamily conflict that may arise. The following section describes important cultural values and practices that help the Dominican immigrant family to remain resilient and strong while in cultural transition.

CULTURAL VALUES AS STRENGTHS IN ASSESSMENT

Dominican cultural practices have served as protective factors for the Dominican immigrant (Colon, 2001). Shared traditions and values have kept Dominican children and families together as an ongoing, distinctive community.

Value of Dominican Children and Youth

It is evident that social and economic class dimensions, and the stage of acculturation, affects the Dominican immigrant family's ability to provide for the emotional and instrumental needs of its members. Nevertheless, it is also evident that children and adolescents are highly valued within Dominican culture. Dominican families have a strong commitment to socialize the child to engage effectively in interpersonal relationships. Presently, Dominican families continue to have larger families on average than mainstream U.S. families; 65% of Dominican families have three members compared to 57% of U.S. non-Latino families with fewer than two members. Garcia and Marrotta (1997) note that within the total Latino population in the United States, Latinos have three times as many families with six members compared to the majority population. The strong commitment of Dominican families to the development of their children is a strength that may provide an avenue for assessment of family issues and planning family-centered interventions.

Human Collectivism

A second Dominican value that provides a strengths perspective is collectivism. Dominican families are willing to seek mutual empathy, to sacrifice self-chosen goals in favor of the interests of the group, to conform to group expectations, and, generally, to trust members of their own family and the community. Marin (1993) contends that among Latino cultures, compared to the individualistic, competitive, achievement-oriented cultures of non-Latino groups in the United States, Dominican culture is oriented toward mutuality and interdependence.

Familism

Finally, an important Dominican value closely related to that of collectivism is familism. Characteristics of *familism* (family centeredness) in Dominican culture, strong orientation and obligation to the family produces a kinship structure qualitatively different from that of other groups. The emphasis is on the needs of the family as a unit.

Ramirez and Arce (1981) describe familism as a multidimensional concept that comprises aspects of structure, behavior, norms and attitudes, and social identity. Dominican immigrants are a source of strength for family members. Social workers and other helping professionals engaged in the assessment and intervention-planning process need to consider the strength inherent in these families.

INDIGENOUS STRATEGIES AND WESTERN INTERVENTIONS

Western intervention strategies rely on a rational, medical model, linear approach to understanding the immigration experiences of recently arrived groups. An indigenous approach to understanding Dominican families' immigration experience must rely on a more transactional, multilinear view of the immigration experience. This view must take into account the reasons for migrating to the United States and the stresses affecting Dominican immigrant families. In addition, indigenous intervention-planning strategies must recognize the instrumental value for clinical planning of the legal status of the family while in the country. Legal status may be a significant force in molding the immigrant family's experience in this country. The difficult adjustment process experienced by many Dominicans alerts the social work practitioner that an indigenous approach to intervention planning considers that, upon their arrival, many Dominican families are disappointed in the reality that awaits them (Paulino, 1994).

Moreover, effective indigenous intervention planning must consider the help seeking behaviors and social service needs of the Dominican families. Drachman and Ryan (1991) suggest that U. S. health and human service systems have not adequately addressed the social service needs of these families. In summary, an indigenous lens is required to address the critical acculturation experiences of these families.

While engaged in the development of an indigenous assessment and intervention-planning process, the helping professional must consider these migration readjustment experiences, which are natural and inherent aspects of the traditional immigrant family that result in a normal degree of acculturation stress (Thomas & Wilcox, 1987). However, given the unique culture, emotions, and behaviors of Dominican people, acculturation stress can disrupt the ability of the Dominican immigrant family to manage changing intrafamily task demands (Powell, 1995). For example, Dominican children and parents attempting to meet the demands of cultural transition, and therefore social adaptation, may experience interpersonal and intergenerational conflicts.

The social work practitioner and other helping professionals must consider the nature and extent of the acculturation pressures on Dominican immigrant families in American society. They must recognize that the societal push experienced by transitional Dominican families as they strive to maintain their identity, pride, and ties to the homeland affects the success or failure of healthy social adaptation. Helping professionals are reminded that Dominican youth are at particular social risk for psychological and emotional distress. The process of social adaptation for Dominican youth requires movement away from the influence of empowering traditional Dominican values toward American beliefs and values not congruent with a strong Dominican sense of personhood. Consequently, these youth may not develop a "goodness of fit" within their constantly evolving American social environment.

Finally, the practitioner must engage in a practice approach that demonstrates an understanding of the important relationship of theory to practice and the interrelatedness of alternative economic, political, and personal perspectives within an ecological framework. The goal of such an approach must also reflect the need for multisystem analysis and action on individual, group, organizational, community, and societal levels. In addition, because social workers and other helping professionals have their own biases, they need to examine them in shaping their professional self-concept and perception of the social realities of others (Green, 1999).

PRINCIPLES OF CULTURALLY APPROPRIATE PRACTICE

The development of effective strategies for a culturally appropriate assessment and intervention-planning process with Dominican immigrant children and families requires consideration of intervention strategies to enhance the following:

- Understanding both the effects of acculturation on the Dominican immigrant family and the struggle to achieve social adaptation in what the family may perceive as a hostile, racist society.

- Understanding how to help clients identify and harness the strengths inherent in the values and belief systems of the Dominican immigrant family. Social worker participation in this active work is a powerful avenue for the engagement of family members in the helping process.
- Understanding the importance of advocacy work for the development of culturally appropriate health and human service programs to address the psychological and emotional stresses confronting Dominican immigrant families.
- Understanding coalition-building activities to ensure that social agencies provide adequate levels of bilingual and bicultural personnel that can provide culturally sensitive interventions to the Dominican immigrant individual, child, and family.
- Understanding alternative paradigms for knowing the social reality of immigrant Dominican families. The achievement of such an understanding enhances the practitioner's skill at promoting the families' telling of their stories.
- Understanding how to identify and develop indigenous intervention strategies that consider the unique help-seeking behaviors of Dominican families. The development of such strategies provide opportunities for helping professionals to understand the impact of issues of social isolation and loss experienced by the family system.

CASE VIGNETTE

The case vignette illustrates the adaptation issues faced by a Dominican family that arrived in the United States during the "*Marielito*" immigration wave. The Dominican family came to the United States to seek better educational and employment opportunities. The family comprises the father, 30 years old, the mother of 27 years, and an 8-year-old son. The family came to live with relatives in a predominantly Dominican population in the Upper West Side of Manhattan, New York. The first 4 years of their life in New York City were difficult ones for the family. The father had to take a low-skills, low-paying job as a clerk in an area Dominican grocery store. The mother did not work, because the father felt that she should be watching over their son as he reached a difficult age in his development. During their fifth year in the United States, the father began to associate with a group of Dominican men who were using intravenous heroin. As he became more hopeless about his life and that of his family in the United States, he began to use the drugs.

Sadly, by the second year of his heavy use of heroin, the father began to feel ill. An area physician diagnosed him with AIDS. The father and the family reacted to the diagnosis with secrecy and great shame. As a proud family, they refused to seek help from the government. Unlike members of other Dominican immigrant waves, this family refused any professional help.

This Dominican immigrant family has unique needs and varying attitudes toward seeking help from human service professionals. Therefore, the social worker practitioner engaged in working with this family must individuate the assessment and intervention planning process to account for the unique needs of each family member.

Given the complex and unique response of this family to helping systems in the United States, the social work practitioner must ensure that he or she engages in an indigenous approach to intervention planning. The intervention plan must consider the unique behaviors, emotions, and culturally congruent coping strategies of this family. It is important to assess the severity and extent of psychological and emotional stress affecting each family member.

CONCLUSIONS

Dominican immigrant families are at risk for social, economic, and political difficulties while residing in the United States because of unemployment and lack of access to educational opportunities. The rapidly growing Dominican population is a young one, within the 20- to 30-year age range, with many single parents living in poverty conditions. U.S. helping systems must develop program services that take into the account the cultural values, beliefs, and demographics of Dominican immigrant children and families (Georges, 1990; Torres-Saliant & Hernandez, 1996).

The social practitioner and other helping professional must consider that whereas many groups of Dominican immigrant families share similar adjustment problems with non-Dominican immigrants residing in the United States, they have unique needs and varying attitudes toward seeking professional help.

Finally, the helping professional must use this awareness to engage in culturally sensitive, indigenous, intervention-planning strategies that will elucidate the dynamics of diversity, social oppression, and social functioning affecting the life experience of Dominican children and families. This is a first step toward working with diverse peoples within a culturally sensitive paradigm.

REFERENCES

Anderson, H., & Goolishian, H. (1992). The client is the expert: A not-knowing approach to therapy. In S. McNamee & K. J. Gergen (Eds.), *Therapy as social construction* (pp. 25–35). Thousand Oaks, CA: Sage.

Aponte, R. (1993). Hispanic families in poverty: Diversity, context, and interpretation. *Families in Society: The Journal of Contemporary Human Services, 36,* 527–537.

Burnette, D. (1997). Grandmother caregivers in inner city Latino families: A descriptive profile and informal social supports. *Journal of Multicultural Social Work, 5,* 121–138.

Colon, E. (2001). Multidiversity and Latino communities. In G. Appleby, E. Colon, & J. Hamilton (Eds.), *Diversity, oppression and social functioning* (pp. 92–178). Waltham, MA: Allyn & Bacon.

Congress, E. (1994). The use of culturagrams to assess and empower culturally diverse families. *Families in Society, 75* (9), 531–538.

Drachman, D., & Ryan, A. S. (1991). Immigrants and refugees. In A. Gitterman (Ed.), *Handbook of social work practice with vulnerable populations* (pp. 618–646). New York: Columbia University Press.

Furnham, A., & Bochner, S. (1986). *Culture shock: Psychological reactions to unfamiliar environments.* London: Routledge.

Garcia, J., & Marotta, S. (1997). Characterization of the Latino population. In J. Garcia & M.C. Zea (Eds.), *Psychological interventions and research with Latino populations* (pp. 1–14). Boston: Allyn & Bacon.

Georges, E. (1990). *The making of a transnational community: Migration development and cultural change in the Dominican Republic.* New York: Columbia University Press.

Giordano, J., & Giordano, G. P. (1977). *The ethno-cultural factor in mental health: A literature review and bibliography.* New York: Institute on Pluralism and Group Identity.

Grasmuck, S., & Pessar, P. (1996). Dominicans in the United States: First and second generation settlement, 1960–1990. In S. Pedraza & R. G. Rumbaut (Eds.), *Origins and destinies: Immigration, race, and ethnicity in America* (pp. 280–292). Belmont, CA: Wadsworth.

Green, J.W. (1999). *Cultural awareness in the human services.* Boston: Allyn & Bacon.

Hayes-Bautista, D., Hurtado, A., Valdez, R., & Hernandez, A. (1992). *No longer a minority: Latinos and social policy in California.* Los Angeles: UCLA Chicano Studies Research Center.

Lee, M. (1996). A constructivist approach to help seeking process of clients: A response to cultural diversity. *Journal of Clinical Social Work, 24,* 187–202.

Lefley, H. P. (1984). Cross-cultural training for mental health practitioners: Effects on the delivery of services. *Hospital and Community Psychiatry, 35*(12), 1227–1229.

Lum, D. (1996). *Culturally competent practice: A framework for growth and action.* Pacific Grove, CA: Brooks-Cole.

Marin, G. (1993). Defining culturally appropriate community interventions: Hispanics as a case study. *Journal of Community Psychology, 21,* 149–161.

Masset, D. S., & Bitterman, B. (1985). Explaining the paradox of Puerto Rican segregation. *Social Forces, 64,* 306–331.

Massey, D. S., & Denton, N. A. (1992). Racial identity and spatial assimilation of Mexican Americans in the United States. *Social Science Research*, 22, 1–27.

Melville, M. B., & Lykes, M. B. (1992). Guatemalan Indian children and the sociocultural effects of government sponsored terrorism. *Social Science and Medicine*, 34, 533–548.

Ortiz, V. (1995). The diversity of Latino families. In R. Zambrana (Ed.), *Understanding Latino families: Scholarship, policy and practice* (pp. 18–30). Thousand Oaks, CA: Sage.

Padilla, Y. (1999). Immigrant policy: Issues for social work practice. In P. L. Ewalt, E. M. Freeman, A. E. Fortune, D. L. Poole, & S.Witkin (Eds.), *Multicultural issues in social work: Practice and research* (pp. 589–604). Washington, DC: National Association of Social Workers.

Paulino, A. (1994). Dominicans in the United States: Implications for practice and policies in the human services. *Journal of Multicultural Social Work*, 3(2), 58–62.

Pessar, P. (1987). The Dominicans: Women in the household and the garment industry. In N. Foner (Ed.), *New immigrants in New York* (pp. 101–110). New York: Columbia University Press.

Pinderhuges, E. (1989). *Understanding race, ethnicity, and power: The key to efficacy in clinical practice*. New York: Free Press.

Powell, D. R. (1995). Including Latino fathers in parent education and support programs: Development of a model program. In R. E. Zambrana (Ed.), *Understanding Latino families* (pp. 85–106). Thousand Oaks, CA: Sage.

Ramirez, O., & Arce, C. H. (1981). The contemporary Chicano family: An empirically based review. In A. Baron, Jr. (Ed.), *Explorations in Chicano psychology* (pp. 3–28). New York: Praeger.

Rosario, J. E., Goris, A., & Angeles, F. (1990). *Political participation of Dominicans in New York City: The case of Dominicans in Washington Heights and Inwood*. New York: Dominican Research Center.

Scott, A. J. (1996). The manufacturing economy: Ethnic and gender divisions of labor. In R.Waldinger & M. Bozoogmehr (Eds.), *Ethnic Los Angeles* (pp. 14–20). New York: Russell Sage Foundation.

Thomas, D., & Wilcox, J. E. (1987). The rise of family theory. In M. B. Sussman & S. Stienmetz (Eds.), *Handbook of marriage and the family* (pp. 81–102). New York: Plenum Press.

Thomas, P. (1967). *Down these mean streets*. New York: Signet Press.

Torres, A., & Bonilla, F. (1993). Decline within decline: The New York perspective. In R. Morales & F. Bonilla (Eds.), *Latinos in a changing U.S. economy: Comparative perspectives on growing inequality* (pp. 85–108). Newbury Park, CA: Sage.

Torres-Saillant, S., & Hernadez, R. (1996). *The Dominican Americans: Profile of an ethnic minority in the United States*. Westport, CT: Greenwood Press.

Tran, T., & Dhooper, S. (1996). Ethnic and gender differences in perceived needs for social services among three elderly Hispanic groups. *Journal of Gerontological SocialWork*, 25(3/4), 21–29.

U.S. Bureau of the Census. (1993, 1995, 1996, 1997). *Hispanic Americans today*. Washington, DC: U.S. Government Printing Office.

U.S. Bureau of the Census. (2001, March). *The Hispanic population in the United States*. Washington, DC: Government Printing Office.

Yinger, J. (1991). *Housing discrimination study: Incidence of discrimination and variations in discriminatory behavior*. Washington, DC: U.S. Department of Housing and Urban Development, Office of Policy Development and Research.

CHAPTER 13

Ecuadorian and Colombian Children and Families

ZOILA TAZI

> When asked why it is difficult for some children to get used to living in this country, 6-year-old Joaquin answered, *"Because when you live in Ecuador you don't know how much you love your cousins and then you come here and you know."*

Preliminary figures for the 2000 census revealed a growth of 38.8% in the numbers of Latinos living in the United States. This dramatic growth is "largely being fueled by immigration" to this country from many Latin American countries, according to the Bureau of the Census. The preliminary census figures also show a shift in immigration patterns in that more and more immigrants are settling in the suburbs rather than the larger cities, where earlier waves of immigrants made their homes. Immigrants continue to seek out enclaves of their own countrymen for their homes, where they begin to alter, enhance, and redefine their communities. The influx of immigrants to our suburbs perhaps forces service providers, agencies, and even citizens to consider how our nation is changing. If the suburbs ever exemplified the culture and comfort of "American" family life, then here, too, we are becoming more diverse, and the term "American" bears redefining.

There is a growing new immigrant population from many Latin American countries in the suburbs outside New York City. Large numbers of Ecuadorian and Colombian families have immigrated from their countries to the suburbs and have begun living in these neighborhoods and schools. Many cultural values are shared among different Latino groups, but the individual groups' political histories, social customs, and patterns of immigration set them apart among Latinos and profoundly affect adaptation and acculturation. The schools, then, must have some understanding of the larger "Latino" group and its values, as well as the individual subsets of Ecuadorian and Colombian values.

HISTORICAL BACKGROUND

Ecuador

A large number of the members of the Ecuadorian community in the suburbs come from the south-central region of the country. Many families now living in New York were neighbors in Ecuador as well, and know each other's extended family members. The community maintains a strong bicultural connection between the two countries.

The south-central region of Ecuador is a picturesque, historic area in the intermontane valley of the Andes Mountains (the Sierra). Colonial architecture and indigenous crafts attract tourists year-round. Historically, the Quichua Indians (among other tribes of the Sierra) populated this region, and many present-day residents are descended from the Quichua. As in other North and South American countries, the native Amerindian groups, including the Quichua, suffered poor treatment from the colonizers. In Ecuador, complex social relationships developed based on race, ethnic affiliation, and social class relegated the Indians to the lowest social and political rank. Indians of all groups, called *indígenas* (indigenous people), were treated as inferior in almost every regard. At the pinnacle of the social ladder were the Spanish, who were regarded as "white." Below the Spanish were the *mestizos* of mixed Spanish and Indian heritage, followed by the descendents of African slaves and, finally, the *indígena*. The *Instituto Nacional de Estadísticas y Censos* (The National Institute of Statistics and Census, 1985) describes these relationships as follows:

> The elite (and middle class) often described itself as *la gente buena* (the good people) or *la gente decente* (the respectable people), contending that it had sufficient breeding, intelligence, and culture to rule others. The subordination of workers, peasants, servants, and all Indians was an essential part of this scheme. In the elite view, gains achieved by subordinates came not as their natural right but through the beneficence of their betters. (p. 49)

This dynamic exists as the backdrop of present-day social interactions between racial and ethnic groups in Ecuador. It then "travels" with the immigrant to the United States and becomes part of the relationships formed with authority figures and service providers, such as the public schools. A parent approaching the public school system with a passive, ingratiating manner is likely to encounter hardship. School systems function best when parents advocate articulately for their children and take some command of critical decisions. When passivity in parents is a cultural value, it is easy for schools to misinterpret this as a disregard for the importance of education. All kinds of interventions that might be designed to reach out to parents who "don't value education" alienate them and perpetuate a defensive stance by the school. However, when we view this deferential attitude in the appropriate cultural context, we can recognize a creative, resilient tactic to combat oppression. In *Ecuador: A Country Study*, Dennis Hanratty further describes the situation:

> Although public deference to other ethnic groups supported stereotypes of Indians as intellectually inferior, Indians viewed deference as a survival strategy. Deference established that an individual Indian was properly humble and deserving of the white's or *mestizo*'s aid and intercession. Given the relative powerlessness of Indians, such an approach softened the rules governing interethnic exchanges" (Hanratty, 1991)

In a society such as ours, which values assertiveness and self-promotion, deference and passivity can be regarded with contempt and can, in fact, lead to oppression. Therefore, one critical initial social work intervention is to make an individual aware of the conflict in cultural values and enhance his or her adaptation to our culture by teaching new advocacy skills.

Colombia

Colombia shares a border and a similar history with Ecuador. Hanratty and Meditz (1990) describe some of Colombia's history in their book *Colombia: A Country Study*, and a brief summary follows. The Spanish colonizers worked so aggressively to dominate the several hundred tribes of indigenous peoples they encountered that little of their lifestyles and customs was absorbed into the emerging Colombian culture. Instead, the indigenous population was used to work the vast tracts of land owned by the wealthy Spaniards.

Colombia has a long history of intermingling between and among its three racial groups—whites, blacks, and Indians. As in Ecuador, the group holding the most power, prestige, and social status was the whites, descended from the Spanish. The influence of Spanish culture and customs touched every aspect of the Colombian society and contributed to a strong Hispanic identification. The worldwide problem of racism also plagues Colombia. Blacks and *mestizos* still tend to be the poorer groups, whereas the whites have more of the country's wealth and political power. Many terms are used to describe precisely a person's color and ancestry. These seem to locate just how close or how far one is from the desired white race.

Despite intermarriage between racial groups in Colombia, the Spanish ideals of family life prevailed as the accepted norms. The father held complete authority and responsibility for the family. The mother, who always deferred to her husband's wishes, was relegated the role of nurturer and protector of the children. These role assignments are more difficult to maintain among poorer families when fathers may not be present, but they are the ideal nevertheless.

Education is greatly valued in Colombia. Public funding for education grows annually, and the country boasts a literacy rate of nearly 90%. Enrollment in universities continues to grow even in a time when students are at risk of harassment by government factions.

Colombia's recent history of violence and political instability affects not only the lives of Colombians but also the perceptions of North Americans receiving Colombian immigrants. Many Colombians have witnessed mass murders in their villages and have many times lost loved ones to the violence. Warring guerilla groups continue to torment villages with their violence, while family members in Colombia and the United States mourn helplessly. Danger and loss at home are often components in the decision to immigrate to this country. Here, we hear so much about drug trafficking in Colombia that it is easy to form an image of Colombians based on the incomplete and negative picture painted by the media. Pride in their heritage and culture often keeps Colombian immigrants from feeling defeated by the vicious stereotypes.

There are more than 300,000 Colombians living in the United States. As the numbers of Colombians now living in the suburbs continues to grow, the importance of understanding the history and values of Colombian culture becomes increasingly important.

ADAPTATION TO THE UNITED STATES

Many definitions for acculturation are offered in the literature. There is general agreement that acculturation is "the psychosocial adaptation made by members of one culture group as a result of contact with another" (Chavez, Moran, Reid, & Lopez, 1997, p. 34). The growing number of new immigrants in the United States has driven some of the research on the levels of acculturation that might serve as predictors of economic, social, or academic success in this country. However, what service providers need most to understand about new immigrants is that the process of acculturation is all-consuming and engages the individual's mind, body, and spirit. It is understandable, therefore, that acculturation might be fraught with complications and setbacks. An individual might not be capable, during a period of intense adjustment, of attending to normal social and psychological demands.

Many Ecuadorian and Colombian immigrants make extraordinary sacrifices to immigrate to this country. Their survival, and even their success, in this country is continually fueled by that powerful, initial drive to immigrate. There are three basic elements, in my experience, that contribute greatly to a new family's adaptation to this country. First is the high regard and support of education for the children. For many parents, completing their own education becomes impossible because of the daily demands of work and family, but parents can ensure a better future for their children when they support their education. Second is the creative use of community and family support. Families develop complex networks among relatives, neighbors, churches, and service providers that truly exemplify the proverb "It takes a village to raise a child." In many ways, this is a reenactment of some of the supports found in the country of origin that evolves and expands with the immigrants in this country. Third is the willingness to take on any kind of work to make a living. The mythology of discrimination would have us believe that immigrants are shiftless and lazy, and that they come to this country because of our generous social programs that allow them to live for free. This could not be further from the truth. Not only are many immigrants ineligible for most government programs, but also, among immigrants, the recognized benefit of this country is the availability of work. In my years as a social worker, I have not met a single immigrant who did not believe this.

PROBLEMS FOR CHILDREN AND FAMILIES

The most difficult sacrifices for an immigrant (or perhaps for anyone) are the sacrifices of relationships and attachments (Smart & Smart, 1995). By its very nature, immigration begins with loss. This clearly becomes a central issue in the helping relationship with a new immigrant family.

Loss and Separation

In my role as a school social worker, I hear the stories children and their families tell of leaving loved ones and beloved homes back in Ecuador and Colombia. Separation from everything familiar is an accepted part of immigrating to this country. Once here, however, the sense of loss and disorientation leads to a period of melancholy. New immigrant children arriving at the school tend to cry more than other children and often display the following symptoms:

1. Separation anxiety
2. Distractibility
3. Overly meek behavior
4. Mistrust of adults
5. Exaggerated fears and sensitivity

The process of mourning their losses can become complicated and lead to depression and adjustment disorders.

Disrupted Maternal Bond

One of the tragedies I have observed in the patterns of immigration among our Ecuadorian and Colombian groups is that mothers are often separated from their young children for long periods of time. Although separation from one's father can also be tragic, the impact of a disrupted maternal bond cannot be underestimated. This has lasting implications for both the mother–child relationship and the developing personality of the child. To facilitate the entire family's survival, mothers sometimes immigrate without their children, leaving them in the care of extended family members. Once in this country, the mothers busy themselves working and saving for the eventual reunion with their children. In the meantime, they have grown detached from their children, and in many cases their children have suffered depression because of the disruption in the maternal bond. When the mother and child are finally reunited, the child then suffers another disruption in the relationship with his or her primary caregiver. Now the child and mother are virtually strangers. The normal parenting tasks of teaching discipline and respect can seem insurmountable to a parent who does not know his or her own child. Parents who have worked so hard to enable their children to have a home in this country face a sense of failure when the reunion is not smooth or pleasant. Many mothers have confided a fear that they have lost affection for their children. This, in turn, provokes guilt and anxiety in the parents; without intervention, this situation puts many children at greater risk for physical abuse. However, the impetus to immigrate to this country is so powerful that some immigrants are willing to endure the sadness and hardship of being separated from their children.

Initial Shock

Anyone who has traveled outside the United States may understand why the first contact with another country can be shocking. Usually, the first noticeable difference is the change in temperature. The body makes quick adjustments. Second, the scenery, the scents, and the sounds are different. The heightened need for observation can be exhilarating if one is on vacation, but what if one is assessing a new home? Many new immigrant children describe feeling overwhelmed with disappointment at how cold, ugly, and smelly our New York airports can be.

Soon after recovering from the physical shock, many children describe beginning mental calculations as to their place in this new world. The embarrassment of inappropriate or shabby clothing distorts children's sense of belonging. Entry ports tend to be grand structures that can signify wealth to the child who arrives with no coat. It does not take long for the child to appreciate how different he or she is.

Trauma

Months (and even years) after arriving, many of the children with whom I have worked continue to describe fear and apprehension about their trip to the United States. Saying good-bye to their homes and families, entering an enormous aircraft, and arriving in a strange place are very intense, disorienting experiences. The pace of change is relentless for a new immigrant, and there is little time to assimilate one's own experiences. For countless new immigrants, the journey to this country begins with an unforgettable trauma. Children, who are not spared these traumatic experiences, suffer the confusion of sorting out their feelings about the trauma from their reactions to a new place. Children who enter the country illegally, either with false documentation or by braving the border, tell terrifying, sad stories, yet the risk of trauma is no deterrent to new immigrants. The poor conditions at home, coupled with the hopes of creating a new life, prove to be a powerful motivation. By the time some new immigrant children begin public school, they have complicated stress reactions to the trauma of their journey. Early intervention and support is critical.

Silence

Teachers are often alarmed when a new immigrant child enters the classroom, then remains silent and docile. Silence is a dramatic symptom that draws much adult attention. The literature on selective mutism reports slightly higher incidence of the disorder among immigrant children. Intervening with support, friendship, and often a therapeutic group experience helps new immigrant children develop confidence and communication skills (James, 1997). However, if school personnel do not understand this aspect of the process of acculturation, it is easy for them to question whether the child is reacting to abuse or mistreatment at home. The school–parent relationship, then, begins with suspicion, and it is often difficult to change that first impression.

Language Acquisition

Language conveys the nuances and attributes of a culture. Language and culture cannot be understood independently of one another. Given that it takes 2 to 3 years to become proficient in a new language, it is evident that the process of acculturation can last many years. English as a second language (ESL) teachers argue that it takes at least 7 years to learn and use the more complex language of academic learning. New immigrants are often judged or criticized for not learning English as their first priority. The idea that employment might be a speedier and more responsible route to acculturation for the new immigrant is sometimes hard to grasp, despite our own work ethic. Once again, service providers might view this as a deficit and fail to recognize a cultural strength and survival mechanism. New immigrant children are often caught between languages and cultures. Clearly this will be reflected in their behavior and academic achievement (Gibson, 1998). It behooves schools to offer bilingual services that ease the transition to a new culture (Holman, 1997).

Resident Status

There is probably no comparable experience in this country that exemplifies the fear and anxiety that undocumented immigrants feel. The very real fear of being caught and deported interferes with every relationship within the school system. We cannot underestimate the significance of resident status to an immigrant. Consider how the process of acculturation is complicated by the fact that the immigrants cannot trust the very people they need to help orient them to this country. Immigration laws continue to limit the numbers of immigrants who can become documented; thus, growing numbers of new immigrant families become "criminals" who violate the law. How can this not profoundly affect a family?

Becoming Mixed

We have the best intentions when we try to "help along" the process of acculturation by encouraging new immigrants to take on more of the values, language, and behaviors of our country. However, the new immigrant who becomes too strongly identified with this culture is often left without supports in his or her native community. Interventions that support biculturalism enable new immigrants to retain their identity, while exploring how they have been changed by contact with the new culture. This is critical for children who are still forming their identities and run the risk of rejecting their own heritage. If we view acculturation as becoming more "mixed" with two cultures rather than becoming more "American," we can support the more difficult aspects of acculturation while we preserve an individual's strengths.

CULTURAL VALUES AS STRENGTHS IN ASSESSMENT

An ample understanding of the issues involved in the process of acculturation is critical to assessing a new immigrant family. In the school, the presenting problems for a new immigrant child are likely to be delayed academic achievement and/or behavioral concerns. A comprehensive history of the family's immigration experience can guide the assessment and ensuing interventions. The clinician's understanding of acculturation can help normalize the experience for the family and can serve to assess the gravity of the presenting problem. Without this understanding, the clinician might intervene with more typical "Western" strategies and begin to look for possible learning disabilities or poor child-rearing practices. This fosters a negative view of Ecuadorian and Colombian families (or Latinos in general) and, inadvertently, perpetuates discrimination.

As in other Latino groups, the Ecuadorians and Colombians employ a complex social network called *compadrazgo*. Literally, this means there are "co-parenting" responsibilities for parents and godparents in raising a child. Each child in a family has his or her own godparent, so this extends a family's support system to several other "co-parents." This is an effective native support system and an immediate strength in assessing a family. How readily a family utilizes *el compadrazgo* signals to the clinician the level of support available to a family, as well as the level of social skills and aptitude required to reciprocate within this system.

Both Ecuadorian and Colombian groups also give much importance to the social graciousness and conduct of their children. Termed *el niño bien educado* (the well-educated child), this is a great cultural strength. The expectations involved in being *bien educado* become allies to the clinician intervening with a family. The child who is *bien educado* understands about cooperation, respect for authority, and personal effort. In working with a family, it becomes imperative to appeal to these principles in solving behavior problems and family conflicts.

These two examples of cultural values, *el compadrazgo* and *el niño bien educado*, represent powerful strengths within any family. It is critical to incorporate these native strengths in the helping relationship with Ecuadorian and Colombian families. These values also serve as readily accepted models the clinician can utilize to help strengthen family functioning.

INDIGENOUS STRATEGIES AND WESTERN INTERVENTIONS

The new immigrant seeking help relies on the clinician to orient him or her to the values and customs of the new country and to teach new skills with which to negotiate the new environment. These basic principles of empowerment guide most social work interventions. To facilitate adaptation, the clinician relies on indigenous strategies that "speak" to the new immigrant in his or her cultural "language." A comprehensive understanding of the backgrounds and values of the Ecuadorian and Colombian groups serves as the basis of these indigenous strategies. For example, a group modality to address parenting issues tends to be very effective, because addressing a child's upbringing among a group of concerned adults is familiar and culturally relevant (*compadragzo*). Children also tend to be oriented toward a group experience (Pabón, n.d.) and prefer to attend sessions in the company of their peers. When it is imperative to intervene with a child or family individually, one of the most critical factors in the success of the intervention is the how the role of helper is employed.

The Helping Relationship

Despite many similarities between the Ecuadorian and Colombian groups, there are striking differences as well. Although Latina myself, I am Caribbean; there are many differences among the three Latino groups. The insight and understanding I developed with the Ecuadorian and Colombian groups are the result of working together many years. I learned from the very families how to truly connect with them.

In my experience, Ecuadorian families are initially more reticent and often take longer to engage. It seems to be that Ecuadorian families are comfortable observing the procedures of the school and my role within it, prior to enlisting my help. For this reason, I tend to introduce myself to Ecuadorian parents early in the school year and continually remind them of my "just stop by" office policy. It tends to take more calls and visits with an Ecuadorian family to begin our work together. Once trust has been established, the Ecuadorian groups respond best when I assume a role of *confidant* and *supporter*. Exploring feelings, memories, and experiences becomes an important aspect of the work with the family. As a "supporter," I am a constant and ready link between the family and the school. Parents are better able to express their concerns to teachers through this intermediary support.

By contrast, Colombian groups tend to be straightforward. However, in approaching Colombian families, I must first establish my expertise to begin our work. Parents need the reassurance that I understand their situation and am adequately prepared by training and experience to intervene. In the initial contacts, I take great care in presenting my perspective and the principles (of psychology or child development) that guide my assessment. Once trust has been established, the Colombian groups tend to respond best when I assume the role of *advisor*. Families "check-in" for advice when there is a question or crisis, then tend to prefer solving problems independently.

PRINCIPLES OF CULTURALLY APPROPRIATE PRACTICE

One of the basic principles of good social work is to learn from the client how to be most helpful. This is particularly important in serving clients from diverse cultures. The history of a country is the first and most overt introduction to its culture. The values of the culture are most often understood through behavior and social institutions. Developing culturally appropriate practices for Ecuadorians and Colombians in a school, in an English-speaking suburb of New York, requires a lot of lessons from the client.

The insights garnered from the history of Ecuadorians and Colombians new to this country suggest that interventions are most culturally appropriate when the following factors are defined and understood:

1. The immigration experience.
2. The process of acculturation.
3. The history of oppression or discrimination in either country.
4. The interpersonal dynamics with authority figures.
5. The prominence of the family and its social context.

For instance, it is critical when working with the Colombian family to engage the father. The role of the father is provider and decision-maker; without the father's approval, the family will not proceed with recommendations. This is often true even if family members do not all live in the same country. The opinions of "missing" family members (who remained back home) must be included in the assessments and practices we develop.

In working with Ecuadorians, it is important to recognize the history of maltreatment of the indigenous peoples (Hanratty, 1991). Not all groups within Ecuador have a similar history. The subsets of Indian groups living in New York suburbs have their own cultural values that may differ from those of another Ecuadorian group. With this group, however, it is important to understand the history and significance of deferring to authority and not confuse this with disinterest.

The group modality predominates in developing culturally appropriate practices with Ecuadorians and Colombians, in my experience. The larger groups of Latinos, to which both Ecuadorians and Colombians belong, tend to be oriented toward a group experience. In the literature, this is often described as allocentrism, or "collectivism."

One example of culturally appropriate practice for new immigrant children from Ecuador and Colombia is acculturation groups that aid in the adjustment to a new culture and school.

Acculturation Groups

The first contact with new immigrant families in the schools should be a gracious welcome and orientation in their own language. This is the opportunity to form an alliance with a child's parent. It can be the basis of a sustained engagement in the helping relationship with the social worker. It is also a critical opportunity to assess a family's needs and normalize their experiences. Children receive the message that they can be successful when their entrance is celebrated.

The groups comprise six play-therapy sessions conducted in Spanish. The children play games that enable them to process their recent experiences in a nonthreatening and age-appropriate manner. The goals of the group are as follows:

- To empower children to articulate their experiences through the use of play.
- To facilitate adjustment to school.
- To teach the words/language of emotions.
- To enhance social functioning.
- To encourage mutual support.
- To screen for depression and/or adjustment disorders.

The games and activities offered to the children all relate to the experiences of new immigrants. These have been prepared with an understanding of the nature of acculturation guided by play-therapy techniques.

CASE VIGNETTES

Although a typical acculturation group at this elementary school includes children from various countries, for this discussion, the case examples are children from Ecuador and Colombia.

Marco, Age 5

Identifying Data

Marco arrived at the elementary school midyear and soon began the spring group. Marco's family immigrated years before his arrival, and he spent his early years with his maternal grandmother. He was his grandmother's darling and his mother's pride. Always a little gentleman, Marco exemplified the model of the *bien educado* Latino child. His mother often commented that he had been "raised properly," although he had not been raised by her. Marco always smiled and always offered appropriate greetings in a very adult manner. Even among other Latino children described as *bien educado*, Marco was exemplary.

Observations

Superficially, it was hard to say there were any problems. Certainly, Marco was cooperative and well behaved; his teachers adored him. However,

Marco tended to prefer the company and attention of adults, and he had not one single friend his age. The history of maternal absence, the recent separation from his grandmother who raised him, and his inability to make friends with his peers seemed to suggest that his compliant behavior might mask some depression or loneliness. The cultural value of raising a child who is *bien educado* is endemic in the child-rearing practices of most Latino groups. As the clinician, it was important for me to remember that remaining *bien educado* in his mother's eyes was healthy and appropriate for Marco. It would have been misguided to attempt to move Marco toward the North American cultural values of assertiveness, where he might have lost a positive self-image and become difficult for his mother to understand. The clinical task was to introduce new social skills that allowed Marco to develop friendships and rely less on adult attention.

Group Progress Summary

Marco was very uncomfortable in the first few sessions of the group. He seemed at a loss in a situation in which he was invited to relax and play. He tended to direct all his comments to me rather than to the group members. He was always the model of good behavior by raising his hand and waiting for turns. As he observed the other children, he began displaying interest and pleasure in their stories. When all the children were asked to choose from several "feelings faces" and tell their feelings about arriving in the United States, Marco listened intently as other children described sadness and anger about all the changes. Marco talked to the group about his own feelings of happiness and sadness, and he presented his feelings faces—a happy face for the mother he came to see, a sad face for the grandmother he left behind. As the group progressed, Marco became increasingly comfortable and genuinely friendly. He laughed wholeheartedly when the group imitated the animal sounds of pets they left behind in the countries. As he became more sociable, Marco was able to relate to his group mates. He continued to utilize new social skills after group ended and became more comfortable in his classroom as well, and began exhibiting leadership qualities.

Yesenia, Age 5

Identifying Data

By the time Yesenia was 5 years old, she had had a series of separations and reunions with her parents. She separated from her father when she and her mother immigrated to the United States from Colombia. Her mother had come to the United States, planning to make a life here after Yesenia's father abandoned her for another woman who also had his child. The struggle to find work and a home proved too difficult for Yesenia's mother, and she opted to send her daughter back to Colombia to live with her father, until life here was more stable. Yesenia then returned to live with her mother in the United States shortly before beginning kindergarten. She was a silent, morose little girl who seemed difficult to reach. Teachers were not aware of the multiple separations but were very concerned about her silence and slow rate of learning. In preparation for the fall acculturation group, I met with Yesenia's mother and discussed these concerns. The marital relationship continued to linger as a problem, although the parents were separated by thousands of miles. Yesenia's mother was very susceptible to anything the father did or said, all the way from Colombia. Because the extended family members on both sides were neighbors in Colombia, everyone took part in solving the marital problems. In the midst of this confusion, Yesenia longed for her father and her country. As her mother grew to understand how her daughter was affected by so many physical separations with emotional entanglements, she was able to set limits with her family and support her daughter's attachment to her father. We made a plan whereby Yesenia would have ongoing contact with her father by sending him drawings and letters. The mother agreed to shield her daughter from negative comments about her father and instead remind her that "Papi" loved her very much.

Observations

Yesenia's silence was the typical response of an overwhelmed child. The initial stage of melancholy upon arriving in this country was complicated by the fact that she did not know her mother well when she was reunited with her, and the attachment with the father had been severed abruptly. All that she had to understand and assimilate distracted Yesenia from her learning. Without intervention, she was at risk for academic failure and an entrenched mutism. The difficulty Yesenia's mother had in separating effectively from the father may have been due to cultural values that give great significance to the role of the husband and father in the family. It proved helpful to support this cultural value in a healthy manner by encouraging a normal attachment and relationship between Yesenia and her father.

Group Progress Summary

Group members were very upset by Yesenia's silence during our sessions. Their interpretation seemed to be that if Yesenia would not share her feelings or stories about coming to this country, it must be because they were particularly grim. Everyone took notice of her drawings, which were her primary form of communication. In the group session following the first snowfall of the year, the children discussed differences in temperature between countries and wondered who had ever seen snow. As an activity, the children colored and pasted drawings of sweaters and swimsuits, snow-covered scenes, and beach scenes in a collage entitled "What it feels like in my first country and what it feels like here." As usual, Yesenia remained quiet, but she took great care in composing her collage. It became apparent to everyone in the group that Yesenia was very interested in the topic of this session. She did not speak to her group mates; Yesenia smiled and looked away when she was complimented, but she did comment to me as she was leaving that she would be sending this collage home to Colombia. Yesenia's progress in school was slow but constant. Her mood improved, and she began to speak in her classroom in the weeks after the end of group.

Samuel, Age 5

Identifying Data

Like Marco, Samuel was a sweet, polite little boy whom anyone would call *bien educado*. There were no reported problems with his behavior, but he clearly needed time and support to process recent traumas. In the summer before beginning kindergarten, Samuel and his mother entered the United States on foot across the border. Samuel repeatedly told the story of standing alongside the river before crossing, his mother placing her hands on his shoulders and saying, "I hope you don't die." Samuel's real concern was that his mother would not survive the trip herself. No one else in his family was traveling with them. In every retelling, Samuel ended the story by saying, "We didn't die."

Observations

The trip to this country was terrifying for Samuel and his mother. Anyone in the school listening to this story almost felt traumatized as well. The realization that Samuel could have been orphaned or injured evoked an intense protective response in the adults at the school. This helped him to regain some sense of security. His mother reacted to the experience in a very different manner. She preferred to not discuss the crossing, perhaps out of fear of being discovered or simply an unwillingness to stir up any feelings. It was difficult for her to understand that this might not be the best way to help her son. Always deferential and polite, Samuel's mother agreed to talk with him about their experiences but never reported whether this was helpful.

Group Progress Summary

Samuel's story frightened some of the group members, but he was quickly accepted and well liked. Speaking of his experience allowed the other children to recognize some of their own fears during the journey to this country. It proved helpful to the group to listen to what Samuel had endured. However, the constant repetition of this frightening story had to be controlled. Samuel was encouraged to draw pictures of what he remembered, then draw pictures of his family now. During Thanksgiving, the children were introduced to this North American holiday and asked to consider how even the country's founders were immigrants. In an activity about the first Thanksgiving meal, the children played with a miniature table and chairs, and were asked to describe the first people to help them when they arrived in the United States. These first helpers (like the Native Americans who helped the Pilgrims) were invited to the little table and chairs to celebrate the child's arrival in the United States. Samuel could not identify any helpers at first, but he clearly thought the topic was of critical importance. He thought and thought, and finally offered a long list of names of aunts, friends, and teachers who could sit at his little table. Samuel's resilience endears him to adults and caregivers. His ability to form loving attachments is likely to continue to help him in the process of acculturation.

Joaquín, Age 6

Identifying Data

Joaquín and his mother separated when he was a young child. He remained with his maternal grandmother when his mother immigrated. Years later, his mother attempted to bring Joaquín to the United States by having him pose as the child of another woman. He was told to use a different name, if he were ever questioned. The woman with whom he traveled was a stranger who remained mute and disinterested throughout the trip. Once they landed in the United States, the woman told Joaquín to wait while she entered the restroom. He never saw her again. Hours later, frightened and crying, Joaquín was taken to a detention center for children. He did as he had been told and gave his false name to the authorities, prolonging the search for his mother. Eventually, the truth was discovered, and Joaquín's mother was notified. Joaquín was restless and often aggressive. He had difficulty adjusting to the routines of a typical school day. He often requested bathroom breaks only to wander the halls. He tended to boss other children and had few real friends. Like Samuel, Joaquín told his story to anyone who would listen. This terrified his mother, who feared repercussions with the authorities. Joaquín and his mother underwent a series of deportation hearings that, thankfully, ended in permanent residence in the United States.

Observations

Like many Ecuadorian mothers at the elementary school, Joaquín's mother politely listened to my suggestions. Despite seeming agreeable, she avoided contact with me and other school staff. After several attempts, she finally felt comfortable to confide her current legal situation and was relieved to receive some support to handle her fears and her son's increasingly unruly behavior. She accepted the suggestion to implement a behavior plan at home that would address some of Joaquín's defiant behavior. The school also implemented a behavior plan using visual cues that aided in the interaction between Joaquín, who spoke no English, and his teacher, who spoke no Spanish.

Group Progress Summary

Joaquín approached his group mates with the same aggressive, bossy manner he exhibited towards others at the school. He defended against any feelings of vulnerability or fear. When he heard other children's frightening stories, he waved them away and laughed that anyone should be so frightened. He offered everyone hints and suggestions about managing dangerous situations, particularly in the session dealing with airplanes. Joaquín found it easier to admit to sadness when the group discussed family members left behind. He lamented the loss of freedom to run and play in this country and talked at length about the games he played with his cousins in Ecuador. This seemed a good beginning to help Joaquín develop healthy social skills in this country. However, he needed ongoing intervention after the group was over. His mother's preoccupations with legal problems, his own traumatic memory of abandonment at the airport, and the complication of being reunited with a mother he had not seen in years sometimes overshadowed his adjustment. Joaquín's mother did not maintain contact after he moved on to another school. By that time, he had been awarded permanent residence, and it is my hope that this victory has afforded Joaquín and his mother genuine psychological benefits.

Catalina, Age 5

Identifying Data

Catalina was a new immigrant from Colombia. Her father's family had never accepted her mother. As a result, Catalina, her siblings, and parents had to live with little support from the extended family. This proved so difficult in a country where family connections are essential that they opted to immigrate. Catalina's mother stated, "We figured if we're going to have nobody but ourselves in Colombia, it couldn't be so difficult to have nobody here." The children and their father came to the United States, while the mother remained behind. The father was overwhelmed caring for the children and intervened little in their misbehavior. He worked into the evening, and Catalina was left in the care of a local babysitter who cared for several children. Catalina was very active and verbal, and the babysitter often found cause to punish her. Her punishment was that she had her pants and undergarments removed until she "composed herself," and Catalina had to endure the embarrassment of the other children's ridicule. When the mother arrived in the United States 6 months later, the babysitter informed her that Catalina was punished in this manner. Catalina's mother quickly removed her daughter from the situation. The mother and father worked opposite shifts, so that one of them was always with the girls. However, the mother had to work many long hours, and the father was not able to provide the consistent discipline they needed. As a result, Catalina was learning little about managing her own behavior. In school, she was mischievous and disrespectful. She instigated problems between students and promptly denied having done so.

Observations

This family that had become accustomed to receiving little support may not have known when to ask for help. The father's inability to set limits suggested that he was beleaguered by the demands on his time and attention. The parents admitted that it was unusual, in their experience, for fathers to assume so much responsibility for the children. They saw this as one of the many sacrifices they were forced to make because of the rejection of his family. Catalina's family needed concrete suggestions about forming a support system and establishing basic rules in the home. In conversations with the mother (the father could not attend), alternate ideas about Catalina's behavior were explored. The mother began recognizing some of her own qualities in her daughter and was better able to acknowledge her daughter's strengths. Both mother and father agreed to implement a behavior plan at home that would help the father establish a daily routine for Catalina. Because the mother recognized how humiliated Catalina had been by the babysitter, she was able to reassure Catalina that she would never be punished this way again.

Group Progress Summary

Catalina was the comedienne of the group. She interrupted with comments and stories that often made her group mates laugh. Perhaps fearful that she would once again be humiliated among her peers by an adult, she quickly acquiesced to group rules provided that she was acknowledged and addressed individually. A bright, verbal little girl, Catalina quickly understood the "point" of the group's games and explained to everyone that they were to talk about what they *felt*. During one game entitled *Lo Último, Lo Primero* (The Last Thing, The First Thing), the children were invited to play a card game with two sets of cards. One set had pictures representing the five senses (eyes, mouth, nose, hands, ears). The other set simply stated "The Last Thing" or "The First Thing." The child would pick a card from both sets and then respond to the group with "The first thing I saw (or smelled, or held, or ate) in this country" or "The last thing I saw (or smelled, or held, or ate) in my first country." Catalina became very attentive during this game. Her responses were filled with nostalgia for what must have been a safer, more tranquil time for her. She remembered great details about Colombia, and her significant verbal skills aided in the telling of long, involved stories about pets, neighbors, and friends. This game remained a favorite for Catalina, and she could often be persuaded to cooperate with the promise of one more turn.

CONCLUSIONS

All interventions and services designed for new immigrant children are most effective when they support the idea that the child must integrate and value the two cultures he or she has experienced. The clinician must be aware of the tendency to perceive a family's cultural values from a deficit perspective when there are complications in the process of acculturation. We support biculturalism when we work within the cultural framework of the new immigrant. When it becomes essential to teach new skills to facilitate adapting to this country, it is helpful to explore with the immigrant the experience of immigrating to illustrate North American cultural values. The new immigrant's unique perspective on our own values reflects back to us what it means to be "North American."

The process of acculturation is an irreversible, indelible process of change. If ever the new immigrants return to their first country after living here, countrymen will find them changed. Ecuadorians and Colombians living in New York suburbs and attending the public schools are irrevocably changed by that experience. The school is also changed and enhanced by the diversity they bring. Children, who represent the future of any country, deserve our best efforts to create a compassionate, hopeful world in which the arrival of a child is more important than his or her nationality.

REFERENCES

Chavez, D. V., Moran, V. R., Reid, S. L., & Lopez, M. (1997). Acculturative stress in children: A modification of the SAFE Scale. *Hispanic Journal of Behavioral Sciences, 19*(1), 34–44.

Gibson, M. (1998). Promoting academic success among immigrant students: Is acculturation the issue? *Educational Policy, 12*(6), 615–633.

Hanratty, D. (Ed.). (1991). *Ecuador: A country study.* Washington, DC: U.S. Government Printing Office. Available at the Library of Congress website: *http:// lcweb2.loc.gov/cgi-bin/query/r?frd/cstdy:@field(DOCID+ec0041)*

Hanratty, D. M., & Meditz, S. W. (Eds.). (1990). *Colombia: A country study.* Washington, DC: U.S. Government Printing Office for the Library of Congress.

Holman, L. (1997). Meeting the needs of Hispanic immigrants. *Educational Leadership, 54*(7), 37–38.

Instituto Nacional de Estadísticas y Censos. (1985). *IV Censo Nacional de Población y III de Vivienda, 1981. Resumen Nacional: Breve Análisis de los Resultados Definitivos.* Quito, Ecuador: Author.

James, D. C. S. (1997). Coping with a new society: The unique psychosocial problems of immigrant youth. *Journal of School Health, 67*(3), 98–102.

Pabón, E. (n.d.). *The cultural context of child development and its implications for treatment of Latinos.* Yorktown Heights, NY: M&P Latino Consultants.

Smart, J., & Smart, D. (1995). Acculturative stress of Hispanics: Loss and challenge. *Journal of Counseling and Development, 73*(4), 390–403.

FURTHER READING

Barnam, J. (2000, September). Trouble in the Andes. *LatinFinance*, pp. 26–34.

Chavkin, N. F., & Garza-Lubeck, M. (1990). Multicultural approaches to park involvement: Research and practice. *Social Work in Education, 13*(1), 22–33.

Curtis, P. A. (1990). The consequences of acculturation to service delivery and research with Hispanic families. *Child and Adolescent Social Work, 7*(2), 147–159.

Keller, J. D., & McDade, K. (1997). Cultural diversity and help-seeking behavior: Sources of help and obstacles to support for parents. *Journal of Multicultural Social Work, 5(1/2),* 63–78.

Mayo, Y. (1997). Machismo, fatherhood and the Latino family: Understanding the concept. *Journal of Multicultural Social Work, 5*(1/2), 49–61.

Portes, A., & MacLeod, D. (1996). Educational progress of children of immigrants: The roles of class, ethnicity, and school context. *Sociology of Education, 69,* 255–275.

Vañó, A., & Pennebaker, J. (1997). Emotional vocabulary in bilingual Hispanic children: Adjustment and effects. *Journal of Language and Social Psychology, 16*(2), 191–200.

Winkelman, M. (1994). Cultural shock and adaptation. *Journal of Counseling and Development, 73*(2), 121–131.

CHAPTER 14

Nicaraguan and Salvadoran Children and Families

FLAVIO FRANCISCO MARSIGLIA
CECILIA MENJÍVAR

The term "Central America" awakens equally strong emotions in progressive and conservative political circles in the United States. The general public also has its own ideas about Central America, fed by images ranging from army men murdering Catholic nuns to guerillas confiscating homes and businesses. Despite the Hollywood-type portrayals and the often polarized views presented by the different political factions, Central America, as a region, is undoubtedly diverse and complex. Countries such as Costa Rica, for example, have enjoyed long-lasting decades of peace, without a disruption in their strong democratic institutions, whereas other countries have suffered the consequences of prolonged proxy wars and recurring natural disasters. This chapter focuses on the unique challenges and remarkable resiliency of migrant children and their families fleeing two such nations: Nicaragua and El Salvador. From an ecological perspective, we situate the struggles of these immigrant groups in their historical and political context, and propose working with these families and children from a strength perspective. Nicaraguan and Salvadoran immigrants have endured many forms of persecution in their countries of origin and in the host society; social workers are called upon to assess the strengths and legacy of war and natural disasters of these families within the context of their culture. Culturally specific social work practice recommendations are provided for U.S.-based agencies providing social services to immigrant/refugee families and children.

HISTORICAL BACKGROUND

El Salvador and Nicaragua began to attract the attention of the general public and policy makers of the United States. In 1979, when long-standing dictatorships in their respective countries were ousted and both countries began a long period of turmoil and political violence that ended at about the same time: 1990 in Nicaragua, and 1992 in El Salvador. Various policies and direct actions sponsored by the U.S. government have fueled a politically charged migration process into this country. This experience appears to have impacted them in ways that more closely parallel the experiences of Vietnamese refugees than the experiences of other Latin American migrants. A noteworthy feature in the migration of Salvadorans and Nicaraguans to the United States is that, contrary to popular belief, the origins of were not just these flows internal to the respective countries but were the result of the exacerbation of internal political conflict by external support to feuding factions. In an effort to contain what was perceived as the "Soviet/Cuban expansion," the United States became deeply entangled in both countries and, with a massive financial package and military buildup, supported the armies that aligned with its ideological leanings. During its 12-year civil war, the Salvadoran government fought leftist guerillas with substantial U.S. support. In Nicaragua, the intent of the United States was to overthrow a democratically elected government friendly to Cuba and the former Soviet Union (the Sandinistas), so it supported and trained a militia, popularly known as the "Contras," that was to topple it.

U.S. foreign policy and military intervention not only shaped the political and economic conditions that Salvadorans and Nicaraguans fled but also helped to enhance the close social, economic, and cultural links that already existed between the United States and both of these countries, through which the immigrants made their way into the United States (Rumbaut, 1994). At this particular historical juncture, the United States emerged as the destination of choice for the thousands of Salvadorans and Nicaraguans who fled the conflicts.

The refugees and their advocates understood that their migration to the United States fell within the parameters established by international law. In 1968, the United States accepted the United Nations Protocol Relating to the Status of Refugees, which also included the principle of nonrefoulment, the prohibition against returning a refugee to a territory where his or her life or freedom would be threatened. This clause was intended to eliminate ideological bias in U.S. law, which had previously given preference to persons fleeing communism and/or the Middle East. However, in practice, the United States continued to admit only those groups it regarded as most deserving, that is, best able to promote U.S. national interests (Menjívar, 2000).

Thus, it should not be surprising that, given U.S. policy in these countries during the peak years of migration, Salvadorans and Nicaraguans who arrived in the United States during the 1980s and into the 1990s (for Salvadorans) were not recognized as refugees by the Reagan and first Bush administrations. Most became undocumented immigrants, even though their situation was more akin to that of people from other countries formally designated as refugees than to that of regular or economic immigrants. These immigrants were denied the "structure of refuge"; in other words, they did not have access to the government resettlement aid available to officially recognized refugees, and were thus left on their own to cope with the consequences of political flight (Rumbaut, 1989). Moreover, because they were categorized as undocumented immigrants, they were also at risk of deportation and unable to work legally in the United States.

The United States recognized that the political turmoil was generating huge population movements in El Salvador, but it refused to admit any of these displaced individuals to its own soil. Thus, although the U.S. State Department reported innumerable cases of political deaths and disappearances, the Immigration and Naturalization Service (INS) not only refused to recognize as legal refugees those fleeing such violence, but it continued to deport Salvadorans (Menjívar, 2000) and thus violated the principle of *nonrefoulment* in the U.N. Convention on Refugees.

The U.S. government could have granted Nicaraguans refugee status in a symbolic gesture, as it had done with other groups fleeing communist regimes (Menjívar, 1999). However, the ideological side that the United States supported, the "Contras," were going to apply pressure to the Sandinista government, with their base of operations located in Honduras, as close to Nicaragua as possible (Pitt, Portes, & Stepick, 1993). Granting these Nicaraguans refugee status, meaning a place to settle and aid with which to do so, would therefore have dissuaded them from continuing their guerilla warfare against their elected government in Managua (Menjívar, 2000).

The civil wars ended in both countries with somewhat different outcomes. Nicaragua, the country subject to the strongest security guarantees (such as resettlement of former guerillas) has been the least stable of the two. El Salvador, in contrast, experienced a more successful conflict resolution despite the lack of any forceful security guarantees by the international community (Peceny & Stanley, 2001). The stream of immigrants into the United States is expected to continue as both societies adjust to peacetime and additional economic challenges.

ASYLUM SEEKERS AND REFUGEES

Many Salvadorans and Nicaraguans entered the United States during the years of political turmoil in their countries. Once on U.S. soil, they could apply individually for political asylum. To be granted asylum is not the same thing as having refugee status. Refugees are processed outside the United States, whereas to apply for political asylum, one needs to set foot on U.S. soil. The benefits the two categories of immigrants receive are also different. Refugees receive resettlement aid that often consists of cash assistance, vocational training, and English-language instruction. Those who qualify for political asylum are only granted protection from deportation and permission to work. After a period of time in the United States, both can apply for permanent residence and, eventually, for naturalization.

Throughout the 1980s, less than 3% of Salvadoran applicants were granted asylum. Immigrants' rights groups lobbied on the Salvadorans' behalf, and Congress eventually granted temporary protection from deportation to all Salvadorans who arrived prior to September 19, 1990. This special dispensation, known as Temporary Protected Status (TPS), allowed Salvadorans to live and work in the United States for a period of 18 months, a provision that was extended a few times, until it expired in December 1994. Also, as of 1990, Salvadorans whose asylum applications had been denied could resubmit them under the *American Baptist Churches v. Thornburgh* (ABC) settlement. Initially their success rate increased to 28% in fiscal year 1992, but has since leveled off and declined to about 3% (Immigration and Naturalization Service, 1995).

Some Salvadorans were included as beneficiaries of the 1997 Nicaraguan Adjustment and Central American Relief Act (NACARA). Designed for Nicaraguans, it also included Cubans and nationals of former Soviet-bloc countries. Salvadorans who entered the country before September 19, 1990 (the same cutoff date established for TPS) and registered under the ABC settlement, or who had filed an asylum application before April 1, 1990, could be granted a "cancellation of removal." Unlike Salvadorans, Nicaraguans are not required to appear before an immigration judge to be granted the benefit. Nicaraguans who can prove that they have continuously resided in the United States since December 1, 1995, can be considered for adjustment of status to permanent residency. Immigrants' rights groups have been lobbying to bring to parity the benefits conferred to these two groups, because the cutoff date for Salvadorans was almost 2 years before the war officially ended, and the cutoff date for Nicaraguans was 5 years after the civil turmoil ended in that country.

During the 1980s, about one-fourth of the Nicaraguan applicants were successful in regularizing their immigration status (Menjívar, 2000). Under pressure from the Cuban American constituency in Miami, where the majority of the Nicaraguans live, the U.S. government stopped deporting Nicaraguans in the period between 1987 and 1988. But when Congress froze military support for the Contras in 1988, the number of Nicaraguans entering the United States increased substantially (Pitt et al., 1993). To stem this flow, the U.S. government reversed its policy, and Nicaraguans once again were treated as undocumented immigrants (Menjívar, 2000).

More recently, natural disasters in both El Salvador and Nicaragua that have prompted temporary changes in U.S. law to protect the victims of these catastrophes. Late in the 1998 hurricane season, Central America was slammed by a devastating hurricane. Most Central American nations were greatly impacted by Hurricane Mitch, one of the deadliest storms to affect the region in the past 200 years (Glantz & Jamieson, 2000). Nicaraguans (along with Hondurans) were granted TPS for a period of 9 months, a time frame that was extended. When three powerful earthquakes hit El Salvador at the beginning of 2001, the Bush administration (at the petition of the Salvadoran president) granted Salvadorans TPS for 18 months.

ADAPTATION TO THE UNITED STATES

The ecological approach looks at the people's strengths, their innate push toward health, continued growth, and release of potential (Germain & Gitterman, 1995). When working with communities facing innumerable obstacles, it is important to look for their strengths as we develop interventions, without overlooking the risks or unique environmental challenges they face (Saleebey, 1997; Weick, Rapp, Sullivan, & Kristhardt, 1989). In the case of Salvadoran and Nicaraguan immigrants, leaving their home countries was a survival strategy. The act of immigration itself reflects strength and resourcefulness. The journey many Central American immigrants undertook was hardly a straight line from their country of origin to their points of entry into the United States. Many had to travel by land, mostly because visa requirements to travel to the United States (and later to Mexico as well) became so stringent that they were beyond the reach of most potential travelers. These land journeys are usually plagued with robberies, assaults, rapes, and even murder. Immigrants often fall prey to unscrupulous immigration officials in Mexico, who extort them to allow them to continue north. Some of the most dangerous people that immigrants encounter along their journeys are their own coyotes (smugglers) whom they hired to bring them into the United States. Children, whether alone or accompanied by adults, have similar experiences during their journeys; they also face extortion, beatings, and—in many instances, particularly the girls—rape. For many, the traumatic episodes during the journeys exacerbate the trauma of political violence in their home countries. For some, harrowing experiences during the journey leave even more lasting marks than the violence of their homelands.

A key challenge for Salvadorans and Nicaraguans has been the ambivalent reception they have received in the United States, which at different points during the peak of their migration even turned hostile. Given the conditions of turmoil under which many left their countries, they could have received assistance for their resettlement or, at least, legal recognition of their presence, perhaps as a gesture of responsibility on the part of the United States for prolonging the civil unrest through military aid to their governments or opposition guerilla groups. Instead, many of these immigrants have joined the ranks of undocumented immigrants, a status that has serious repercussions for their adjustment to life. The INS (1997) has estimated that close to 60% of Salvadorans and approximately 40% of Nicaraguans in the country are undocumented.

The status of undocumented immigrants is characterized by constant stress and a lack of access to basic social services (Pitt & Marsiglia, 2000). For example, Salvadorans are one of the immigrant groups with the lowest rates of health insurance. Even among those working full-time, only half have employer-sponsored coverage, compared with 81% of nonimmigrant full-time workers. Legal status was identified as one of the main variables accounting for this disparity (Carrasquillo, Carrasquillo, & Shea, 2000). These statistics have great impact on the well-being of children whose families cannot access basic social services because of their immigration status.

In addition, Central Americans, as a group, have one of the lowest wage rates in the country. They enter the U.S. economy earning low wages and have a more difficult time than other immigrant groups catching up with U.S.-born workers (Schoeni, 1997). Lower educational levels, immigration status, and traumatic experiences in their countries of origin account for these differences.

Many Nicaraguan and Salvadoran children and adults carry within them a legacy of war. War trauma has had serious repercussions on the lives of these immigrants (Aron, Corne, Fursland, & Zelwer, 1991; Guarnaccia & Farias, 1988). This situation has especially affected children, many of whom have been diagnosed with posttraumatic stress disorder (PTSD), which has seriously impaired their incorporation in U.S. society (Espino, 1991). Children report as many psychiatric symptoms as their parents in clinical trials (Rousseau & Drapeau, 1998).

Although the legacy of war affects the whole family, it has a more acute and long-lasting impact on children. During the years of the conflict in their home countries, Central American children were exposed to political violence, such as the murder and disappearance of family members and friends, sightings of mutilated or tortured bodies, and widespread intimidation by armed groups, as well as harsh economic conditions. Children also faced forced recruitment by combatant groups; children as young as 12 years old were sometimes enlisted. In the Central American region as a whole, with about half of its population under age 20, children represented a major element of the Central American political drama in the 1980s (Urrutia-Rojas & Rodríguez,1997). Once in the United States, many of these children struggle in schools, sometimes because war-related trauma still permeates their lives, a condition compounded by the circumstances in which they now live (Espino, 1991). For instance, Nicaraguan adolescents have been found to experience greater acculturation stress than their Cuban peers (Gil & Vega, 1996).

Exposure to the war affected Salvadoran immigrants' cognitive appraisal of their current life circumstances. Many were found to experience greater stress in their resettlement process than other Latino groups, such as Mexicans (Salgado de Snyder, Richard, Cervantes, & Padilla, 1990). Salvadoran torture survivors show higher levels of PTSD, psychosomatic impairment, and stress response disturbance than other nontorture/trauma refugees (Thompson & McGorry, 1995). In addition, Salvadoran women were found to have experienced high rates of child sexual abuse during the civil war (Barthauer & Leventhal, 1999).

The traumatic past, in addition to uncertainty with respect to their legal status, has acutely affected the resettlement of Salvadorans and Nicaraguans in the United States. Their legal limbo, coupled with generally low educational levels, particularly among Salvadorans, limits their job opportunities and, consequently, their access to the better paying jobs that provide security and social mobility. Importantly, their lack of access to job retraining and language instruction—-which comes with resettlement aid packages provided to officially recognized refugees—-has had a homogenizing effect on these immigrants' job prospects, because professionals have been unable to find jobs commensurate with their human capital potential. For instance, a Nicaraguan chemist with extensive work experience was only able to work for an hourly wage and without any benefits, even though he performed the duties of a professional chemist. In his view, un certain legal status was the greatest impediment to getting ahead (Fernández-Kelly & Schauffler, 1994).

Undocumented Salvadoran youth and children are often able to receive an elementary and secondary education but cannot register for college without the proper papers. The knowledge that college is not an alternative because of their legal status affects younger children's overall disposition toward planning for a postsecondary education and gives them a sense that their opportunities of advancing socially are limited.

A comprehensive comparative study of immigrant groups in south Florida revealed that Nicaraguans have slightly higher levels of marital stability and educational attainment than other groups, and that they are more likely to have been professionals before arriving in the United States. However, they are significantly worse off financially than other groups (Fernandez-Kelly & Curran, 2001). Although Nicaraguans in Southern Florida have been identified as a model of entrepreneurship among Latino immigrants (Zsembik, 2000), Nicaraguan parents are more likely to view their opportunities for advancement as diminished compared to other groups (Fernández-Kelly & Curran, 2001). This perception is particularly prevalent when they compare themselves to their main reference group, Cuban Americans in south Florida, who receive not only government protection but also, usually, assistance from the local community.

Such views affect the children, because their parents are not always equipped to offer them opportunities that they see as unreachable. In the host schools and neighborhoods, Nicaraguan youngsters often feel the sting of discrimination by other children, which affects their academic performance. Although parents place a high value on education and try to instill it in their children, such efforts are counterbalanced by the children's dim views of their futures, the impoverished environments in which they come to live, and the troubled schools they attend (Fernández-Kelly & Curran, 2001). Thus, these children, rather than becoming American by following a path toward upward mobility, become American by following a trajectory toward downward mobility, and their experiences resemble those of native-born groups that have been marginalized and subjected to prejudice.

PROBLEMS FOR CHILDREN FAMILIES

Many Central American families travel together and face the struggles of resettlement in the new society together. But just as many (or perhaps even more) are separated by the migration of one or both parents. The children stay home with a grandparent or a relative, then sometimes reunite, maybe even years later. Such separations are the direct result of immigration policies that, as observed earlier, have made it extremely difficult for Central Americans to settle in the United States. These family reunifications can be painful, because parents and children, after being separated for many years (for most of the children's lives in many cases), often no longer recognize one another as family once they reunite. Sometimes parents and children do not even recognize each other physically, as happened to a Salvadoran woman who, when she went to pick up her son at the smuggler's house, hugged and kissed the wrong man, thinking that it was her own son (Menjívar 2000).

During these separations, different family members are exposed to widely different experiences and find it difficult to live together again as a family, or the parent or parents bear other children, who are U.S. citizens. This gives rise to families with different combinations of legal status: whereas one parent can be applying for political asylum, another may be a permanent resident; whereas one child can be a U.S. citizen, another is undocumented. Such unevenness is common and can present serious challenges for families, because these different statuses confer different rights and benefits to those who hold them.

Sometimes these separations are voluntary, but, in other cases, they are the result of decisions made by parents—who live in dangerous neighborhoods (that offer affordable housing) and witness the lure of gangs and the easy money coming from drug trafficking—to shield their children from the social ills of the inner cities in which they live. These separations are, in fact, common to other immigrant groups and such people have been referred to as "transnational families," because decisions to raise children in the immigrants' homelands, as well as the financial resources to support them, are made by the parents (or parent) in the United States. Attempts to romanticize these family separations in the context of transnational conceptualizations should be tempered by the numerous costs, anxiety, dislocation, and alienation that these separations often produce (Hondagneu-Sotelo & Avila, 1997).

In many cases, it is couples that are separated, which gives rise to divorces (when the man and woman are legally married) and to the formation of different family forms, with different combinations of stepchildren and stepsiblings. In other cases, older parents are brought in to help with the care of children, or because their offspring in the United States worry that the parent(s) are alone in the homeland. These older immigrants sometimes feel out of place when they come to the United States to join their children; they cannot fully participate in the labor force, even though they would like to contribute economically to their families; they neither speak the language nor do they have the same social support, friends, and, importantly, respect that they enjoyed as older adults back home (Menjívar, 2000). This does not mean, however, that these adults do not make important contributions to their families and the communities they join (Wallace, 1992).

Families can also disintegrate when women become exposed to and adopt less rigid gender roles. An ethnographic study conducted in Canada identified some dissatisfaction in men who note undesirable changes among the women since resettlement. Women were found to desire an opportunity for education, employment, and a less restricted life (Kulig, 1998). These changes are resisted by men, because they feel left behind. Sometimes men express their frustration with the changes through violent means, such as spousal and child abuse (Van Hightower, Gorton, & DeMoss, 2000). A multiethnic study revealed that Central American immigrants are more likely than any other Latino subgroup to be arrested for violent and domestic violence crimes (Gil-Rivas, Anglin, & Annon, 1997). A natural tendency of many social workers is to work solely with the women and neglect the men. Involving the whole family, including the children, in prevention and educational programs will probably produce better results and reduce the need for later intervention. All family members sooner or later feel the stress of a legacy of war, acculturation, and the pressures of living in two worlds. These people are often left alone, without any support as they struggle with the many pressures and adjustment problems.

CULTURAL VALUES AS STRENGTHS IN ASSESSMENT

The cultural values and strengths generally associated with Nicaraguan, Salvadoran, and other Latino cultures are dynamic and fluid. Although it is difficult to generalize and apply a specific set of norms and values to a very heterogeneous group of people, the specialized literature tends to stress strong intergenerational family ties and other expressions of cooperation and collectiveness among Nicaraguans and Salvadorans. The list of cultural values summarized in Table 14.1 was adapted from selected literature on norms and values, and from the practice experience of the authors (Comas-Díaz & Minrath, 1987; Harrison, Wodarski, & Thyer, 1992; Mayers, Kail & Watts, 1993; Smart & Smart, 1995). This list of cultural values is just a starting point, a preliminary tool to be used with caution.

The values listed in Table 14.1 are connected to strong kinship networks encompassing members' deep sense of obligation to each other for economic assistance, encouragement, and support. The greater kin-centeredness of Latino families (*familismo*), as opposed to the strong ethos of independence common among European American families, may intensify the natural helping processes and outcomes among Salvadoran and Nicaraguan families (Cantor, Brennan, & Sainz, 1994). Latinos tend both to rely on relatives more often than European Americans for emotional support and to regard familial support for emotional problems as superior to all other types of support (Keefe, Padilla, & Carlos, 1979). While conducting an assessment of families or individuals, social workers need to be flexible in their understanding and definition of "family." More than family structure, the assessment will look for family functions. There is a need to identify those who provide family-like support, regardless of blood relationship.

Traditional values and norms such as relying on kin first (or other family-like relationships) provide invaluable support to immigrant children and families, but they may have other unintended consequences in the United States. For example, traditional support systems may delay family members' access to needed social services, or access to them as a last recourse, only when all traditional venues have been exhausted.

Family support has also been found to produce mixed effects on the immigrants' social advancement. For example, a Los Angeles-based study established that strong family ties affect the status and wages of Salvadoran immigrants, with remarkably different consequences for women and for men (Greenwell, Valdez, & DaVanzo, 1997). Working with relatives was associated with higher wages for male workers and lower wages for female workers. Thus, for Salvadoran women, having non-coresident relatives in the United States was associated with higher wages. The researchers explain these effects as a consequence of effective social networks among Salvadoran women living in working-class communities (Greenwell et al., 1997).

TABLE 14.1. Summary of Cultural Values and Strengths

Value/strength	Definition
Familismo (family orientation)	The centeredness of family in the life of its members. Value in trusting entire network; family/extended family valued as center of social support, solidarity; family not limited to blood relatives. Includes *compadrazgo*, a ritualistic form of kinship of choice.
Marianismo and *Machismo* (traditional gender roles)	*Marianismo*: Strength of women to cope with adverse situations and suffering inflicted upon them by men; modeled after the virgin Mary in the Catholic tradition.
	Machismo: males as providers and protectors of the family; becomes confused with abusive behavior toward women in contemporary consumer society.
Respeto (respect)	Giving deference to persons of status or acknowledging their position, avoiding humiliation of others or direct public confrontation.
Dignidad (dignity)	Value placed on self-worth as demonstrated through behaviors; a value to be protected.
Personalismo (personal treatment)	Preference for being treated on a personal basis rather than according to categories, rules, or policy.
Simpatia (niceness)	Creating pleasure in others by actions, kindness, and grace in personal treatment, regardless of the person's status.
Hechos (action orientation)	Emphasis on evidence of one's intentions through his or her actions.
Espiritualismo (spirituality)	The belief in the existence and reliance on other forces beyond the human experience. Expressed through organized religion or most commonly through domestic rituals and practices such as *altares* (altars) and *curanderismo* (traditional healing practices).
Fatalismo (fatalism)	Related to *espiritualismo*. A sense that one is not in complete control of one's destiny. In adverse situations, one does not attempt to gain control; instead, one gives oneself to stronger forces, such as God or destiny.

Polarized gender roles (machismo and marianismo) seem to be working against immigrant women, whose work appears to be undervalued or equated with nonremunerated household labor by their relatives. Other researchers who studied the influence of transnational families on gender relations have found that transnational factors are a significant but not singular agent for change in the support of other women in El Salvador or in the United States, and it appears to be the strongest source of effective assistance for women (Mahler, 1999). There is a need to support these female-to-female support systems. Men need support connecting back to the true meaning of *machismo* by regaining a positive sense of themselves as providers and protectors of the family.

Younger people integrate social norms and behaviors from the host society faster than do their parents (Marsiglia, Kulis, & Hecht, 2001). Some children lose their Spanish fluency and exhibit disinterest in their heritage (Marsiglia & Navarro, 1999). Often, as a means to regain control over their children, it is common for parents to discipline their children in ways that can be construed as emotional or physical abuse (Kulig, 1998). These issues present important challenges for assessment and service delivery in these communities. Parents accustomed to the value of *respeto* (respect) find themselves confronted and sometimes denigrated by their children. Their sense of *dignidad* (dignity) also suffers as they interact with larger social systems, such as schools and health care facilities. Social workers can mediate among all these systems and become cultural interpreters for the children and their parents. Families often need help in learning ways to reconcile their traditional values and norms with the new values and behaviors.

Social workers can develop a stronger rapport with their clients by keeping in mind the values of *personalismo* and *simpatia* (see Table 14.1). The social worker needs to learn how to convey to the client that he or she is recognized as a person of worth and that the social worker truly cares. One effective means of demonstrating a true interest in the family is to inquire about the children and learn their names. *Hechos* (actions) on the part of the social worker also promote credibility. Although social workers believe in the healing effects of words, immigrant children and their parents facing extreme situations often need to see some results before they truly engage in an intervention.

Spiritualism and fatalism are easily misunderstood by Western practitioners. Many immigrants facing extreme trauma have survived in part due to their belief and reliance on the spiritual world. Spiritualism needs to be seen as a strength and a resource. Fatalism, on the other hand, needs to be understood within the context of the clients' biographies. Knowing that one does not have control over everything gives peace to some clients. However, when taken to an extreme, fatalism can stop change and may work against empowerment.

Differences in acculturation between Nicaraguan parents and adolescents were found to be associated with lower levels of family cohesion, increased parent–child acculturation conflicts, lower adolescent self-esteem, and adolescent perceived teacher derogation (Gil & Vega, 1996). In addition, once in the United States, many Salvadoran and Nicaraguan children come to join other inner-city youth and end up attending troubled schools with increasingly restricted budgets. There, these children are exposed to crime, gangs, and low academic standards. Such schools do not offer many opportunities, for these children often do not even learn the proper English-language skills that would help them in the local labor market or further their education, as is the case with some Nicaraguan children in Miami (Fernández-Kelly & Schauffler, 1994).

Given the conditions in which their parents live, many children feel pressured to start earning a living. Thus, they start to work full-time at an early age, often dropping out of school. The cases of three very smart teenagers in San Francisco who had to start working in construction and cleaning houses to help their parents, thus sacrificing what could have been a better future, come to mind (see Menjívar, 2000). Many Central American adolescents face the triple burden of entering adolescence, a new society, and reconstituted families that often seem strange (Hondagneu-Sotelo & Avila, 1997). In these situations, the social worker may play an important role in presenting alternatives to the youth and providing a structure in which young people can meet and discuss issues of concern and together look for solutions.

INDIGNEOUS STRATEGIES AND WESTERN INTERVENTIONS

Given the void of a formal structure for resettlement, many community organizations were formed to aid Salvadoran and Nicaraguan immigrants in their resettlement in the United States. Churches, Catholic and other Christian denominations alike, were vital in helping immigrants with a range of services, from legal assistance to finding jobs; to provision of food, shelter, and health care; to English-language instruction. A good example is the Sanctuary movement, organized to protect from deportation the Salvadoran and Guatemalan immigrants whose lives would have been in danger if they returned to their countries in the early 1980s (Wiltfang & Cochran, 1994). Religious workers, basing their actions on religious conviction, acted in ways contrary to U.S. policy, often denouncing not only U.S. immigration policy toward these Central Americans, but also U.S. policy in the Central American region in general.

Local, nonprofit organizations also joined forces with religious communities to provide services to the newcomers. Importantly, the immigrants themselves organized a web of support for their compatriots who followed them that alleviated greatly the painful process of resettling in an often-inhospitable society. Most of these community organizations, such as CARECEN (formerly Central American Refugees Center), created by the immigrants themselves have now been formalized, and persons requesting their services must now pay a nominal fee. With the end of the war in El Salvador, and with more Central Americans staying in the United States longer, these community organizations have switched strategies and even their names, as in the case of CARECEN, which now is called Central American Resource Center. Those in charge of these organizations point out that Central Americans are no longer refugees, but immigrants, which changes the organizations' orientation from temporary strategies (such as providing initial help for resettlement) to more long-term objectives, such as lobbying for better conditions for these immigrants, including immigration amnesties.

Similarly, Nicaraguan newcomers organized to help their compatriots, concentrating their efforts on obtaining legal protection for them. Like Salvadorans who worked with the Sanctuary workers, Nicaraguans, mainly in Miami, have joined forces with local residents to lobby on behalf of their compatriots. Political ideology has played an equally important role in establishing these alliances among the Nicaraguans as well, only in reverse. For instance, many of the Nicaraguans who settled in Miami found their ideological twins in the powerful Cuban community there. Sharing important political affinities, as well as resettlement experiences in the United States, linked to the establishment of pseudo-Marxist regimes in their respective countries, has been an important point of convergence. The alliance with Cubans produced important victories for Nicaraguans, such as being able to reverse temporarily the practice of deportation of Nicaraguan nationals in the mid-1980s, and the passing of the NACARA in 1997. The high levels of entrepreneurship found among Nicaraguans have been identified as an important contribution to the growth of Florida's economy (Zsembik, 2000). At the same time, the vast majority of Nicaraguans interviewed in a large south Florida study reported having received little or no assistance from government or charitable organizations for their resettlement (Fernández-Kelly & Curran, 2001). Although intra- and cross-immigrant group cooperation is real, cultural differences based on national origin, and most importantly, class, as well as ideology, are strong factors challenging the development and maintenance of coalitions. The examples given are meant to illustrate important efforts undertaken by certain sectors of these immigrant communities.

The end of the war in El Salvador and the defeat of the Sandinistas in Nicaragua, however, have not stopped the influx of Central Americans into the United States. Many of these newcomers arrive in need of a range of assistance, not only material and financial but also emotional aid. A community worker in San Francisco, for instance, commented that she often doubles as a counselor, even though she is not trained as one, because of the great need for counseling that she sees among Central American clients that come to her organization (Menjívar, 2000).

A key point to keep in mind is that once a migration process starts, important networks between families and friends in the receiving and in the sending country develop, and migrations then become autonomous, or independent of the conditions that initially gave rise to them (Massey, Alarcón, Durand, & González, 1987). So when natural disasters occur in those countries, more immigrants leave and go where they have relatives and friends. Friends and family, although present, are not always in a position—financially and otherwise—to receive newcomers in need, and such networks do not always prove to be as strong and resilient as one might expect (see Fernández-Kelly & Curran, 2001, on Nicaraguans, and Menjívar, 2000, on Salvadorans).

Salvadoran immigrants residing in San Francisco, for example, were found to receive a great deal of help from kinfolk to make the journey north, but these networks often failed to provide assistance at the point of destination (Menjívar, 1997). Even if newcomers sometimes find it difficult to obtain help from those they had expected to assist them, they are seldom on their own, because they can turn to other relatives, other friends, and to community organizations for help. Salvadorans and Nicaraguans follow similar patterns of natural helping identified among other Latino groups (Patterson & Marsiglia, 2000). Networks for Central American immigrants tend to be strong and provide a great deal of support, but they have been found to have an insulating effect that diminishes immigrants' interaction with the larger community (Leslie, 1992). It is expected that higher socioeconomic-status (SES) immigrants are more connected to the larger society than lower SES immigrants. Educational level and immigration status emerge as key factors in explaining levels of insertion into the host society.

Macro-structural forces in the host society and cultural/SES variables from the society of origin shape network dynamics among immigrants in significant ways. The forces in the receiving context include immigration policies, the pressures of a consumer society, and the effects of acculturation on family dynamics. The forces of the society/culture of origin include characteristics of the immigrant community such as its resources, migratory history, the legacy of war, and unique cultural norms (Menjívar, 1997). More research is needed to sort out all these different variables and gain a better understanding of how Nicaraguan and Salvadoran immigrants/refugees reconcile these differences forces. More research is needed to identify the strengths and challenges that make the fabric of their social experience in the United States. Within this context, social workers in dialogue with the communities continue to define their role more adequately.

PRINCIPLES OF CULTURALLY APPROPRIATE PRACTICE

The described experiences and values of Salvadoran and Nicaraguan immigrants and refugees require a culturally appropriate social work response. Some guiding principles to consider from practice and policy perspectives are listed as follows:

1. The adjective "Central American" needs to be questioned as part of the client, family, group, or community's assessment. We need to

gain an in-depth understanding of the etiology of the migration process. Country of origin, date of departure, reasons(s) to migrate, migration alone or with other family members, and possible effects of war, natural disasters, and the migration experience need to be assessed.

2. We need to assess for undocumented status to assist the client in fully benefiting from existing legal venues available. Due to fear and mistrust, this area needs to be explored after the social worker has developed a strong bond and sense of trust with the client.

3. We need to assess for PTSD in adults and children. If PTSD is present in the family, appropriate treatment plans and/or referrals need to be developed. Identifying culturally and language-appropriate services is vital. In addition, it is important to consider ideological and political factors. For example, it would be counterproductive to place a former guerilla from El Salvador in treatment with the wife of a former Salvadoran general.

4. We need to work with the whole family and be open to defining "family" in a broad sense, identifying and working with the strengths and the challenges. Issues of acculturation, transnational families, and changing gender roles need to be considered and addressed.

5. We need to recognize the past social status of clients as not only a resource but also as a source of frustration. For example, a Nicaraguan medical doctor may be working in a clerical job. She may gain self-esteem and pride from her past professional life but at the same time be grieving the lost status and professional identity. We need to listen to the stories as they are being told and assist the clients to change the content of their narratives from frustration and despair to action and empowerment.

6. We need to be open to working separately with men, women, and children. Changing acculturation statuses and gender roles requires provision of a safe space where the different members of the family can express themselves freely. Once they have identified the issues and developed the language to express them, whole-family sessions would be appropriate. Group work appears to be the appropriate venue for age- and gender-specific interventions. In group, women and children can normalize their situation as they learn from other group members, and provide and receive effective support. Multifamily groups allow for support and behavior modeling among the different families.

7. Community-based efforts need to be supported to affect policy regarding immigration, access, and equity issues. Coalition building and lobbying have proven quite effective in attaining important goals for these two communities. Social work practitioners and students need to be educated about the different political issues the immigrant communities value to avoid alienating themselves or offending certain groups.

8. We need to identify the unique acculturation stresses children face and attempt to identify and work on intergenerational conflicts when

they exist, respecting the difficulty families face in sharing "family problems." Intervention should come early.

9. We need to engage community resources but maintain confidentiality at all times. Closely knit communities often experience difficulties understanding the concept of confidentiality. We need to utilize familiar images, such as confession, to explain the concept.

10. We need to use the language in which clients feel more comfortable communicating. Often, children feel more comfortable speaking English; we should not force Spanish on them. Rather than make assumptions, we should assess for language proficiency. When a client is bilingual, Spanish is probably the language of emotions and feelings, and he or she may switch to English to speak about practical issues. We need to be flexible and open to such integration.

The multilevel nature of the experiences of Nicaraguan and Salvadoran refugees and immigrants in the United States requires constant retooling. Civil wars and natural disasters are not mutually exclusive. The newer immigrants and refugees may be bringing with them the sequelae of civil war, although their reason to immigrate may have been a natural disaster. Newer immigrants may encounter in their host communities former political enemies, and uninformed social service agency personnel may force them to act as members of the same community based merely on national origin. As long as we remember the incredible resiliency of these clients, we can walk with them as they enter a new phase of their journey. Listening to their stories is our most effective compass.

CASE VIGNETTE

One of the most difficult challenges of immigration is that it alters age-related expectations, and culturally accepted roles are often reversed within families. Often, children take on responsibilities reserved for adults, and their status is enhanced, because they generally learn English and to navigate the sociocultural environment around them before their parents do, and must perform the role of "cultural brokers" between their families and local institutions (Menjívar, 2000). Also, parents work long, back-breaking hours in low-paying jobs and often have little time to devote to the children.

Take the case of a Salvadoran couple in San Francisco (Clara and José), whose two children (Tony and Esteban) are left alone almost all day, because the parents must work long hours to generate income that is barely adequate to survive (see Menjívar, 2000). They are relatives of Lolita, a woman who left El Salvador on short notice after being released from a prison, where she had been held (and tortured) because of her political activities. Lolita came to live with Clara and José, and when she saw that the children were misbehaving (answering back to their parents, not obeying, etc.), tried to reprimand them; according to her, this simply was not done. The children, who were well aware of their new authority and knowledge about the new society, did not keep quiet. They threatened to call the police and to have her deported if she ever scolded them again, and when they translated for her, Lolita suspected that they purposefully made mistakes to get her in trouble. Lolita was simply appalled; she could not understand how the "law doesn't let you educate [the children]."

Social workers can be called to intervene in such situations. Lolita only reprimanded the children verbally. However, in other, similar situations, various means of disciplining children practiced in the country of origin are used. Role reversal, the legacy of war, and different cultural understandings about disciplining children converge to create a delicate situation. A risk that English-speaking, monolingual social workers face is to reinforce the role reversal by speaking only with the children and asking them to serve as interpreters. Giving power to the children cannot be achieved by taking the power away from the adults. A balance needs to be found, but a lack of mastery of the language and understanding of the culture by the social worker could prevent this balance. To be culturally competent, we need to listen to the stories and assess clients within their cultural and historical context. The better listeners we become, the better we can serve the needs of immigrant children and their families.

REFERENCES

Aron, A., Corne, S., Fursland, A., & Zelwer, B. (1991). The gender specific terror of El Salvador and Guatemala. *Women's Studies International Forum, 14*(1/2), 37–47.

Barthauer, L. M., & Leventhal, J. M. (1999). Prevalence and effects of child abuse in poor, rural community in El Salvador: A retrospective study of women after 12 years of civil war. *Child Abuse and Neglect, 23*(11), 1117–1126.

Cantor, M. H., Brennan, M., & Sainz A. (1994). The importance of ethnicity in the social support systems of older New Yorkers: A longitudinal perspective (1970 to 1990). *Journal of Gerontological Social Work, 22*(3/4), 95–128.

Carrasquillo, O., Carrasquillo, A. I., & Shea, S. (2000). Health insurance coverage of immigrants living in the United States: Differences by citizenship status and country of origin. *American Journal of Public Health, 90*(6), 917–923.

Comas-Díaz, L., & Minrath, M. (1987). Psychotherapy with ethnic minority borderline clients. *Psychotherapy, 225*, 418–426.

Espino, C. (1991). Trauma and adaptation: The case of Central American children. In F. L. Ahearn & J. L. Athey (Eds.), *Refugee children: Theory, research, and services* (pp. 106–124). Baltimore: Johns Hopkins University Press.

Fernández-Kelly, M., & Schauffler, R. (1994). Divided fates: Immigrant children in a restructured U.S. economy. *International Migration Review*, 28(4), 662–689.

Fernández-Kelly, P., & Curran, S. (2001). *Nicaraguans: Voices lost, voices found*. Unpublished manuscript, Department of Sociology and Office of Population Research, Princeton University, Princeton, NJ.

Germain, C. B., & Gitterman A. (1995). Ecological perspective. In R. L. Edwards (Ed.), *Encyclopedia of social work* (19th ed., pp. 816–824). Silver Spring, MD: National Association of Social Workers.

Gil, A. G., & Vega, W. A. (1996). Two different worlds: Acculturation stress and adaptation among Cuban and Nicaraguan families. *Journal of Social and Personal Relationships*, 3(3), 435–456.

Gil-Rivas, V., Anglin, M. D., & Annon, J. J. (1997). Patterns of drug use and criminal activities among Latino arrestees in California: Treatment and policy implications. *Journal of Psychopathology and Behavioral Assessment*, 19(2), 161–174.

Glantz, M., & Jamieson, D. (2000). Societal response to Hurricane Mitch and intra- versus generational equity issues: Whose norms should apply? *Risk Analysis*, 20(6), 869–882.

Greenwell, L., Valdez, R. B., & DaVanzo, J. (1997). Social ties, wages, and gender in a study of Salvadoran and Filipino immigrants in Los Angeles. *Social Science Quarterly*, 78(2), 559–577.

Guarnaccia, P. J., & Farias, P. (1988). The social meanings of Nervios: A case study of a Central American woman. *Social Science and Medicine*, 26(12), 1223–1231.

Harrison, D. F., Wodarski, J. S., & Thyer, B. A. (Eds.). (1992). *Cultural diversity and social work practice*. Springfield, IL: Thomas.

Hondagneu-Sotelo, P., & Avila, E. (1997). "I'm here, but I'm there": The meanings of Latina transnational motherhood. *Gender and Society*, 11(5), 548–571.

Immigration and Naturalization Service. (1995). *Statistical yearbook of the immigration and Naturalization Service*. Washington, DC: U.S. Department of Justice.

Immigration and Naturalization Service. (1997, February 7). *INS releases updated estimates of U.S. illegal population*. [News release]. Washington, DC: U.S. Department of Justice.

Keefe, S., Padilla, A. M., & Carlos, M. L. (1979). The Mexican-American extended family as an emotional support system. *Human Organization*, 38(2), 145–152.

Kulig, J. C. (1998). Family life among El Salvadorans, Guatemalans and Nicaraguans: A comparative study. *Journal of Comparative Family Studies*, 29(3), 469–478.

Leslie, L. A. (1992). The role of informal support networks in the adjustment of Central American immigrant families. *Journal of Community Psychology*, 20(3), 243–256.

Mahler, S. J. (1999). Engendering transnational migration: A case study of Salvadorans. *American Behavioral Scientist*, 42(4), 690–719.

Marsiglia, F. F., Kulis, S., & Hecht, M. L. (2001). Ethnic labels and ethnic identity as predictors of drug use and drug exposure among middle school students in the Southwest. *Journal of Research on Adolescence*, 11(1), 21–48.

Marsiglia, F. F., & Navarro, R. (1999). Acculturation status and HIV/AIDS knowledge and perception of risk among a group of Mexican American middle school students. *Journal of HIV/AIDS Prevention and Education for Adolescents and Children*, 3(3), 43–61.

Massey, D. S., Alarcón, R., Durand, J., & González, H. (1987). *Return to Aztlan: The social process of international migration from western Mexico.* Berkeley: University of California Press.

Mayers, R. S., Kail, B. L., & Watts, T. D. (1993). *Hispanic substance abuse.* Springfield, IL: Thomas.

Menjívar, C. (1997). Immigrant kinship networks: Vietnamese, Salvadorans and Mexicans in comparative perspective. *Journal of Comparative Family Studies,* 28(1), 1–12.

Menjívar, C. (1999). Salvadorans and Nicaraguans: Refugees become workers. In D. Haines & K.E. Rosenblum (Eds.), *Illegal immigration in America: A reference handbook* (pp. 232–253). Westport, CT: Greenwood Press.

Menjívar, C. (2000). *Fragmented ties: Salvadoran immigrant networks in America.* Berkeley: University of California Press.

Patterson, S., & Marsiglia, F. F. (2000). "Mi casa es su casa": A beginning exploration of Mexican Americans' natural helping. *Families in Society,* 81(1), 22–31.

Peceny, M., & Stanley, W. (2001). Liberal social reconstruction and resolution of civil wars in Central America. *International Organization,* 55(1), 149–158.

Pitt, R., & Marsiglia, F. F. (2000). Like oil floating in water: The narrative of an undocumented worker. *Reflections,* 6(4), 18–23.

Pitt, R., Portes, A., & Stepick, A. (1993). *City on the edge: The transformation of Miami.* Berkeley: University of California Press.

Rumbaut, R. G. (1989). The structure of refuge: Southeast Asian refugees in the U.S., 1975–1985. *International Review of Comparative Public Policy,* 1, 97–129.

Rumbaut, R. G. (1994). Origins and destinies: Immigration to the United States since World War II. *Sociological Forum,* 9(4), 583–621.

Rousseau, C., & Drapeau, A. (1998). Parent–child agreement on refugee children's psychiatric symptoms: A transcultural perspective. *Journal of the American Academy of Child and Adolescent Psychiatry,* 37(6), 629–636.

Saleebey, D. (1997). *The strengths perspective in social work practice* (2nd ed.). New York: Longman.

Salgado de Snyder, V., Richard, N., Cervantes, C., & Padilla, A. M. (1990). Gender and ethnic differences in psychosocial stress and generalized distress among Hispanics. *Sex Roles,* 22(7–8), 441–453.

Schoeni, R. F. (1997). New evidence on the economic progress of foreign-born men in the 1970s and 1980s. *Journal of Human Resources,* 32(4), 683–740.

Smart, J., & Smart, D. (1995). Acculturative stress of Hispanics: Loss and challenge. *Journal of Counseling and Development,* 73, 390–396.

Thompson, M., & McGorry, P. (1995). Psychological sequelae of torture and trauma of Chilean and Salvadoran migrants—a pilot study. *Australian and New Zealand Journal of Psychiatry,* 29(1), 84–95.

Urrutia-Rojas, X., & Rodríguez, N. (1997) Unaccompanied migrant children from Central America: Sociodemographic characteristics and experiences with potentially traumatic events. In A. Ugalde & G. Cárdenas (Eds.), *Health and social services among international labor migrants: A comparative perspective* (pp. 151–166). Austin: University of Texas Press, Center for Mexican American Studies.

Van Hightower, N. R., Gorton, J., & DeMoss, C. L. (2000). Predictive models of domestic violence and fear of intimate partners among migrant and seasonal farm worker women. *Journal of Family Violence, 15*(2), 137–154.

Wallace, S. P. (1992). Community formation as an activity of daily living: The case of Nicaraguan immigrant elderly. *Journal of Aging Studies, 6*(4), 365–383.

Weick, A., Rapp, C., Sullivan, W. P., & Kristhardt, W. (1989). A strengths perspective for social work practice. *Social Work, 34,* 350–354.

Wiltfang, G. L., & Cochran, J. K. (1994). The sanctuary movement and the smuggling of undocumented Central Americans into the United States: Crime, deviance, or defiance? *Sociological Spectrum, 14*(2), 101–128.

Zsembik, B.A . (2000). The Cuban ethnic economy and labor market outcomes of Latinos in metropolitan Florida. *Hispanic Journal of Behavioral Sciences, 22*(2), 223–236.

CHAPTER 15

Balkan Children and Families

MELISSA GOODMAN

People from the Balkans come to the United States to seek refuge from the ethnic conflicts of these regions. The Balkans consist of several countries and many republics, but in this chapter, I focus on the former Yugoslavia, which comprises Slovenia, Croatia, Bosnia–Herzegovina, Montenegro, Serbia, Macedonia, and Kosovo Autonomous Province. Albania is also relevant to this discussion. The three main religions in the Balkans are Roman Catholic, Orthodox Christian, and Muslim (Klain, 1998; Mooren & Kleber, 1999). To best assist Balkan immigrant children and their families, it is important to understand the history and problems of the many beleaguered subgroups from this region. This understanding is especially important, because Western interventions often conflict with the prevailing views of life among members of these subgroups. This chapter covers historical background, problems and issues, cultural strengths, indigenous strategies, and a case about a Bosnian woman that highlights culturally competent practice principles.

HISTORICAL BACKGROUND

This brief history of the Balkans is designed to show that military actions in this region have created an artificial union of people with diverse cultures and religions. These artificial groupings have given rise to bitter wars and antagonism among these groups. In the Middle Ages, the Turks defeated the Serbs in the Battle of Kosovo (1389), giving rise to Turkish domination of the region (Klain, 1998; Mooren & Kleber, 1999). Over the centuries,

Austria, Germany, and Hungary fought off the Turks and governed various sections of the Balkans. World War I began in Bosnia–Herzegovina, when a rebel representing Serbs and Muslims assassinated Archduke Ferdinand, thus ending the rule of Austria and Hungary.

Between 1918 and 1941, Serbians dominated the Croatians and Slovenians in Yugoslavia. Next came the Nazis, who occupied Yugoslavia during World War II. Josip Broz, commonly known as "Tito," launched a revolution against German rule during the Nazi occupation in the 1940s. President Tito, who ruled Yugoslavia until his death in 1980, instituted a type of socialism that made him a hero to some, an enemy to others (Mooren & Kleber, 1999). Under his rule, factories and businesses were run collectively, relying heavily on loans. When Tito died, economic problems, notably, poverty and unemployment, revitalized ethnic hostilities. Hostility among subgroups was transmitted transgenerationally based on the memories of the atrocities committed by religious and ethnic groups during earlier times (Klain, 1998).

The year 1991 marked the beginning of a decade-long war that changed the face of the Balkans and resulted in a substantial influx of Balkan immigrants and refugees to the United States and other safe havens. Slovenia and Croatia declared their independence from the former Yugoslavia that year. Bosnia–Herzegovina followed the next year. Civil war ensued, in which Serbs tried to destroy the Albanians, most of whom were Muslims. In addition, Bosnian Serbs and the Serbian military occupied Bosnia. Conflict began between Bosnian Muslims and Bosnian Croatians.

The civil war officially ended in 1995 with the Dayton Peace Agreement but, for most people of the region, no peace followed. In March 1999, the North Atlantic Treaty Organization (NATO) intervened after much debate among its constituents to prevent genocide of Albanians by Serbians. Albanians in Kosovo were forced from their homes and sought refuge in Macedonia and Albania, in one of the largest movements of people since World War II (Brusin, 2000). This displacement of Albanian Muslims and other subgroups continues, as does the effort to pinpoint accountability of war criminals at international trials at The Hague. Many people fled to the United States. Some bought false documents; others were sponsored by family members; still others sought refugee through international organizations such as the International Rescue Committee.

ADAPTATION TO THE UNITED STATES

Adaptation of the children and families from the Balkans to the United States depends primarily on (1) the experiences they endured back home before emigrating, and (2) their stage of life when they arrived.

Wartime Experience

People from the Balkans, especially those who survived the last decade of war and internal conflict, had to live surrounded by enemies, while having inadequate food, water, electricity, and heat (Filipovic, 1994; Karcic & Karcic, 2000). The widespread shelling and bombing created anxiety about whether they and their loved ones would be tortured or killed, as the young teenager Zlata Filipovic so poignantly described in her diary (Filipovic, 1994). Zlata, often called the "Anne Frank of Sarajevo," was a bright, middle-class, preteen, who chronicled the change from a happy, normal life in 1991, to an existence filled with death and uncertainty after the Serbians invaded this cosmopolitan city.

Van der Kolk, McFarlane, and Weisaeth (1996) have described the permanent changes in physiobiology that can result from such intense wartime stress. Children forced to witness their parents killed or tortured, for example, may forever lose their ability to modulate their response to stress. This is especially true for children younger than 8 years old, whose neurological systems are still developing. Garbarino and Vorrasi (1999, p. L2-2) point out that "each number in the body count of war represents a hole in the life of a child." Many children from the Balkans have witnessed many war events. The intrusive memories of violent episodes can trigger massive anxieties in Balkan children. Each subsequent threat to their sense of stability then sets off a new spiral of terror.

Many displaced Balkan adults and children spent time in refugee camps before being allowed to come to the United States. The children's anxiety level tends to be proportional to the disruption in the social structure of their lives (Garbarino & Vorrasi, 1999). Sometimes Balkan children could not go to school because of wartime conditions and their displacement; their fathers and brothers might have left home to fight; and their mothers were less likely to be available emotionally; thus, their developmental growth may have been impeded.

Adults run a high risk of profound depression as they face existential losses such as shattered faith, disillusionment, loss of trust, and dashed hopes for the future (Kasnar, 2000). Men and women leaving the Balkans and adapting to the United States had to cope with many losses. Some gave up hope and interest in living; others lost faith in humanity. Their feelings of loss may have hindered the adaptation to their new life in the United States and influenced their children's perspective.

For example, according to their developmental needs, children's sense of safety depends on access to competent, emotionally available parents or their own ability to make use of surrogate nurturing figures (Garbarino & Vorrasi, 1999). Art therapists Kalmanowitz and Lloyd (1999) showed that orphaned Bosnian children living in refugee camps without responsible adults created prolific work marked by a pervasive sense of barrenness. On the other hand, Bosnian Muslim children, who spent time in camps where women tended to communal needs, displayed retained hope for the future in their artwork.

In general, Muslims faced the most severe persecution, although Muslim refugees in Croatia, who lived outside of the refugee camps, fared somewhat better (Karcic & Karcic, 2000). One of the latter, a courageous 19-year-old Albanian Muslim, spent 10 years indoors in her home with her schizophrenic mother and schizophrenic grandmother as the war raged. Only her father dared venture out to work; the women and girls dared not go out, because they feared that Serbians would rape and torture them. In addition to missing out on the normal experiences of school and work, the 19-year-old suffered severe panic attacks that rendered her speechless at times. But she was spared the torture and rape to which other women were subjected thus faring better than others of her gender.

At greatest risk for depression and posttraumatic stress disorder (PTSD) are those who were tortured in the primitive, horrific ways characteristic of this war. Torture is designed to destroy the soul and spirit. The experience changes the way people communicate with one another and the patterns of relationships by which they define themselves and give meaning to their lives. Torture breaks off important emotional and social connections, weakening survivors' ability to extend themselves, even when they find a safe haven.

Because of the war crimes trial of Slodoban Milosevic at The Hague, many people know that Serbian rebels and the Serbian army tortured children and the elderly. In addition, Serbian women married to non-Serbs were victimized by both their husbands' ethnic group, because they symbolized the enemy, and by women in their own Serbian ethnic group, because they married outside the ethnic group and belonged to the enemy side (Stevanovic, 1998).

But the greatest insults, including mass rape and torture, befell Muslim women. The raped women felt guilt, shame, and loss of self-respect (Klain, 1998). They knew that their rape was a means to degrade their husbands, so they refrained from talking about their experiences and often developed psychosomatic reactions, depression, and suicidal tendencies. Men were also raped in this cruel war and seldom sought help for their problems (Klain, 1998). These are only a few examples among the numerous tragedies bestowed upon Balkan men, women, and children.

Thus, many Balkan refugees come to the United States having been multiply traumatized and therefore at risk for PTSD and other mental illnesses. They face the challenges of living in an English-speaking, capitalistic country after their coping skills have been taxed to the maximum.

Stage of Life

Generally speaking, adapting to the United States is easier for young people than for their parents. For example, Weine et al. (1995) and Becker, Weine, Vojvoda, and McGlashan (1999) studied 12 Albanian Muslim teenagers, who survived the war in Bosnia–Herzegovina, in their first year in the United States and 1 year later. Because they saw in the United States social, educational, and work opportunities unavailable back home, they adjusted more rapidly than did their parents. They learned English quickly and worked hard in school, held part-time jobs, and deferred going away to college in favor of living at home and attending local colleges. These actions reflected, in part, their decision to protect their parents from the demands of the new culture. The parents of these teens, with the aid of refugee resettlement workers and church sponsors, obtained jobs but lagged behind in learning English. They tended to isolate themselves within their own community. Their priority was to create opportunities for their children (Weine et al., 1995).

Many senior citizens who came to the United States in the 1950s and 1960s, when Tito ruled, resisted learning English, remained isolated, and longed to go home. When they do venture home, the grief they feel can be unspeakable. For example, in the 1960s the parents of one Croatian American social worker immigrated to the United States when they were in their 30s. They declined to be interviewed, because they felt that dragging up old memories would serve no purpose. "There were no jobs then [in the 1960s]," their daughter says. "And there are no jobs now, because there is no money to rebuild the country."

She and her parents returned to their old neighborhood in Croatia, in 1999, and grieved over its destruction. Next door to a beautiful home owned by a Croatian family was rubble from a building that had been bombed just because the family who lived there was Serbian.

PROBLEMS FOR CHILDREN AND FAMILIES

Surviving and trying to find certainty about housing, jobs, schooling, and support networks in the heterogeneous culture of the United States creates major challenges for the Balkan families. Furthermore, because of differences in cultural values around male dominance and patriarchal practices, the issue of domestic violence, for example, may cause Balkan immigrants to clash with their newly adopted culture.

Survival

Survival is uppermost in the minds of people who come to the United States from the Balkans. Many obtain assistance through humanitarian organizations, such as the International Rescue Committee (IRC) and religious groups. Among the types of assistance such organizations provide are (1) English-language classes; (2) initial housing and furnishings, food, and clothing; (3) cash assistance and medical evaluations; (4) food stamps; (5) help with school registration for children; (6) orientation to the community; (7) social security cards; and (8) employment information (Velazco, 1999).

Also of concern to many are visa problems, fear of deportation, derailed careers or education, and uncertainty about family members back home (Karcic & Karcic, 2000). Children, for example, who must first master English, may find themselves behind their classmates. In addition, their parents may have brought them to the United States to enable them to have a better life. But this is small consolation to a child who is very close to grandparents, and the beloved grandparents remain in danger back home. Children may feel powerless and question their parental values, because these parental values may appear to them to have caused suffering for themselves and their families.

Immigrant and refugee families often face ethnic discrimination in the United States. They frequently live in high-crime areas because of their low wages or to be near others of their ethnicity. They usually need job retraining despite prestigious work statuses held in the home country. Because of language deficiencies in English, there are often intergenerational conflicts between parents and children, whose roles may become reversed, and tensions arise (Bijelic, 1998).

Isolation may add to the adjustment problems of families. Because of phobias and agoraphobia, one Balkan family may be unaware that someone from their native city lives within a few minutes' walk, because they fear traveling even a block from home (Kasnar, personal communication, December 5, 2000). This fear may also be reinforced by differences in cultural norms and beliefs between the Balkan countries and the United States.

Domestic Violence

For many Balkan immigrants and refugees, the concept of domestic violence may be alien to them because of different understandings and expectations of the role of men in each culture. It is particularly important that first responders and other clinicians who deal with disclosures about domestic violence understand the belief systems of the subgroups. The subcultures of many of the Balkan people who made it to the United States are highly patriarchal. Thus, men dominate women and are authoritarian in their treatment of children. Although not conventionally labeled as such in the cultures of the Balkan countries, domestic violence permeates daily life (Klain, 1998). Despite the fact that it is unacceptable in the United States, Balkan women and children are beaten, abused, and marginalized.

For example, a teenage Kosovar Muslim related to me her flight from the former Yugoslavia on the eve of a wedding that her father had arranged. Rather than submit to this practice of an arranged marriage, she bought a false passport, traveled to Mexico alone, then sought political asylum in the United States. She spoke not one word of English. There are adjustments for Balkan families to make in adapting to their new social environment, particularly for the men, who find that these former behaviors of arranging marriages for daughters and abusing their wives are challenged and forbidden in the United States.

What mental health workers in the United States think of as domestic violence may represent "business as usual" to women from the Balkans. As Mrsevic and Hughes (1997) point out, women fear that more violence will result if they try to leave. An Albanian woman came for treatment because of disabling panic attacks coupled with agoraphobia. She described as "an accident" the fact that her husband threw her headlong across a room and into a wall. Family traditions hold women responsible for holding the family together "for the sake of the children." Economic necessity also binds women to their husbands and partners. Leaving their husbands may create a sense of isolation from their community and the subsequent loss of comfort a family provides. In a recent research study among 40 Bosnian refugee couples (Spasojevic, Heffer, & Snyder, 2000), wives' marital satisfaction was best predicted by the level of their husbands' PTSD and acculturation, and, finally, their own level of PTSD. Their husbands' marital satisfaction was not predicted by any of these factors. Thus, the wives saw their lives primarily in terms of their husbands' happiness, thus negating their own worth.

Providing information about obtaining police reports and orders of protection, relocating to shelters and safe houses, and getting the locks changed may be culturally dystonic. The abused Balkan woman may very well feel that she is fulfilling her lot in life, according to her cultural beliefs, by staying in an abusive relationship. However, when children are the objects of abuse, families may be shocked to find themselves face-to-face with child protection workers in the United States. Considering the negative experiences many immigrants have had with government officials in their country of origin, inquiries are likely to be met with suspicion, lack of cooperation, and intense resentment. Just as the grassroots organization Sahki arose to meet the needs of South Asian women who suffered domestic violence, one could hope to see a similar effort among the Balkan immigrants run by and for each other. Counseling efforts must focus on a gradual understanding of the patients' views of the world. Only then can they gain an inkling into alternative lifestyles.

CULTURAL VALUES AS STRENGTHS IN ASSESSMENT

Balkans hold family life, community, and nature as some of their important cultural values. A key cultural strength among Balkan families is the core value of family life, especially when headed by a dominant man. Related to this is the importance of community and sharing rather than the competitiveness of American culture. This is especially true for people from the former Yugoslavia, who, for the most part of their lives, experienced ethnic tolerance before the strife of recent years. There in the former Yugoslavia, Serbs, Croatians, Bosnians, and Muslims lived side-by-side and mingled as friends and coworkers, and intermarried. Finally, as former farmers, fishermen, and shepherds, they share a strong sense of nature.

In working with Balkan clients, social workers and other professionals might ask the following questions to assess the strengths and needs of children and their families. These questions reflect the Balkan value of family life, the stressful situation of war and conflict, and the acknowledgment of the diversity of religions:

"Who do you live with?"

"Where is the rest of your family?"

"What are your mother, father, sister, brother, grandmother, grandfather, etc., like?"

"Do you know other people who have come to the United States from your part of the world?"

"How does life differ here from your life back home?"

"Is religion an important part of your life?"

"Where do you worship?"

"Who is your best friend?"

"What is that person's family like?"

"What are your goals?"

"What was the best thing about living back home?"

"What is the best thing about living in the United States?"

The answers to these questions provide information about how intact the cultural values remain for the family.

Most people from the Balkans assume that people from the United States do not know about their culture. Armed with an understanding of the history of this tempestuous region, social workers can help Balkan clients feel understood. If photos have survived the trip, then men, women, and children may find it meaningful to share these symbols from a time when their lives were, if not better, at least less alien. American counselors/social workers who show that they care about the Balkan culture pave the way for an easier assessment of cultural strengths and determination of culturally appropriate service needs.

INDIGENOUS STRATEGIES AND WESTERN INTERVENTIONS

Most people from the Balkans whom mental health professionals encounter have had little or no contact with psychotherapy, psychotropic medications, or psychiatrists. The most common indigenous approach for most Balkan people involves solving a problem within the family, without interference from strangers. Counseling is considered unlikely to change anything and is highly stigmatized. Hard work and "God's help" are believed to solve life's difficulties and personal problems.

Here in the United States, psychiatrists Stevan Weine and Ivan Pavkovic, cofounders of the Project on Genocide, Psychiatry, and Witnessing in Chicago, work within the cultural value system of the immigrants. Specifically, they focus on a family and community framework to make Balkan refugee families stronger (Friedrich, 1999). Their program CAFES (Coffee and Family Education and Support for Bosnian Families) supports family strengths rather than identifying individuals with mental health problems. Half a dozen Bosnian families meet for nine sessions over a 15-week period to talk about what they experienced during the war and the challenges they face in their new lives in the United States. The sessions enable families to improve communication within the family and to connect with other refugees who have endured similar experiences. Other advantages of the groups are that members helped each other find jobs. In addition, psychoeducation about the impact of traumatic experiences on healthy people encourages individuals in need to avail themselves of mental health services (Friedrich, 1999).

As the number of Muslim Kosovar immigrants has increased in Chicago, Weine's group has turned its attention to determining the best way to help this population. Kosovar society is highly patriarchal, gender-rigid, and authoritarian, Weine reports (Friedrich, 1999). Many generations tend to live together under the rule of one man, the designated head of house. If one fails to engage that man in treatment planning or implementation, all interventions are likely to fail, Weine notes.

Failure to help Balkan family members who have endured various forms of torture is possible. To prevent this, professionals have to take into account the history of the breakdown of the former Yugoslavia. The various tragedies imposed internally on small groups because of religious wars and cultural conflicts contribute to the problem.

Helping those who have been tortured is usually beyond the purview of most clinicians. However, organizations staffed by specialists in this area can help restore survivors' sense of dignity after their dehumanizing experiences (Refugee Resources, 1999). Balkan families and other immigrants in New York City, for example, can access Doctors of the World-USA, Inc., The Bellevue/NYU Program for Survivors of Torture; New York Association for New Americans (NYANA); and Safe Horizon/Solace (Refugee Resources, 1999; Solace, n.d.). All of these organizations have trained staff who deal with intense anger, grief and losses, fears and phobias, and other PTSD issues related to traumas and tragedies.

PRINCIPLES OF CULTURALLY APPROPRIATE PRACTICE

Children from Balkan families often need help in adapting to their new environments in the United States. Teachers and other helping professionals in the schools play a key role in helping children process their prior trauma, adapt to their adopted country, and grow in developmentally appropriate ways. One intervention involves understanding racism and affirming a child's ethnicity (Northwood & Nielsen, 1998). Other interventions may involve dealing with feelings of betrayal and abandonment.

Children and adults alike may need to "postpone" dealing with their intense emotions until they feel safe in their new environment (Garbarino & Vorrasi, 1999). One of the most painful issues for Bosnian teens was the attempt to reconcile feeling betrayed by friends, neighbors, and even relatives back home (Becker et al., 1999; Weine et al., 1995). Before the war, multiculturalism was a natural part of their environment. This concept of the world as a place with many cultures coexisting clashed with their experiences of being persecuted by Serbs. Teens need to understand how multiple cultures can peacefully coexist and be respectful of religion, philosophy, and politics.

Also important is helping Balkan young people find role models in persons such as Zlata Filipovic, the model of the modern-day Anne Frank, and Croatian sports figures, who can enhance self-esteem and inspire youth. Teens can also be encouraged to write for local newspapers, those designed for both their own community and the public. They can describe their experiences in scholarship applications. In Astoria, Queens, children from the Balkans alternate with children from other ethnic groups in displaying their dance and music to others in Athens Square park. Giving testimony or telling one's story has been a powerful therapeutic tool among oppressed people (Kasnar, personal communication, December 5, 2000). This is similar to narrative therapy in which the stories told "are powerful because they determine what [people] notice and remember" (Nichols & Schwartz, 1998, p. 198).

Encouraging children to create art that describes their early experiences back home provides a means of channeling complex emotions constructively (Northwood & Nielsen, 1998). As Kalmanowitz and Lloyd

(1999) have described, while playing, refugee children whose homes had been destroyed repeatedly built and rebuilt houses. Some were made from objects from the town dump. If local children knocked them down, the refugees rebuilt them as many times as necessary. This posttraumatic play is typical of preschool and school-age children (Webb, 2003).

One way to overcome learning and behavior problems that develop after children have lived through periods of chronic danger is to provide opportunities for them to succeed in nonacademic or nontraditional ways. Families, community leaders, and mental health providers can all contribute to this effort. Children with goals tend to have a sense of purposefulness that gives renewed meaning to life (Garbarino & Vorrasi, 1999). They feel empowered by their ability to affect situations around them (Garbarino & Vorrasi, 1999). Some of the Bosnian children planned to send their parents back to Bosnia and visit them often; others thought far ahead, planning to retire there themselves. The teens in the Becker et al. study (1999) chose to bear witness by talking about their experiences with others, writing about them, and engaging in political activism here in the United States.

A method of helping adult refugees cope with their massive losses is to encourage them to return to their homelands to fight for human rights (Kasnar, personal communication, December 5, 2000). Others serve as witnesses for Amnesty International and other organizations. Balkan families can be empowered, with the help of the community. They can be encouraged to address and take pride in their differences, along with generations of immigrants before them. They can address traumatic experiences verbally and nonverbally, and honor themselves as survivors.

CASE VIGNETTE

Nada volunteered to tell her story so that "people will know the truth." A woman in her early 40s, she was born in a small city of about 60,000 people in Bosnia. She lived there with her parents and siblings during high school, then traveled to Sarajevo to attend a specialized high school to become a medical pharmacy technician. Nada remembers this as a safe and comfortable time for her family, when a young woman could safely travel by herself without a second thought. She graduated, obtained a full-time position as a pharmacy technician for the government, and lived in employee housing. "When Tito ruled, it was the perfect time," she reminisced. Two years later, she married and moved in with her in-laws for 4 years, until she and her husband were able to find housing, which was in short supply. She and her husband had two children, a boy and a girl, who were part Serbian Orthodox Christian and part Bosnian Muslim.

Then, in 1991, when the war began, the peaceful life she and her multicultural family had known disappeared before her eyes. "People were like animals," she stated. Most families had no money and were jealous of anyone who had anything. She remembered vividly an experience in which a woman in the village was the only person who had a green pepper, and surrounding people demanded to know who had the pepper because they were all hungry. Nada and her family lived for 3 years with no electricity and running water. Food was in short supply.

One evening during this time, bombs exploded nearby. "For a fraction of a second, I thought I was dead," she recounted. "But God saved us." After that, she shook constantly and suffered from diarrhea. She would conceal her children with covers and blankets, no matter what the temperature. Her husband, she noted, warned her that she might smother them if she were not careful. Rationally, she knew that her son and daughter did not need the covers, but Nada felt that if she could cover them up enough, she could protect them from harm. They spent most of their time at home when they were not in school.

At one point, when life had become especially treacherous, Nada's family urged her to take the children to Serbia for a week or two. They thought the hostilities would be temporary. They had to stay for months, Nada says angrily, with no contact with the rest of her family. Her town in Bosnia, where her husband and his parents lived, was surrounded by enemy factions. With a pen in hand, she stabbed the map in all the places where she was stopped as she tried to return home with her children, which took 4 months.

Two years later, an incident occurred that caused her heart to beat fast just telling the story. It was a school day, and no bombs were falling. As her children were heading out through the courtyard leading from their apartment, Nada heard a bomb fall and could no longer see her children. Instinctively, she felt an urge to jump from her third-floor balcony in a superhuman effort to save her children. Fortunately, she then heard them running up the stairs to find her.

Nada suffered from chronic headaches, a feeling of numbness, and depression during the war years. Resources were so scarce that "people lived from the air," she reported. Ultimately, as their financial situation worsened, Nada and her family registered in Belgrade to emigrate. Although her husband had a brother in the United States, he would have preferred to stay in Bosnia. However, he has recently given up his desire to retire in Bosnia because of the desperate financial problems there, where jobs are few and far between.

The International Rescue Committee helped the family settle in the United States. They provided free rent for 3 months, essential furniture, $160 for household items, and help in finding work. Nada's husband began packing costume jewelry; she became a cashier and ultimately landed a job doing the work for which she trained. Her husband now works in a meatpacking plant.

"We came here for our children," Nada says. But her children suffered greatly when separated from their grandparents. Her elementary school-age daughter, Irma, came home crying day after day, when she could be pushed to go to school at all. Some days, Nada got a call from school that Irma was crying in school because she wanted to go home. Nada, fearing that child protective services would take Irma away, begged the child to be strong. Ultimately, a Croatian American teacher took Irma under her wing and discovered that the child cried because she "felt stupid," because her English was not good enough for her to excel in school as she had back home.

Five years later, Irma excels academically and teaches tai kwon do in a local academy. She drinks bottled water, and prefers Chinese food and McDonald's to her mother's cooking. Irma also has many friends and wants to be a lawyer. A dispute in the family centered on her desire to shave her legs when she was 10. Her brother, however, has not adapted to life here and saves all the money he earns from a part-time job to return home to Bosnia to be with his friends and family. He is not academically oriented and wants to learn a trade. Although athletically oriented, he has given up sports now that he is in the United States. He does not feel safe walking around alone in New York City because of tough kids who attend the same school. He rarely goes out if he does not have to, and he does not date. His few friends come from the former Yugoslavia.

The children spent the summer of 2001 back home in Bosnia. Their parents sent them primarily "to bring joy to their grandparents." Nada and her husband also felt that the children were better off there rather than in New York City during the summer. The children enjoyed being in the country with their grandparents and their friends.

Nada and her family hope to move to Upstate New York eventually. In one town in particular, a large population of Bosnian immigrants has established a community. Together, they build homes cooperatively and live a lifestyle more like the environment to which they are accustomed. For now, "anything but war is OK," Nada says.

Nada last spoke to me in September 2001, about 2 weeks after terrorists flew two commercial aircraft into the World Trade Center. She was anxious and depressed about the added uncertainty in her family members' lives. Her children had returned from Bosnia on September 7, just 4 days before the attack. Nada's son will turn 18 soon, and she fears that he will be drafted. "We came here to escape the war," she said, "but now we are afraid all over again."

CONCLUSIONS

Culturally competent social workers who work with children and families from the Balkan countries need to be aware that, because of internal strife

in that region, there is tension among the ethnic subgroups due to historical, cultural, and religious differences. Nada and her family represent many
multiethnic families from this region. Their wartime experience was highly
stressful and filled with privation, but they were spared torture and rape.
Their family also remained intact. Because of stage-of-life issues and her
natural personality structure, the young daughter adapted more readily to
life in the United States. Other Balkans families may not have fared as well.

Nada's daughter Irma's early unhappiness was alleviated by a mentor-
ing teacher, who understood and respected her culture. Social workers and
other professionals are exhorted to be like the teacher and learn about the
different cultures and norms of the former Yugoslavian countries. With
some Balkan youth, such as Nada's son, who was 4 years older than the
daughter and found it more difficult to flourish in the United States in the
tough world of teenage boys, social workers need to try more persistently
to help them establish some supportive social networks.

Nada and her quiet, hardworking husband, a family man who still
struggles to learn English, have had to adapt to the extraordinarily complex
and competitive life in the United States. Although Nada, a resourceful
woman, brought photo albums for me to see of family outings in the beautiful hills of Bosnia, her ethnically diverse coworkers back home, and her
husband on a hunting trip in which catching game played second fiddle to
enjoying the wilderness with friends, she must cope with new anxieties
now. But she still lives and survives by the credo verbalized by many people
from her culture: hard work and God's help will see them through.

Social work practice with war-experienced immigrants requires knowledge of their traumas and fears. Social work skills and interventions need to
be adapted to incorporate cultural beliefs that may be represented in idioms
such as "Hard work and God's help." Culturally competent practice does
occur when preexisting environmental conditions affecting treatment are
honored. Working with Balkan clients, for whom communication barriers
exist as a result of little or no contact with psychotherapy and counseling is
highly stigmatized, the social worker may find that approaches such as role
modeling, narrative, and art therapy may be more culturally appropriate.

REFERENCES

Becker, D. F., Weine, S. M., Vojvoda, D., & McGlashan, T. H. (1999). Case series:
    PTSD symptoms in adolescent survivors of "ethnic cleansing": Results from a 1-
    year follow-up study. *Journal of the American Academy of Child and Adolescent
    Psychiatry, 38*(6), 775–781.
Bijelic, M. (1998). *Refugee youth: School considerations: Working effectively with
    schools to address the needs of refugee children.* Minneapolis: Center for Victims
    of Torture.

Brusin, S. (2000). The communicable disease surveillance system in the Kosovar refugee camps in the former Yugoslav Republic of Macedonia, April–August 1999. *Journal of Epidemiology and Community Health, 54,* 52–57.

Filipovic, Z. (1994). *Zlata's diary: A child's life in Sarajevo.* New York: Penguin.

Friedrich, M. J. (1999). Addressing mental health needs of Balkan refugees. *Journal of the American Medical Association, 282*(5), 422–423.

Garbarino, J., & Vorrasi, J. A. (1999). Long-term effects of war on children. In L. Kurtz (Ed.), *Encyclopedia of violence, peace, and conflict* (Vol. 1, pp. L2-1–L2-15). New York: Academic Press.

Kalmanowitz, D., & Lloyd, B. (1999). Fragments of art at work: Art therapy in the former Yugoslavia. *The Arts in Psychotherapy, 26*(1), 15–25.

Karcic, A., & Karcic, E. (2000). Mental health among Bosnian refugees. *Journal of the American Medical Association, 283*(1), 55–56.

Klain, E. (1998). Intergenerational aspects of the conflict in the former Yugoslavia. In Y. Danieli (Ed.), *International handbook of multigenerational legacies of trauma* (pp. 279–295). New York: Plenum Press.

Mooren, G. T. M., & Kleber, R. J. (1999). War, trauma, and society: Consequences of the disintegration of former Yugoslavia. In K. Nader & N. Dubrow (Eds.), *Honoring differences: Cultural issues in the treatment of trauma and loss* (pp. 178–210). Philadelphia: Brunner/Mazel.

Mrsevic, Z., & Hughes, D. M. (1997). Violence against women in Belgrade, Serbia: SOS hotline 1990–1993. *Violence Against Women, 3*(2), 101–128.

Nichols, M., & Schwartz, R. (1998). *Family therapy: Concepts and methods.* Boston: Allyn & Bacon.

Northwood, A., & Nielsen, L. (1998). *Refugee youth: Classroom considerations.* Minneapolis: Center for Victims of Torture.

Refugee Resources. (1999). *Refugee resources, family enrichment and support, and community development, culture and the arts.* New York: Author.

Solace. (n.d.). *At Solace, reclaim the humanity that is rightfully yours.* Jackson Heights, NY: Victim Services.

Spasojevic, J., Heffer, R.W., & Snyder, D.K. (2000). Effects of posttraumatic stress and acculturation on marital functioning in Bosnian refugee couples. *Journal of Traumatic Stress, 13*(2), 205–217.

Stevanovic, I. (1998). Violence against women in the Yugoslav war as told by women refugees. *International Review of Victimology, 6*(1), 63–76.

van der Kolk, B. A., McFarlane, A. C., Weisaeth, L. (Eds.). (1996). *Traumatic stress: The effects of overwhelming experience on mind, body, and society.* New York: Guilford Press.

Velazco, A. (1999). *Survival and adaptation in the refugee experience.* Washington, DC: Immigration and Refugee Services of America.

Webb, N. B. (2003). *Social work practice with children* (2nd ed.). New York: Guilford Press.

Weine, S., Becker, D. F., McGlashan, T. H., Vojvoda, D., Hartman, S., & Robbins, J. P. (1995). Adolescent survivors of "ethnic cleansing": Observations on the first year in America. *Journal of the American Academy of Child and Adolescent Psychiatry, 34*(9), 1153–1159.

CHAPTER 16

Russian Children and Families

TAMAR GREEN

The Former Soviet Union has a rich historical, cultural, and political background, and its population is representative of multiple ethnic and religious identities. Under communist rule, however, customs and religions could not be openly practiced. The Jewish population was the most politically and religiously persecuted group in the Former Soviet Union. As a result, several waves of Jewish migrant children and families from the Former Soviet Union immigrated to other countries over the past century. New cultural challenges, combined with traditional cultural values and strengths, contributed to the level of adaptability of this immigrant population to the United States.

This chapter reviews the history of the migration and adaptation of the Russian people to the United States. Problem areas and cultural values as strengths are discussed. A review of indigenous strategies and Western interventions is presented, and a discussion of culturally appropriate practice principles precedes a case vignette and conclusions.

HISTORICAL BACKGROUND

The major reason for emigration in 1970, and for the next 30 years, was rooted in anti-Semitism. In response to the religious and political persecution, the United States passed a law in 1973 to facilitate Soviet Jewish immigration. Therefore, in the early 1970s, the Former Soviet Union permitted emigration because of international pressure (Flaherty, Kohn, Golbin, Gaviria, & Birz, 1986). From 1970 to 1981, approximately 125,000

Soviet Jews immigrated to the United States from the European states, encompassing the larger cities and consisting of nonreligious Jews. All the groups of émigrés consisted of large numbers of educated and professional people subjected to anti-Semitism; therefore, lack of opportunity for their children was their main reason for leaving the Former Soviet Union (Flaherty, Kohn, Levav, & Birz, 1988).

The application process for exit visas in the Former Soviet Union in the 1970s introduced an added dimension of persecution toward potential émigrés and their families. Those who left in the 1970s were accused publicly of being traitors to their country. If they were not granted exit visas right away, they were harassed, denied work in their professions and educational opportunities, and had to take lower paying jobs. They reapplied yearly for visas and suffered financially, while they waited year after year for approval to leave. These people were treated like social outcasts, and their citizenship was revoked once they left the country. There were also repercussions for extended family members of émigrés who remained in Russia. They, too, were harassed, and denied promotions and other privileges; consequently, they suffered financially and socially. Thus, those who left the Former Soviet Union and embarked on new lives of freedom felt sorrow for leaving their families and guilt for the consequences imposed on those left behind.

The Afghanistan war, in 1979, and the gradual decline in Soviet–U.S. relationships in the early 1980s markedly reduced the number of Jews leaving the former Soviet Union. From 1981 through 1986, less than 1,000 Jews left each year (Flaherty et al., 1988). In the late 1980s, they emigrated because of anti-Semitism, the consequences of Chernobyl, and economic and political problems in the Former Soviet Union. Despite the difficulties encountered in the Former Soviet Union, this group was less motivated to immigrate than the group in the 1970s and more discouraged by the difficulties of resettlement. These immigrants were less likely to receive refugee status and would come to the United States with parolee status instead. Parolees could enter the United States, but they could not receive benefits (i.e., health insurance, financial aid). This meant that families either had to leave members behind in the Former Soviet Union, or parolee members had to be dependent on others if they chose to come to the United States as a family unit.

The Immigration Reform Act of 1990 increased the refugee ceiling for immigrants from the Former Soviet Union to 50,000 per year. This legislation prioritized applications based on family reunification and job skills needed by the U.S. economy. In 1992, over 20% of this population was 65 years of age or older, making this one of the oldest groups immigrating to the United States (Brod & Heurtin-Roberts, 1992). Between 1989 and 1995, Soviet Jews came not only from the former European Soviet Republics of Russia and the Ukraine but also from the Former Asian Soviet

Republics of Uzbekistan, Tadzhikistan, and Turkmenistan. This latter group, known as Bukharan Jews, is an ancient Jewish community that has completely different customs, practices, and language than the Jews from other parts of the Former Soviet Union. With the collapse of the Former Soviet Union, Bukharan Jews in the newly independent Muslim countries of Uzbekistan, Tadzhikistan, and Turkmenistan were subjected to increased anti-Semitism, political and economic chaos, beatings and looting of property, kidnapping, blackmail, and harassment in school and at work. Whereas only 3,000 Bukharan immigrants came to the United States between 1981 and 1988, 19,000 arrived between 1989 and 1995. Today, Bukharan communities are very culturally and religiously active in the United States (Halberstadt & Nikolsky, 1996).

During the final decade of the 20th century, following the fall of the communist regime, political and economic upheaval became major factors in the decision of Former Soviets to emigrate. Émigrés came to the United States to flee religious persecution, to reunite with their families, to improve their economic status, and to escape political chaos as the Former Soviet Republics struggled to maintain themselves as independent countries. In the United States, in recent years, the more frequently granted status of parolee has made the option of immigration less enticing and more frightening than the refugee status. Immigration rules are now stricter; that is, many Former Soviets who want to join family members need to wait until their family members become citizens. People have been entering the United States with working visas, some with the intention of earning money and returning to the Former Soviet Union, and others with the hope of obtaining residency status and remaining. Since this wave of immigration began, immigrants from the Former Soviet Union have settled across the entire United States.

ADAPTATION TO THE UNITED STATES

The Soviet Jewish immigrant population is an extremely heterogeneous group (Belozersky, 1990). The diverse cultural, religious, socioeconomic, and educational backgrounds of these immigrants have contributed in some instances to a positive adaptation to the United States, and in others to a less successful adaptation. Age factors, as well as individual and family dynamics, have also added to the adjustment process. One of the major transitions across the board for this population has been of a political nature. Immigrants from the Former Soviet Union have had to acclimate from a communist society to a capitalist society, and some of them have had great difficulty in this transition. The reception, degree of knowledge, and cultural sensitivity of the United States to this immigrant population, as well as the location of settlement in the United States, have also factored into the adaptation process. Generalizations about this immigrant population are made, although there are multiple differences and nuances among the various members of this immigrant population.

"Language" is the first and foremost response of every Former Soviet who is asked about problems of adaptation. Lack of language skills builds a barrier on all levels, from the concrete to the psychodynamic. Without knowledge of English, people have difficulty obtaining employment, shopping for food, filing applications for benefits or any other services, and communicating with schoolteachers about a child's educational progress or behavior. Children, who learn the language more quickly than their parents, carry the burden of translation, until their parents catch up to them. This may mean missing school to accompany family members to appointments. Basic English as a Second Language (ESL) classes are offered to refugees upon arrival, but émigrés often pursue more advanced classes at local colleges or adult education programs. Those adults who find jobs and are open to friendships outside of the Russian community develop a higher language capacity and have access to more options.

"Employment" is the second response when émigrés are asked about problems of adaptation. People who come to the United States believing that they will automatically become financially well off need to make some adjustments. Many of the émigrés who were educated and worked in professional capacities in the Former Soviet Union start off in the United States working at low-paying jobs and, with acquisition of language and skills development, move on to higher paying jobs and new professions. Some émigrés are fortunate enough to have family members to support them financially while they pursue their studies and training. Immigrants who cannot successfully learn the English language, will not allow themselves to work at lower level jobs, or are close to retirement age and cannot find employment are at risk for greater financial, emotional, or medical problems.

Refugees report to specific agencies set up to assist with "resettlement," the term most frequently used to describe the adaptation process for the immigrant population. These are federally funded private agencies. Medicaid, public assistance, and supplemental security income (SSI) are arranged until refugees are able to find work and support themselves. ESL classes, vocational training, and job referrals are offered free of charge, but services are time-limited. Parolees need to rely financially on family members, because they are not eligible for benefits until they are granted residency status by the United States. They need to learn English and find employment on their own. Immigrants from the Former Soviet Union are "community-oriented," so they often help one another; however, the stress of not having benefits or an income, and the need to depend on others, does impact negatively on adaptation level.

The majority of Soviet immigrants are Jewish but have very little Jewish awareness (Goldstein, 1979). The Jewish person belongs to both a nationality and a religion; these come with birth. Soviet Jews raised in Russian culture, and under Soviet rule, were forced to lose their connection to Jewish culture, to give up their Jewish identity, yet they were also forced to be identified as Jews on their passport. Even those who achieved high professional status were not fully accepted into Russian society. Being labeled "Jewish" led to internal conflicts about social competence (Goldstein, 1979), causing a sense of both exclusion and exclusivity. Soviet émigrés have conflicts about their Jewish identity and work toward resolution when they reach the United States.

When Soviet Jews immigrate to the United States, they have multiple choices as to how to approach the Jewish religion. They can choose not to acknowledge the religion, they can choose to observe some practices and not others, or they can choose to become Orthodox Jews and observe all religious practices. Often, nonreligious families put their children in religious schools either because these schools in some cities are known to provide better education than the public schools, or because these families want their children to learn about the religion. Children in these schools often come home and confront parents about why they are not practicing various religious rituals, and conflict may arise. At times, parents compromise and practice some of the religious rituals; other times, they remove their children from the schools to alleviate conflict. In instances in which teenage children want to become religious and cannot overcome differences with their parents, they leave their family and move into a religious community with a religious family.

Adults have a more difficult time than do children in adapting to religious ideas and concepts to which they were not exposed while living under communist rule. Some admit that they have difficulty simultaneously adjusting from a communist society to a capitalist society, and from a nonreligious environment to a more traditional/religious one. When given a choice, they sometimes opt not to deal with the latter. Because they were not allowed to acknowledge the Jewish religion, some Soviet Jews from the European republics never felt a connection with the Jewish religion and feel more connected to Russian Orthodox customs and traditions. Others consider themselves atheists or agnostics.

The transition from communism to capitalism, from a life of compliance and fear to a life of autonomy and freedom, sounds, in theory, like a "dream come true." But in reality, it can be a difficult journey. Preconceived notions are quickly abated when émigrés realize that the United States has social problems such as poverty, unemployment, expensive housing, crime, and costly medical care. The elderly have the most difficult time adapting. The younger and middle-aged adults and the adolescents struggle but succeed; the children have the least amount of trouble adjusting to this change.

In the Former Soviet Union, everyone was entitled to medical benefits, housing, education, employment, and a pension. Former Soviets relied on these without realizing it (Goldstein, 1979). In the United States, only education is guaranteed. Not all people have medical benefits, and even with benefits, there are restrictions regarding medical consultations and procedures to which the émigrés are not accustomed. Housing is expensive in the United States, and there are waiting lists for subsidized and public housing. The government does not take responsibility to ensure housing; often, people are left homeless. Expensive housing is less of an issue for families with close intergenerational ties, who may adjust well to living together in one home. This was typical in the Former Soviet Union, in cities where housing was limited and three generations often lived under one roof, or in republics in which this was a tradition rather than a necessity.

In the United States, individuals are responsible for finding employment on their own and need to "sell" themselves to potential employers. This is a foreign concept to émigrés from the Former Soviet Union, who were taught to be modest. Soviets were brought up to feel uncomfortable about their needs for competition, assertiveness, achievement, and success (Goldstein, 1979). In the United States, jobs and salaries are competitive, and assertiveness and aggressiveness are the only way to succeed. Soviets struggle as they try to seek and maintain employment, and still comply with their own cultural standards. Professional status in the hierarchy of society is part of a Soviet émigré's identity, and the loss of status that often occurs with emigration becomes a threat to this identity (Goldstein, 1979).

Elderly people have fewer choices in terms of employment, housing, and medical benefits. They may not have the ability to start over, and may need to rely on others. Whereas depending on the government is an acceptable concept for older Soviets, depending on children and friends is not. In the Former Soviet Union, children depended on the parents. The role reversal is difficult for elderly persons to accept. They are not prepared for the economic and psychological burdens imposed here (Brod & Heurtin-Roberts, 1992). Although the Soviet system encouraged dependency and compliance on government, Former Soviet émigrés have proven themselves to be adaptable and independent here in the United States. Extended families and communities find ways to take care of each other. They share homes, lend each other money, and find jobs for one another. They do not allow other émigrés to be left in the care of a system that will leave them homeless and hungry.

Freedom of expression, and freedom of options are new experiences for Former Soviet immigrants. In the Former Soviet Union, choosing whether to travel or buy a new car, wondering how to provide a better quality of life for one's family, returning to school to further one's career, pursuing better employment opportunities, and changing lifestyles were not within the realm of possibility. Life was accepted for what it was.

In the United States, where autonomy and initiative are valued, freedom can also be overwhelming. "A Soviet immigrant carries within himself a totalitarian state, a system of 'inner dictates' " (Goldstein, 1979, p. 258). Soviet immigrants often struggle with the conflict between dependence and a quest for freedom (Goldstein, 1979, p. 259). Even in the United States, they are afraid to take chances and pursue the multitude of opportunities available. Inner dictates interfere with a successful adjustment to this country. Adaptation to freedom is a great challenge.

PROBLEMS FOR CHILDREN AND FAMILIES

Married Couples

In the Former Soviet Union among the European republics, women had equal rights in the workforce and earned pay almost equal to men. At home, they had traditional roles of wife, mother, homemaker, and money manager. Men's traditional role was only to earn a steady income; at home, men had no responsibilities. In the United States, during resettlement, as couples study English and train or look for employment, wives continue to run their households, but the men find themselves without a role until they find employment. Given their experience with multiple roles, wives often become successful before their husbands, which means that they master the English language, find a job, and still maintain the household. The husbands become demoralized, angry, and are at risk for depression. This can strain a marital relationship, especially one that was already strained (Belozersky, 1990).

In the Bukharan community, families are patriarchal. Husbands are often the sole financial providers, although it is not unusual for women to work. The Bukharan male controls the family finances. His self-worth in the Bukharan community is determined by the family's financial security; if he does not succeed financially in the United States, he loses standing in the Bukharan community. Women are subordinate to their fathers, brothers, and husbands; Bukharan men expect obedience from the women. The status of women is low, regardless of education or profession, and increases only with age and number of children; elderly grandmothers are the only women treated with respect. Verbal and physical abuse of women is acceptable in the Bukharan community. It is also acceptable for a man to have premarital sex and extramarital affairs. Emigration often exposes such affairs. Emigration is also known to trigger other types of marital conflicts when extended families are reunited. The most frequent scenario in this conflict is the rejection of the wife by the husband's family if the wife is from a different social stratum or ethnic group, is better educated, or comes from a different city. Separation among Bukharan families is not acceptable, because it jeopardizes status in the community, as well as marriageability of children (Halberstadt & Nikolsky, 1996).

Young couples with no children, or with one young child, adapt more easily to resettlement than do older couples with more and older children. The developmental task for young couples is adjustment during the early years of marriage, so beginning life in a new country becomes part of the adjustment process. Developmental tasks for older couples with adolescents should be a time for reaching professional potential, financial stability, and guiding adolescents toward separation. Instead, they face unemployment or entry-level positions and feel overwhelmed, incompetent as professionals and as parents, and are unable to offer their children the guidance that they need (Belozersky, 1990).

All immigrant families go through a period of disruption of established family roles during the immigration and resettlement process. Families that did not function well in the Former Soviet Union face a significant intensification of their problems. Those who functioned well in the Former Soviet Union have an easier time adapting to the United States (Belozersky, 1990). Those who are open-minded and appreciative of their new life adapt better than those who cannot adjust to their preconceived notions about life in the United States.

Elders

In the Former Soviet Union, parents of adult children played a significant role in the intergenerational family life. Even if they did not live with their adult children, they assisted with finances and with child care. Elderly persons emigrated because their children needed them or earlier laws stated that families had to emigrate as a unit. Aging parents were also forced to leave with their children if no family members remained in the Former Soviet Union to care for them (Brod & Heurtin-Roberts, 1992). These reluctant émigrés came to the United States feeling displaced even before meeting the challenges of being new immigrants, and this placed them at risk for depression, medical problems, and family discord.

Regardless of whether they came willingly, once in the United States, the status of elderly persons changes on many levels. They are no longer financially independent. They either receive financial benefits or have lower paying jobs than those to which they are accustomed, and lose their role as financial supporter of their children. Lack of understanding of the English language makes elders dependent on their children and grandchildren, so they lose their autonomy. If the family lives together because of financial necessity and not from choice, then the parents are experienced as a burden to the children. If adult children choose to westernize and live separately, then the parents are extremely hurt. If intergenerational relations were poor in the Former Soviet Union, then they deteriorate further in the United States. As a result of living separately, having less interaction between generations, and the weakening of their formerly central roles in the family, elderly persons experience loss of self-esteem (Brodsky, 1988). The resulting stress intensifies problems, such as increased animosity between in-laws and physical symptomotology in the elderly parents (Belozersky, 1990). Elderly émigrés, especially those reluctant to come to the United States, do not always adapt successfully.

Children

From the parents' perspective, Former Soviet children and adolescents adjust more quickly and easily to life in the United States than do adults. They minimize any problems children might have during resettlement and find that children acculturate easily and readily. Children and adolescents learn the English language more quickly than do adults, and superficially, they adjust better than adults. Children often become parentified and do all the translating and/or negotiating, until the parents become proficient in English. Children and teens report that they cannot always turn to their parents for emotional support after they emigrate, and parents supported this fact. Parents who are overwhelmed by the demands of resettlement are less available.

Adolescents, in general, test limits of parental authority, but among immigrants, that authority is often temporarily lost while parents adjust to their new surroundings and roles. Unless parents are able to resume their role of protector and provider quickly, children and adolescents become disrespectful of the parents and grandparents. Teens, more often than children, struggle with parents as they try to acculturate. They want to adopt the same language, clothes, and music as their American peers. Parents want children to maintain their Russian language and customs. In the Bukharan community, the period of adolescence is short. Marriage is arranged at a young age, and courtship is only a few months long, curtailing adolescent revolt and sexual explorations (Halberstadt & Nikolsky, 1996). Unlike teens from the European regions, although Bukharan teens feel peer pressure to join American culture, they are very fearful of losing acceptance in their traditional community.

When asked directly, some children and adolescents volunteered that initially resettlement caused a major disruption in their lives. They suffered significant losses, such as relationships with family members, teachers, friends and classmates, and participation in extracurricular activities. Social and cultural activities and lessons (music, dance, etc.), which are a big part of a child's life in the Former Soviet Union, cost a lot more money in the United States, and families generally do not have much money when they relocate. Among the child and adolescent émigrés from the European regions, there are mixed preferences in terms of friendships. Some children and teens gravitate primarily toward Russians. Others want only to be with Americans and distance themselves from the "old country" and the old ways. In the Bukharan community, child contacts are limited to immediate and extended families. Marriages among cousins are common (Halberstadt & Nikolsky, 1996).

Children and teens report that they looked and felt different when they first came to the United States, especially when they started school. Their clothing was different, their names were different, and, initially, so were their accents. School was difficult for the first few days, but all said that, in general, they adapted to their school environment. The most difficult adaptation was not to the lack of language, but to the feeling of being "singled out" to take the ESL classes. Some felt ESL classes were too basic, and that they could have learned English just as well if they had remained in a regular classroom. Children and parents agree that the level of education in the Former Soviet Union is more difficult than in the United States, and that Former Soviet students are more advanced than American students in the equivalent grade level. Among the European Soviets, students are generally motivated and focused to learn, because they come from a background that stresses education. Among Bukharans, however, schoolwork is a low priority; traditional family roles are stressed instead, and it is acceptable for boys to drop out of school to help the family financially. Many children have learning disabilities and/or behavioral problems at school. Obtaining cooperation to evaluate and test the children is difficult, because parents do not understand the source of the problem or the resources available (Halberstadt & Nikolsky, 1996).

Health Care

Issues regarding health care have been problematic for both Soviet émigrés and American health care workers. Perceptions of health care in the two countries are very different. In the Former Soviet Union, health care was free. Treatment was not constrained by cost-effective regulations and health care contracts, as it is in the United States. Repeated visits to the doctor were acceptable for the same ailment, and repeated tests and procedures were permissible. In the former Soviety union, hospital stays were provided for illnesses treated on an outpatient basis in the United States. Approved sick days from work and hospital stays were for longer periods than those allowed in the United States. When émigrés seek services in the United States, they do not understand financial constraints, limitations on the number of approved visits, and why they are not admitted to the hospital for certain procedures. Lack of understanding results in demanding patients and frustrated doctors.

In the Former Soviet Union, so many patients sought treatment per day that it was common for them to exaggerate their symptoms to ensure that they received services. They also exaggerated symptoms to obtain optimal care, such as admission to a better hospital (Wheat, Brownstein, & Kvitash, 1983). Former Soviet patients exaggerate the same way in the United States, catching doctors in a web of either trying to treat symptoms that they do not realize are exaggerated, or feeling frustrated by patients who deliberately exaggerate. Former Soviets lack appreciation for preventive health care, because none existed in the Former Soviet Union. They were used to being given directives by doctors, not recommendations for self-management of illness (i.e., diet and exercise). The concept of treatment options is new and often frightening to the Soviet émigré, because options fall under the American values of autonomy and self-reliance.

Mental Health Services

Emigrants from the Former Soviet Union are extremely resistant to mental health services. In the Former Soviet Union, inpatient psychiatric care was forced on political nonconformists treated with forced commitment to psychiatric hospitals. Psychotropic medications were administered punitively. Psychiatrists prescribed medication for depression on an outpatient basis, but no counseling or emotional support accompanied this biochemical approach. Goldstein (1984, p. 117) wrote that the whole notion of exposing one's personal feelings to a stranger under a contractual agreement with payment is a foreign concept to the Soviet spirit. Émigrés prefer to see their primary care physicians for psychosocial support and assistance. In fact, émigrés see the medical setting as the gateway to all social services needs. Among the Bukharan communities, stigmatization is so great that if word of seeking mental health services leaks out, the social standing of the family is jeopardized and the marriageability of children is in danger. Because marriages are arranged and dating is unnecessary, the diagnosis of mental illness is often concealed. Families continue to minimize the illness even after it is found out (Halberstadt & Nikolsky, 1996).

CULTURAL VALUES AS STRENGTHS IN ASSESSMENT

Possibly, the most outstanding cultural values of the immigrants of the Former Soviet Union fall into a cluster under the heading of survival skills. Under communist rule, and throughout the adjustment to a capitalist society, this population has demonstrated resilience and perseverance. Despite discrimination and persecution, war and political conflict, this population successfully survived. Following arrival to the United States, in the face of culture shock, complete with language and professional barriers, financial and often medical hardship, and potential for a variety of family conflicts and self-esteem issues, this immigrant population has demonstrated determination and adaptation, and, in general, has successfully acculturated without losing its own culture. Most émigrés have learned English, many have moved out of their communities to seek employment; many socialize outside their community, and, to their credit, are able to move back and forth successfully between their Russian community and the general community.

   Family and *community* are cultural values that have aided this population in both the Former Soviet Union and the United States. In the former, financial and emotional supports were frequently sought and given within the family or community. The elderly parents assisted their children with finances and child care. Colleagues and neighbors served as confidantes in times of trouble. In the United States, where immigrants often have less than the minimum basics, families and the Russian community often need to open their doors even wider, and they rise to the occasion. It is not unheard of for more acclimated immigrants to pay a few months' rent, to share an apartment, or to offer or help find a job, until a newcomer "gets on his feet."

Higher education, especially among immigrants from the European regions, was always very important. Professional and societal status, and self-esteem, were based on level of education. Immigrants have represented a variety of professions, including doctors, teachers, college professors, engineers, and so on. Immigrants cannot always automatically become employed in their careers in the United States; they often need to return to school to fulfill requirements, so they can continue practicing their professions in the United States. Some return to school and pursue a different career. This value of education has become a good resource for the United States in general.

Immigrants from the Former Soviet Union have a *strong work ethic*, as demonstrated by pursuit of professional aspirations through higher education. Immigrants employed in consumer-related jobs (i.e., manicurists, shoemakers) and business owners are also known to work long hours and to be reliable and responsible. In the Bukharan community, the work ethic is more valued than education, and boys are given employment responsibilities at a very young age. Stories vary in terms of financial and job satisfaction. Although the work ethic itself remains the same, the purpose of the work ethic has changed somewhat in the adaptation process from the Former Soviet Union to the United States. Social status is no longer the primary focus of the Former Soviet émigré. Earning a living and supporting a family, so that future generations can achieve in the future, have become the primary purpose.

For some, though not all, Former Soviet Jews, *religion* and *religious identity* are cultural values. Some practiced their religion secretly, because their faith helped them survive their adverse experiences. Others survived their adverse experiences because they hoped someday to have the opportunity to practice their religion openly. Still others, introduced to religion for the first time when they arrived in the United States, found that it held meaning for them. Judaism is a family- and community-oriented religion that addresses faith, as well as laws and customs for day-to-day living. People can immerse themselves in the religion on a variety of different levels and draw strength from each. For those who desire more structure, there are daily rituals and practices and congregational prayer. For others who desire less structure, there is the option of individual prayer. This cultural value can be as significant or insignificant, personal or public, as an individual or family wants or needs it to be.

"Immigration, with its accompanying feelings of uprootedness, vulnerability and numerous losses, acts as a powerful stressor" (Belozersky, 1990, p. 124). But the function of values as strengths in the lives of this immigrant population has greatly aided Former Soviets in adapting and resettling in the United States.

INDIGENOUS STRATEGIES AND WESTERN INTERVENTIONS

Talking about problems is not culturally valued among émigrés from the Former Soviet Union, so psychosocial stressors and psychodynamic issues are not addressed. Lifelong macro-social stressors (Brod & Heurtin-Roberts, 1992) encountered by the elderly in the Former Soviet Union, and losses and stressors encountered by all generations as a result of emigrating, provide only a framework of the problems that are somatized. The Bukharan culture is especially nonverbal, "so somatization of psychological discomfort is widespread" (Halberstadt & Nikolsky, 1996, p. 249). This is especially true of women, who are not able to oppose the domineering men in their families. "[They] frequently complain of headaches and stomachaches. Physical and emotional vulnerability of women is accepted by the Bukharan culture," and "it is often the woman's way to attract the attention from her family or to moderate conflict" (Halberstadt & Nikolsky, 1996, p. 249).

In the Former Soviet Union, medical care consisted of a mixture of Western medicine, natural and home remedies, and even magic. Repeated visits for the same medical complaints were not considered excessive and inappropriate use of services, as they are in the United States. Often, patients were not aware that complaints, or severity of complaints, stemmed from emotional causes. Patients just knew that they found relief in periodic conversations with the doctor, although the real problems were never addressed.

Soviet patients repeatedly return to the doctor with the same complaints. They present with the same illnesses and symptoms as other populations (i.e., arthritis, diabetes, and heart disease), but émigrés from the Former Soviet Union "emphasize their symptoms out of proportion to disease activity" (Wheat, Brownstein, & Kvitash, 1983, p. 900). The degree of impairment that they report "is above and beyond the influence of age, disease severity, or duration of illness" (Brod & Heurtin-Roberts, 1992, p. 335). They have greater difficulty coping and perceive more pain, with general feelings of unwellness and many somatic complaints that are difficult to evaluate. Their multiple, chronic complaints often turn out to be manifestations of depression and anxiety (Brod & Heurtin-Roberts, 1992).

Mental health services were rarely pursued. Nonmedical interventions were used for emotional stress and somatization. An acceptable and common form of treatment in the Former Soviet Union was balneotherapy, utilizing mineral springs, mud baths, sulfur, and other natural resources. Visits to spas were common for both children and adults, and treatments were offered for a variety of medical problems, as well as for neuroses (Grabbe, 1996). Multiple folk and home remedies were also utilized for pains and illnesses. *Znakharstvo*, or magical healing, was a primitive practice subscribing to supernatural forces. *Znakarki*, or wise women, used "magic water and whispered charms" (Grabbe, 1996) to treat illnesses that did not respond to ordinary medicine. *Znarkarki* can be found in some Russian neighborhoods in the United States as well.

In the United States, émigrés are still bringing their somatic complaints to the doctors. Often, primary care physicians are not equipped to handle emotional problems, and the mental health issues are not addressed at all, but in many instances, the emotional component of somatization is now being recognized. Some primary care physicians prescribe antidepressant and other psychotropic medications, without discussing the psychosocial or psychodynamic problems causing the depression. These physicians and their nurses realize that patients would be better taken care of with counseling than by medication, but they are not trained in counseling; therefore, they repeat the cycle of unnecessary medical visits perpetuated in the Former Soviet Union. From the patient's perspective, the physician is a high-status person satisfying the needs of people "whose own status and social identity have been compromised by emigration" (Brod & Heurtin-Roberts, 1992, p. 335).

For treatment of depression and somatization, Western interventions would be more beneficial than the indigenous strategies utilized by this immigrant population. Ideally, individual therapy would address psychodynamic and psychosocial issues that led to somatization and its underlying emotional distress. Support groups that target the Soviet immigrant population would address common experiences and issues, and lead to the resolution of some of the physical, if not emotional, symptoms. Clearly, in both forms of treatment, there would be a great deal of discussion, storytelling, and resistance before treatment would begin to take place. However, engaging clients and joining resistances are areas of expertise of mental health professionals, who, with a little knowledge about Russian immigrants, could treat this population.

PRINCIPLES OF CULTURALLY APPROPRIATE PRACTICE

The social work profession does not exist and has never existed in the Former Soviet Union. Volunteers trained by the Soviet government to help coordinate government benefits are perceived by Soviet citizens as government agents (Stutz, 1984). Former Soviet émigrés do not understand that, in the United States, employees of voluntary agencies or even municipal and federal social service agencies are not government officials to be feared and avoided. Russian émigrés would greatly benefit from the services of social workers and mental health professionals, but before they accept any such services, they need to be educated about the multifaceted roles of these professionals and the different types of help they provide.

Immigrants from the Former Soviet Union turn to the medical profession as the primary source of assistance of any form (medical treatment, benefits applications, housing). Social workers who speak the Russian language and/or are knowledgeable about Soviet immigrants should work closely with physicians and other health care providers. In hospitals, they should be prepared to do outreach in emergency rooms and medical clinics. Ideally, private doctors should have access to these social workers as well, at least for consultation. Communications between the various agencies offering services to this population would be beneficial, so that a referral network could be set up. As part of their provision of care, social workers would educate clients about the services offered. Brochures explaining services in the Russian language could be printed and handed out for immigrants to browse through at their convenience and share with others. Clients should be encouraged to share positive experiences with others in their community. Community hospitals and clinics can sponsor health fairs, lecture series, or other programs that educate immigrants about social work, preventive health care, and so on, and Russian-speaking social work and health care professionals should be present to address the needs of the Former Soviet Union population. Placing social workers at sites where immigrants are most likely to seek help will enable these people to obtain services on an as-needed basis. Until immigrants seek services on their own, this approach could extend social work services to a larger number of Soviet immigrants (Brodsky, 1988).

Obviously, Russian-speaking social workers and mental health and health care professionals would be most helpful to immigrants who speak little English. "A social worker from the same community is trusted to understand the client's way of life and values" (Halberstadt & Nikolsky, 1996, p. 254). Concerns about confidentiality are high, because this population is so community-oriented, and there can be ramifications if problems are found out. A social worker who speaks the same language but comes from another part of the Former Soviet Union might be more trusted because of shared culture and life experience, but distance from the community. Adolescents and young adults who speak some English might choose to speak with an English-speaking social worker and use him or her as a role model (Halberstadt & Nikolsky, 1996).

To engage successfully, it would benefit the professional to understand the Russian client's attitude toward his or her profession ahead of time. According to Smith (1996), nurses and social workers need to solicit support from the doctor to validate their roles for clients from the Former Soviet Union. When engaging Soviet immigrants, key issues to explore include the client's motivation to emigrate, what family members are in the United

States, the quality of the relationship with these members, and comparison of the family's social status in the Former Soviet Union and in the United States. These factors can help determine the degree of culture shock and re-settlement issues.

Professionals need to "become well versed in the culture, customs and general attitudes" (Stutz, 1984, p. 188) of émigrés from the Former Soviet Union, and, in the case of more recent immigrants, the republics or countries from which they come. Social work, mental health, and health care practitioners need to understand the Former Soviet immigrant's "past experiences of health care and be sensitive to their different attitudes to health" (Grabbe, 1996, p. 205). They need to know how history, psychosocial, and cultural factors impacted on the immigrant's life. Rather than challenge traditions, they should understand that behaviors learned during a lifetime spent in a different cultural and political reality are ingrained. "For American health care professionals, these behaviors may be difficult to understand" (Brod & Heurtin-Roberts, 1992, p. 336). In turn, émigrés need to be educated about health concepts and the American health care process. "A vicious cycle," according to Brod and Heurtin-Roberts (1992), "is set into motion between patients who feel the medical system is unresponsive to their needs and physicians who feel they are forced to deal with difficult patients" (p. 336).

A variety of beneficial services can be offered to elderly Soviet émigrés. Senior citizen centers and adult day care centers that service multicultural clients could hire a Russian-speaking social worker, translator, or receptionist. These centers could offer services such as health and nutrition, disease prevention, and safety programs; ESL classes; assistance with translating documents and letters; and exercise classes. Larger cities in the United States have centers that cater specifically to the Russian community in the Russian language.

There are many creative intervention options for children and adolescents. The lack of parental support and participation is usually the issue. If Russian-speaking teachers or guidance counselors are available in schools, then, when indicated, early interventions can take place without issues of language barriers. Preventive interventions and effective communication about emotional issues can take place without waiting for children and parents to learn English. In terms of behavioral and mental health–related issues, parents tend to respond to the schools when they are called about behavioral or emotional problems. According to discussions with school guidance counselors and therapists in mental health clinics, parents do not always comply with the next step of bringing children to a mental health clinic or emergency room. There are enough services, both voluntary (guidance counselors, mobile outreach workers) and authoritarian (child protective services, police) available that, ideally, children eventually should receive the necessary services. Successful outcomes vary.

Some schools in New York City organize workshops for parents to educate, acculturate, and support them. Topics include discipline (with emphasis on positive strategies and laws on child abuse), stress management, test preparation, resettlement issues, and so on. Schools or community centers can set up support groups exclusively for new émigré children and teens to discuss resettlement experiences. In addition, children and teens should be encouraged to participate in afterschool clubs and activities that would aid with acculturation, help maintain the daily structure and support that existed in the Former Soviet Union, and prevent the social isolation that some children experience because the family cannot afford to pay for extracurricular lessons or recreational activities.

CASE VIGNETTE

Dina, a 14-year-old Bukharan girl, came to the United States from Uzbekistan 3 years ago with her parents, her older brother, and her younger brother. Her maternal grandparents accompanied her family, and in the United States, they reunited in New York City with her father's parents and his brother's family. Dina's father had many extended relatives around New York City, and family was a major social support. Her father's brother found Dina's family a two-bedroom apartment in his neighborhood. Dina's uncle paid the security deposit and first few months' rent, until Dina's father could establish a small business for himself, like the one he had in the Former Soviet Union. Many tenants in the building, as well as in the neighborhood, were from Uzbekistan, and most were Bukharan Jews. Dina's family was very traditional. Her father was in charge of all the decisions, her mother was a homemaker, and her older brother helped in her father's business after school and was expected to drop out of school and work when business increased. Dina came home after school every day to do her homework and help her mother clean and cook, and look after her younger siblings when her mother was not home. The grandparents were elderly, and Dina and her mother took care of their nursing and daily needs at home. Dina had always lived with her grandparents, so the crowded space and lack of privacy was not new to her. The family joined the local synagogue but spent most of their time with extended family. Dina's brothers received average grades, and Dina herself did very well in school, though this was more important to her than to her parents. Teachers and guidance counselors supported and encouraged her, and Dina secretly hoped to go to college. She was often invited to join afterschool activities, but Dina declined, explaining her strict and traditional upbringing to her teachers, including the expectation that she return home right after school.

In the beginning of the ninth grade, Dina's grades began to drop. Her homework was not always handed in, her class participation decreased, and she barely passed her exams. A concerned teacher sent her to the guidance counselor, but Dina denied having any problems. Her parents were called in, but they did not seem concerned. Her father said her grades were adequate for her future role as a wife and mother.

In the middle of the school year, Dina met with her guidance counselor to discuss high school applications. Because of her low grades, she could not apply for the specialized schools that she had originally hoped to attend. Dina became very upset and tearful. The counselor was finally able to engage her and find out what had precipitated the change in behavior. Dina explained that life in her home was not as perfect as it appeared. It was customary in the Bukharan culture for men to be domineering and abusive toward their wives and children, but her father's recent verbal outbursts toward her and her mother had become more frequent. He did not hit his children in the United States, because he had been educated about child protection laws at his younger son's school, but he did hit his wife. Dina believed that she was the cause of his increased abuse toward her mother and felt very guilty. She felt that she could no longer live under the traditional constraints in her household, and that she needed to have more time out of her home for personal space and growth.

Apparently, Dina had asked her parents for permission to join the clubs at school, and her father forbade her to join. Her mother supported her wishes, and in response, her father became more abusive and violent toward her mother for disagreeing with him. In an attempt to individuate and, admittedly, to rebel, Dina defied her father by coming home late after school and sometimes staying out at night; in response, his abuse toward her mother worsened. Dina's concentration and grades dropped as she spent more and more time out of the home to avoid hearing her father's abusive outbursts. Although she knew her behavior was not a solution, she did not know any other way to cope. She was too embarrassed to bring her problems to the school and had therefore denied having any when approached by the people who wanted to help her.

The guidance counselor suggested that she meet with Dina and her mother to discuss a referral for counseling. Dina was worried that her mother would be embarrassed and angry with her, but the counselor promised not to confront Dina's mother about the home situation and to frame her recommendations in such a way that they would benefit Dina's well-being. The counselor was tactful with Dina's mother, as she had promised, touching on the abuse in terms of its effect on Dina and only empathizing with but not confronting the mother. Dina's mother agreed to take her to counseling. She understood that in American society, teenagers were encouraged to develop autonomy and creativity, and that life in the household was constricting Dina. The counselor then had a meeting with Dina and both her parents to encourage Dina's father to support the therapy, because he was head of the household. During this meeting, the abuse was not discussed. The discussion addressed Dina's poor grades and her unacceptable behavior of not returning home after school, as well as the difficulties of adolescence and the cross-cultural issues that Dina was trying to resolve. Her father was encouraged to permit therapy, so Dina could resolve the conflict of being caught between two cultures. With some persuasion, he agreed.

Dina met with her therapist weekly, and her mother joined her periodically for family sessions. She stopped staying out late and obtained permission from her father to spend time in the library after school; in a short time, her grades improved. She used her sessions to explore her wishes and to develop strategies of approaching her father without defying him, so that she could get her needs and wishes met. Dina's mother slowly became trustful of the therapist and spoke more openly about her own issues. She agreed to her own individual sessions, where she spoke about her own stagnation due to marriage at an early age, her dissatisfaction with her submissive role in her marriage, and, eventually, the abuse. The therapist provided psychoeducation about the fact that domestic violence is a criminal act in this country, but she did not aggressively pursue separation or shelter placement. She knew this would not be culturally acceptable and that a separation would put her family's reputation and the marriageability of the children in danger. Like her daughter, Dina's mother was caught between the Russian and Western cultures. Because the relationship between her daughter and husband had improved, with the aid of the therapist, Dina's mother decided to invite her husband for a few sessions. The therapist knew that couple counseling was not an ideal treatment plan for domestic violence, but her relationship with the family and the wife's insistence that she could not leave the home persuaded her to agree. During the first session, the husband's opinions about the daughter's progress in therapy were discussed, and the idea of improving verbal communication with his wife was addressed. During the second session, the domestic violence was "gently" discussed (i.e., How did it come about after so many years of marriage without it, what did it accomplish, and was there another way to communicate negative feelings?) The husband agreed to come for one last session, where the therapist continued to explore the issues of violence. He reluctantly agreed to try to curtail acts of violence. Dina had terminated treatment by now, but her mother continued for a few more months. By the end of treatment, Dina's mother reported that the violence had stopped, the verbal abuse occurred less frequently, and, at times, she was able to end the verbal abuse by encouraging discussion.

CONCLUSIONS

Many services are needed by and available to refugees from the Former Soviet Union. There are also many professionals willing to provide these services. Before services can be offered, and before they will be accepted, providers need to understand the cultural background of this population, so that they can make culturally competent assessments and practice interventions. In addition, funding sources need to be convinced to finance programs for this population. Because of the present political and economic changes in the United States, existing programs may not maintain sufficient funds, and additional funding may not be allocated to new programs. Another role that social work, mental health, and health care professionals may have to take on is the education of politicians and funding sources about the needs of émigrés from the Former Soviet Union.

REFERENCES

Belozersky, I. (1990, Winter). New beginnings, old problems—psychocultural frame of reference and family dynamics during the adjustment period. *Journal of Jewish Communal Service*, 124–130.

Brod, M., & Heurtin-Roberts, S. (1992). Older Russian émigrés and medical care [Special issue: Cross-cultural medicine—a decade later]. *Western Journal of Medicine, 157*(3), 333–336.

Brodsky, B. (1988). Mental health attitudes and practices of Soviet Jewish immigrants. *Health and Social Work, 13,* 130–136.

Flaherty, J. A., Kohn, R., Golbin, A., Gaviria, M., & Birz, S. (1986). Demoralization and social support in Soviet-Jewish immigrants to the United States. *Comprehensive Psychiatry, 27*(2), 149–158.

Flaherty, J. A., Kohn, R., Levav, I., & Birz, S. (1988). Demoralization and social support in Soviet-Jewish immigrants to the United States. *Comprehensive Psychiatry, 29*(6), 588–597.

Goldstein, E. (1979). Psychological adaptations of Soviet immigrants. *American Journal of Psychoanalysis, 30*(3), 257–263.

Goldstein, E. (1984). "Homo Sovieticus" in transition: Psychoanalysis and problems of social adjustment. *Journal of the American Academy of Psychoanalysis, 12*(1), 115–126.

Grabbe, L. (1996). Understanding patients from the former Soviet Union. *Family Medicine, 32*(3), 201–206.

Halberstadt, A., & Nikolsky, A. (1996, Summer). Bukharan Jews and their adaptation to the United States. *Journal of Jewish Communal Service* pp. 244–255.

Smith, L. (1996). New Russian immigrants: Health problems, practices and values. *Journal of Cultural Diversity, 3,* 68–73.

Stutz, R. (1984). Resettling Soviet émigrés: How caseworkers coped. *Social Work, 29*(2), 187–188.

Wheat, M. E., Brownstein, H., & Kvitash, V. (1983). Aspects of medical care of Soviet émigrés [Special issue: Cross-cultural medicine—a decade later]. *Western Journal of Medicine, 139,* 900–904.

Culturally Competent Contextual Social Work Practice and Intersectionality

ROWENA FONG

We hope this book will challenge and equip social workers to examine the social environments, cultural values, and indigenous interventions of immigrants and refugees before they came to America and incorporate them into Western therapeutic treatments, creating culturally competent contextual social work practice. As does my text on culturally competent practice (Fong & Furuto, 2001), this book also advocates that, in working with immigrants and refugees, culturally competent practice be strengths-based, empowering, grounded in cultural values, and inclusive of indigenous interventions to create a biculturalization approach. This book, however, furthers the theory and practice model. It includes a contextual/person-in-environment framework (Kemp, Whittaker, & Tracy, 1997) and a proposed, solution-focused therapy approach (Greene & Lee, 2002) with indigenous interventions. Contextual social work practice (O'Melia & Miley, 2002) and person–environment practice (Kemp et al., 1997) are practice approaches that need to be addressed simultaneously with cultural knowledge, values, and skills to create culturally competent contextual social work practice.

Thus, the components for culturally competent contextual social work practice, as stated in Chapter 3, are as follows:

1. *A theoretical framework* of an ecological model incorporating micro-, meso-, macro-levels of person–environment practice.
2. A strengths-based orientation with macro-level societal and cultural values used in *assessments and intervention planning.*

3. The intersectionality of macro- and cultural values and *differential assessments*.
4. An *empowerment intervention* through a solution-focused therapy approach reflecting the biculturalization of interventions.

CONTEXTUAL AND CHANGING SOCIAL ENVIRONMENTS

Immigrants and refugees are forced to transition into multiple environments. Leaving their native countries and familiar social environments, they are often forced to accommodate or adjust to new situations. Relying on their coping skills and resilience, they adapt to new physical, psychological, cultural, and political environments. Seeking the familiar, and trying to find ways to bridge what was formerly known to them, clients look to the previously existing strengths. Unfortunately, some of these strengths may be questioned, and because they are newcomers, immigrants and refugees are forced to change. But as the United States becomes increasingly multicultural with the presence these newcomers, paradigm shifts even in culturally competent practice must occur. Social worker practice is no longer a straight-line journey; it involves concurrently switching from one context to another. Social work practice must become contextual. Culturally competent contextual social work practice needs to become more pronounced in the profession and in the social work curriculum.

In a case example, a refugee from Vietnam may experience several different social environments: the first in Vietnam, a second one in the refugee camps in Thailand, a third with relatives or sponsors in the United States, a fourth with the Vietnamese ethnic community within the United States, and the last with extended family and nuclear members in the United States. Each juncture demands new coping skills and adjustments to these various social environments.

To fully understand the journey, history, and impact of the immigrant and refugee experiences, tools should be developed to assess each step of their journey. Lee (1994) speaks of empowering oppressed people through a "fifocal" lens that includes a history of oppression (p. 22). Frequently, the social worker in the United States knows that the immigrant and refugee have been through a trying experience, but the severity is not always accurately assessed. The multiple layers of trauma need to be explored and addressed in a contextual and culturally competent manner. Trauma, for instance, may produce recurrent behaviors, but if the social worker does not look far enough back into the history and context of the trauma, the incident identified as causing the trauma may not in fact be the cause. What is more, the trauma may be receiving reinforcement without the knowledge of the social worker, if assessments of the various social environments and their contribution to the trauma have not been thorough. Each social environment needs to be examined for interacting variables and their consequences during the adjustment to life in the United States.

Multilevel assessments are needed but are appropriately implemented only after the social worker and client have developed a suitable working relationship. Forcing a traumatized client to divulge information prematurely, without a trusting relationship with the social worker, may compound the trauma rather than alleviate it.

CULTURALLY COMPETENT CONTEXTUAL
SOCIAL WORK PRACTICE AND INTERSECTIONALITY

Culturally competent contextual social work practice is grounded in the belief that multiple variables intersect in clients' lives, and it is the challenge of the social workers to find how these intersections sort themselves out. The concept of intersectionality has been used in disciplines other than social work. Pope-Davis and Coleman (2001), writing for the multicultural counseling field, describe the importance of the intersection of race, class, and gender. In social work, Devore and Schlesinger (1999) advocate for the ethnic-sensitive social worker who considers ethnicity and class. Davis and Proctor (1989) stress the importance of integrating race, gender, and class.

Another recent work on intersectionality is Lum's (2003) categorization of intersectionality in terms of internal and external intersectionality. Lum's definition of intersectionality is " those multiple intersections and cross roads in our lives that are replete with multiple social group memberships that are interconnected and interrelated" (p. 42). Lum cites Spencer, Lewis, and Gutierrez (2000), who identify three factors that define intersectionality: "1) We all have multiple group memberships and identities, 2) the impact of these factors on our daily lives is not simply additive, and 3) that each social group membership cannot be completely extracted from all others" (p. 42). Summarizing Lum, intersectionality focuses on the individuals, families, groups, and social group memberships, such as race, ethnicity, sexual orientation, gender, age, and physical and mental abilities.

In Lum's book (2003), I speak of intersectionality in terms of social services, cultural values, and indigenous interventions and strategies. My chapter, "Cultural Competence with Asian Americans," addresses the need to "grapple with the intersections of ethnicity, sexual orientation, gender and national origins" (p. 276). One approach to intersectionality is to consider the following components that interact in the assessments, intervention planning, and implementation of culturally competent practice: (1) societal-level/cultural values; (2) social environments; (3) ethnicity/gender/religion/politics; (4) legal statuses; and (5)indigenous strategies/biculturalization of interventions. This book contributes to theory building, and skills development in culturally competent practice is achieved by asserting that social environments play a key role in the contextuality and intersectionality of people's social group membership, internal and external variables, and social service delivery system. In working with immigrant and refugee children and families, culturally competent contextual social work practice and intersectionality are the future directions to take in working with this growing and massively diverse population.

REFERENCES

Davis, L., & Proctor, E. (1989). *Race, gender, and class: Guidelines for practice with individuals, families, and groups.* Englewood Cliffs, NJ: Prentice-Hall.

Devore, W., & Schlesinger, E. (1999). *Ethnic-sensitive social work practice.* Boston: Allyn & Bacon.

Fong, R. (2003). Cultural competence with Asian Americans. In D. Lum (Ed.), *Culturally competent practice: A framework for understanding diverse groups and social justice* (pp. 261–281). Pacific Grove, CA: Brooks/Cole.

Fong, R., & Furuto, S. (Eds.). (2001). *Culturally competent practice: Skills, interventions, and evaluations.* Boston: Allyn & Bacon.

Greene, G., & Lee, M. (2002). The social construction of empowerment. In M. O'Melia & K. Miley (Eds.), *Pathways to power: Readings in contextual social work practice* (pp. 175–201). Boston: Allyn & Bacon.

Kemp, S., Whittaker, J., & Tracy, E. (1997). *Person–environment practice: The social ecology of interpersonal helping.* New York: Aldine de Gruyter.

Lee, J. (1994). *The empowerment approach to social work practice.* New York: Columbia University Press.

Lum, D. (Ed.). (2003). *Culturally competent practice: A framework for understanding diverse groups and social justice.* Pacific Grove, CA: Brooks/Cole.

O'Melia, M., & Miley, K. (Eds.). (2002). *Pathways to power: Readings in contextual social work practice.* Boston: Allyn & Bacon.

Pope-Davis, D., & Coleman, H. (Eds.). (2001). *The intersection of race, class, and gender in multicultural counseling.* Thousand Oaks, CA: Sage.

Spencer, M., Lewis, E., & Gutierrez, L. (2000). Multicultural perspectives on direct practice in social work. In P. Allen-Meares & C. Garvin (Eds.), *The handbook of social work direct practice* (pp 139–149). Thousand Oaks, CA: Sage.

Index

313